Spilker
Bahson

THE FOOT BOOK

THE
FOOT
BOOK
ADVICE FOR ATHLETES

by Harry F. Hlavac, M.Ed., D.P.M.

Contributors:
G.S. (Buz) Hamlin, D.P.M.
G. Wayne Jower, D.P.M.
Gerry Kuwada, D.P.M.
Paul Kruper, D.P.M.
Robert Parks, D.P.M.
Steven Wan, D.P.M.

Illustrated by Peter Freund, D.P.M., Stanley Newell, D.P.M.
Photography by Rick Mallamo

World Publications

Dedicated to Connie Gay Kim, without whose love and support this book would not have been possible.

Acknowledgements

Writing a book of this nature is the culmination of my wish to help athletes help themselves. Their own motivation to achieve and their desire to maintain good health will ultimately determine their level of performance in sports. Athletes are those individuals who use their bodies to express themselves. Competition in sports is one measurement of and a reward for excellence, but is not essential for self-actualization of the athlete in his particular sport.

Foot and leg strength, endurance and flexibility are necessary for all weight-bearing sports, and there are consistent principles that podiatrists can now share with the athlete and with other professionals involved in sports medicine.

The Foot Book began with an individual dream and instantly brought support from many colleagues, particularly the contributing authors who are all podiatrists and actively involved as athletes and in the practice of podiatric medicine and surgery: G.S. Buz Hamblin, D.P.M. (Atascadero, Calif.), G. Wayne Jower, D.P.M. (Foster City, Calif.), Gerry Kuwada, D.P.M., and Robert Parks, D.P.M. (Tacoma, Wash.) both completing post-graduate surgical residency programs. I also wish to thank Steven Wan, D.P.M., for his help on initial research and give particular thanks to Paul Kruper, D.P.M., who as a pharmacist as well as a podiatrist has written the sections on drugs, medications, vitamins and electrolyte replacements.

Many individuals and groups have given unselfish support in order to make this book a reality: the American Academy of

Podiatric Sports Medicine, particularly Drs. Bob Barnes, Richard Gilbert, John Pagliano and Steven Subotnick. Special thanks to Dr. Richard Schuster, who is an inspiration to us all, and to Dr. Tom McGuigan, Trenton, N.J., who is doing the things that bring the knowledge that we write about. Other podiatrists have given special help to me: Dr. Felton O. Gamble in Tucson, Ariz., Dr. Ted Clarke in Kokomo, Ind., Dr. Ted Eden, Bay Shore, N.Y., Drs. Mike and Larry Burns of the Burns Podiatric Laboratory in McCook, Neb., and Dr. Sheldon Langer of Langer Laboratories in New York.

The Dean of the California College of Podiatric Medicine, Dr. Paul Scherer, has given support to do research, use unpublished material and college facilities. The biomechanics department, particularly Ron Valmassy, D.P.M., Chris Smith, D.P.M., Northwest Podiatry Labs, and Richard Bogdan, D.P.M., co-director of the Sports Medicine Clinic have been a constant source of help.

I wish to thank my teachers in podiatric biomechanics Merton Root, John Weed and Thomas Sgarlato. The students of the podiatry colleges where I have had the honor to teach have been a constant source of stimulation for me to actually understand the things that I am supposed to be teaching. "Thank you" to the patients who have worked along with me toward the understanding and the resolution of their lower extremity problems.

Kees Tuinzing, exercise physiologist in charge of the Skyline College Fitness Academy, was the man who, along with his wife, Sandy, inspired me to begin a regular exercise program four years ago. He is the president of the Tamalpa Runners who help me to run the trails and hills of Marin County. He and Lori Kristovich are the models for the position and stretching exercises. Thanks also to Rick Mallamo, photographer, and the help of the Audio-Visual Department at Skyline College.

Dr. George Sheehan is a leader in sports medicine who has been a constant source of help to me. He has brought order out of chaos, and common sense to treatment. He has asked the athletes to expect more from their doctors and has changed the attitudes of many people. The American Medical Joggers Association, especially Ron Lawrence, M.D., and Tom Bassler, M.D., have brought worthwhile information to doctors, athletes and doctor-athletes. Rory Donaldson, editor of *The Jogger*, publication of the National Jogging Association, has given both moral and realistic support. The editor of the *Nor-Cal Running Review*, Jack Leydig, has supported my "Podiatric Medical Advice" column since 1974.

The majority of the illustrations for *The Foot Book* were done by Peter Freund, D.P.M., a podiatrist in San Francisco who contributed much time and effort. Stan Newell, D.P.M., a podiatrist in Seattle, gave permission to use his illustrations as well.

Enthusiasm to complete this book has brought friends who in turn have inspired me to further achievements: my associates in Sports Safety, Inc., Dr. Lee Smith, Bill Bacon, Ralph Booze, Ken Coburn and Fred Leopold; friends at the San Francisco Olympic Club, especially Mike Putterman and Jim Stephenson; Joan Ullyot, author of *Women Running*; and Bob Anderson (Englewood, Colo.), author of *Stretching*, the best book of its kind I have ever seen.

I am delighted to see that several of my colleagues, including my associates in practice Rich Schiller and James Dietz, have begun a regular running program since our involvement in sports medicine. Thanks to Dad, Harry V. Hlavac in Tarpon Springs, Fla., who lives by and has taught me the respect for good health.

The people at World Publications have been a tremendous help, first in accepting my ideas and then in carrying them out: Bob Anderson, president, Kevin Shafer, *Soccer World*, and especially Joe Henderson, editor of *Runner's World*, have guided me along the way.

Finally, thanks to Connie Gay Kim for countless hours of typing, editing and review.

Harry F. Hlavac, M.Ed., D.P.M.
P.O. Box 3964
San Rafael, Calif. 94902

Foreword

In 1973, we celebrated the 500th anniversary of the birth of Nicholas Copernicus. We honored the man who first said the earth revolved around the sun, the man who wrote, "If we face facts with both eyes open, finally we will place the sun himself at the center of the universe."

That same year, a meeting was held in San Francisco proposing a theory no less revolutionary. The foot, said this convention, is the cause of most athletic injuries. The athlete, claimed this convocation, revolved around his or her foot. Treatment must begin there, or there would be no beginning at all.

Four years ago, sports medicine was still a surgical specialty. The typical patient was one of Saturday's Heros. The typical injury was the damage resulting from a split-second collision of irresistable force and immovable object. The typical treatment was surgery.

"The sports medicine meetings I attend," a team physician told me at that time, "are really surgical conferences."

The emphasis on surgery to the detriment of orthopedic medicine had been deplored by the surgical leaders. In 1951, the president of the American Academy of Orthopedic Surgeons had issued this warning: "Because operations are spectacular, our residents often complete their training with distorted views as to the importance of surgery in orthopedics. They enter practice with but a vague view of the application of orthopedic principles."

This condition even now has not changed. Recently, I talked to a young orthopedic surgeon with a professional team who told me he had learned more sports medicine from a baseball trainer than he had in all of residency or practice.

"Before that," he said, "I had taken the traditional approach: make the diagnosis; select the appropriate operation."

But even four years ago, the handwriting was on the wall. There were no longer any appropriate operations. We had gone from the sports medicine of trauma to the sports medicine of overuse. The typical patient became a common, garden-variety human being engaged in a running sport, jogging or tennis or handball or basketball or the like. The typical injury was the result of innumerable repetitions of the same action. The typical treatment was medical.

The problem now was too much conditioning rather than too little, overdeveloped muscles rather than underdeveloped ones. The basic cause was a structural weakness in the foot, rather than an act of God in the momentary cataclysmic reaction between two opposing forces.

So orthodoxy failed. Standard practices were not enough. The athlete began to look elsewhere. "It is a well known fact," wrote South African physiotherapist C. Pilkington in 1970, "that a great number of sportsmen lack confidence in the medical profession and turn to quack treatment for a rapid cure." I felt the same way myself.

I began running 15 years ago, before jogging became respectable. And it cost me days and weeks of injuries to learn that I, a physician, knew nothing, and my colleagues knew nothing. In my years of running, I have never been helped by anyone with M.D. behind his name. I learned about feet from a podiatrist, muscles from a gymnast coach, the short leg syndrome from a phys. ed. teacher.

The roads became my teaching laboratory. I learned to use different shoes, different surfaces, arch supports and exercises. I discovered that running on the other side of the road could help, or running with my toes floating or even pigeon-toed. But I never put it all together, never saw that it all came down to maintaining a neutral position of the foot from stride to take-off.

That final illumination came from a most courageous human being, an ex-Marine who ran in what he called "essentially agony" for two whole years with chondromalacia patella, or runner's knee. He had gone through the usual treatments, drugs, cortisone shots, casting, and had experienced no relief.

This was unfortunately the usual outcome with this irritation of the undersurface of the kneecap. An editorial about that time in the *British Medical Journal* had said of chondromalacia patella: "The exact cause of this syndrome remains a mystery." And therefore the treatment remained problematical. The orthopedic surgeons who had taken control of sports medicine on the basis of treating one injury of the knee, the torn cartilage, were about to lose that control due to failure to handle chondromalacia of the kneecap, the most frequent overuse injury.

The ex-Marine was finally cured, but not by the surgeons. He developed some pain in his arch and consulted a podiatrist friend who made an orthotic or support for his foot. And that support not only cleared up the foot pain but, mirable dictu, the knee as well.

Sports podiatry had been born.

The 1973 San Francisco convention on "The Role of the Foot in Sports injuries of the Lower Extremity" met not to announce a new miracle drug or a new miracle operation. It met to announce the birth of sports podiatry.

The cry at San Francisco that year was body engineering, body mechanics, body physics. Butzolidine and cortisone were dead. The foot mold would replace the scalpel. Exercises would take the place of machines. Orthopedic medicine would occupy the center of the sports medical world. The sports podiatrist and the physiotherapist would become the central figures in the athlete's care.

All these were set in motion when runner's knee was cured with a foot support. We learned then that an abnormal foot strike can cause trouble with the knee, and we realized that the way to treat a knee was simple: Ignore the knee and treat the foot.

If this is so, then drugs and shots and operations and even exercises aimed at the knee will predictably fail. And if a foot support can help the knee, what else can it help? We soon found out. An odd foot strike can cause trouble at three levels: (1) the foot itself, with stress fractures, metatarsalgia, plantar fasciitis, and heel spur syndromes; (2) the leg with stress fracture (this time of the tibia and fibula), shin splints, achilles tendonitis and posterior tibial tendonitis; (3) the knee, with tibio-fibular arthralgia and, of course, runner's knee. All begin with a biomechanically weak foot.

So the sports podiatrist who could diagnose and treat these peculiar feet became the new leader. Orthopedic medicine, the non-surgical side of orthopedic care, was in the ascendancy. But the podiatrist and the physiotherapist would lead the way. They would fill the void that the surgeons had chosen to neglect.

As late as 1975 Dr. Paul Lipscomb, the president of the American Orthopedic Association, saw this as a continuing danger. "What can we do," he asked his colleagues "to prevent orthopedic surgeons from becoming technicians with little or no responsibility for preoperative diagnostic evaluations, or post-operative rehabilitation, and for the management of the 80 or 90% of patients who do not require surgical procedures?"

My own feeling is that the present way is the best. Orthopedic surgeons should be surgeons. Surgeons are born, not made. They have a particular personality: dominant, energetic, competitive, courageous, optimistic. It would be boring and out of character for them to occupy themselves with the routine medical care of the athlete.

What we must do is allow every specialist to do what he does best, be it podiatry, physiotherapy, osteopathy, chiropractic or orthopedic surgery. There is a place for everyone on this team. The only requirement that they be effective, and that the treatment be directed at the reason for the injury, not just the result. Nor should we waste time with treatments that have proven time and again to be ineffective.

We must accept, however impalatable, however unexplainable, the therapy that is successful. "Truth," said Williams James, "is what works." And the truth is that sports podiatry works.

George Sheehan, M.D.

Contents

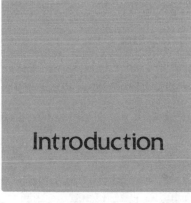

Introduction

A highly trained athlete in good mental and physical condition doesn't suffer injuries. Proper training methods, good equipment, preventive medical procedures (including proper food, rest, individual attention and biomechanical therapy, when necessary) will establish a system of good health. Injuries will be minimized and will be less disabling.

The athlete will feel the emotional and physical support through this approach, and perform at his best. Good health is a lifelong process. Coaches and trainers have the opportunity to share in this development. Their attitudes will determine the achievements and attitudes of the athlete. Performance in sports is based on motivation (desire, attitude), training (conditioning) and genetics (hereditary structure).

Motivation of the athlete and the development of the best training methods long have been goals of physical education teachers and coaches. This book presents positive attitudes toward personal achievement in sports and a review of conditioning methods for fine tissue structure and function. Until recently, genetics or hereditary structure dictated (helped or hindered) athletic ability. Now it is possible to alter structural stability and make the athlete function more efficiently.

Proper function of the foot is essential in almost all sports. The foot is that complex structure which must absorb forces coming up from the ground and down through the body. The foot must control and direct the center of gravity of the body.

The Foot Book describes the mechanics of the foot and leg in different types of sports, and prescribes conditioning activity to prevent injury at points of maximum stress. Our goal is to show the reader what ideal foot structure and function is, how to recognize the abnormal, how the athlete can condition himself to prevent injury and how the athlete can provide initial self-treatment and rehabilitation when injuries occur. We also describe those types of injuries which require professional evaluation and treatment.

Our goal is to keep the athlete in condition during the healing period, and to get him back to participation and competition as quickly as possible within sound medical judgment. We have included a listing and discussion on the value of medications, vitamins, preparations, tapes, padding and supportive materials which are available over the counter. In addition, we have included a glossary of sports and medical terms.

As podiatrists, our specialty includes the medical, mechanical and surgical management of the foot and ankle. Many problems of the limb and body above the foot are related to foot function, and the reverse also is true. The book does not attempt to deal with medical or metabolic problems affecting the foot, but rather the structure, function and reaction of tissues to conditioning, stress and injury.

Before a person begins a new program of athletics, we recommend a physical examination by a physician, and most certainly a complete examination should be performed before any seasonal team participation.

HOW WE GOT INVOLVED

The Foot Book has been written by podiatrists for coaches, trainers, athletes and other professionals and non-professionals. Our training is in a specialized, scientific medical profession.

In our private offices and clinics we have been very satisfied with our results of treatment and with our patients' responses. Each of the people involved with this book has a particular interest in podiatric sports medicine. Each has given time and creative effort unselfishly.

I have been involved with sports medicine only a few years, but I

4

find that the biomechanical principles I use in understanding the structure and function of my "regular" patients apply to athletes as well. I find an understanding of the mechanics of the sport is necessary to successful treatment of biomechanical problems.

Contributors to this book have come from various backgrounds, but each has participated in competitive sports (regular running programs including marathons, college football, college wrestling, karate blackbelt competition, tennis, baseball and swimming competition) and we continue to participate in regular aerobic conditioning activities. We have learned a lot by working together, and still have a great deal to learn about successful treatment of athletes. We feel that athletes deserve our full understanding and our best treatment ability. We all enjoy working with athletes because they want to understand the nature of their problems and to work with us toward solutions.

THE INJURED ATHLETE

Many research studies have established that injuries and pain in the lower extremities are a major area of disability. A survey of runners responding to a *Runner's World* magazine questionnaire indicated that more than six out of 10 runners were disabled during some part of a year because of injury (that percentage was even higher in teenagers, women, ultra-distance runners and racers).

Similar surveys exist for other sports such as football or skiing, but one must simply ask a coach or trainer, or even visit a hospital emergency room on a Saturday afternoon, to know there are many limping athletes. Proper coaching, conditioning methods (including strength, endurance and flexibility training), warmup and cooldown periods as well as good equipment and facilities will prevent many of these injuries.

Most disciplines of medicine consider vital needs of mankind (and they should). The study and treatment of internal or cardiac problems, and the effects stress and trauma on the restoration of health in the average man, are of essential concern. The main effort of American medicine has been the treatment of disease. Little attention has been paid to prevention of disease and still less to the establishment of the healthy individual.

A highly trained athlete has attained this elite state and is approaching an ideal. He is in tune with his body and his body responds to his needs. His body does not function like that of an average man. His pulse (heart) rate is below normal; his total metabolism is not "normal." He often asks his body to do abnormal things, eat abnormally and train under abnormal conditions, such as a variety of surfaces, inclement weather and stress beyond normal endurance. He associates with people like himself who have shared the same experiences.

Those athletes who have not yet attained this elite state have short periods of success, exhilaration, and awareness of this one-ness with body and spirit. They become totally involved. They achieve a positive addiction. A day without activity brings on "withdrawal" symptoms. They become anxious, jittery and obsessed. They need a daily activity "fix."

This attitude is difficult for doctors familiar with average patients to understand. Normal prescriptions of rest, drugs and other medications are not accepted by the injured athlete. The athlete wants to understand the mechanics of the problem and condition himself through it. Many doctors are so involved with the sick that they don't see the importance of treating overly healthy patients.

Podiatric medicine evolved to fill a void. It shares responsibility with the orthopedist for bone, joint and muscle problems, with the neurologist for nerve problems, with the vascular specialist for blood vessel problems and with the dermatologist for skin problems of the foot. Podiatrists also attempt to work with the family doctor, internist or pediatrician when foot problems are recognized. Podiatrists attain the degree of DPM (doctor of podiatric medicine) through a specialized course of medical training and are fully aware of the relativity of the foot to the rest of the body.

We are trained in the recognition of medical disease. Foot and ankle problems, for the most part, are not vital or life-threatening and for that reason are not studied by other medical specialities. Podiatrists generally are concerned with "little things," such as an understanding of the structure and function of the 26 bones in each foot, shoes, supporting surfaces, overuse injuries, pressure points and the integral function of the limb above the foot.

Much of the work of a podiatrist is the simple relief of pressure and pain (through the use of pads and protective devices), the care of people who are unable to care for themselves, and the prevention of foot and leg problems by early treatment of children.

Surgical correction of foot and ankle problems is, for the most part, elective rather than emergency in nature. These surgeries may be performed in hospitals, but many times are performed in a private office for those cases in which the patient may walk immediately after the surgery is performed. Most foot and ankle procedures afford minimal disability. Foot surgery may be performed by a podiatrist, orthopedic surgeon or general surgeon.

When a doctor takes the time to understand the "little things," the mechanics of the particular activity and the emotional effects of lost training, he will then be able to prescribe a series of activities to keep the athlete in condition while the particular injury heals. This satisfies the doctor, coach and trainer, and helps the attitude and performance of the athlete.

TRENDS IN SPORTS MEDICINE

The greatest trend at present is the establishment of preventive medicine as it applies to sports. This entails: pre-season evaluation of individual athletes; specific conditioning programs to establish strength, endurance and flexibility of the mechanically inefficient areas; and education of athletes, coaches and trainers on specific initial treatments. In order for a doctor to apply his knowledge, it is necessary for him to understand the mechanics and ideal technique of a particular sport. It helps if he gains this knowledge through involvement as a participant observer.

Very few doctors specialize in treatment of the injured athlete, and the athlete is fortunate to find an "athlete" doctor. Traumatic injuries with pain, swelling and disability require immediate professional treatment, usually calling for rest and immobilization. But for the most part, injuries to the lower extremities of athletes result from imbalance or overuse.

When injuries occur after sustained activity, or produce recurrent stresses, strains or sprains on muscles, bones and joints, they can be treated mechanically with such devices as pads attached to the foot or outside ankle braces. Physical therapy is used on an

7

ongoing basis to keep inflammation down, and progressive resistance exercises are used when training muscles to overpower injured areas. Through a science of measurement procedures, including studies of the limb off-weight bearing, in stance, and during function, proper casting methods and the construction of a functional orthotic device, we are now able to set up a consistent control between the ground and the foot. This insert can be used in regular shoes, and during vigorous activities.

By preventing the adaptation motion between the foot and the ground, we are able to prevent inefficient motion, directly control action of the foot and indirectly control motion of the knee and hip. Most endurance activities establish strong development of the heart and lungs, but increase stress on the feet and legs. Orthotics help prevent this trauma. Orthotic devices make the body more efficient in sports by preventing wasted motion; they prevent side to side motion in runners and provide inside-edge control in skiers. Orthotic devices do not correct feet; they correct gait, just as contact lenses or eyeglasses do not correct eyes but correct vision.

USING THIS BOOK

Many of the descriptions in this book can be used by the athlete in all sports. Specific recommendations listed under "Forward" activities, "side-to-side" activities, "ballistic" activities and "mixed" activities will apply to many different weight-bearing sports. It will be helpful to use the index and glossary. Our recommendations are meant as guidelines and should be used or adapted by coaches and trainers based on their years of experience.

Young athletes, especially those during the growing years, are prone to injury which could result in permanent damage. They should not be allowed to participate or compete in the presence of injury to soft tissue or bone. They should be encouraged and motivated within their ability, and not "driven" by parents or coaches. This not only produces physical damage, but emotional stress as well. They should be taught the proper training and conditioning methods, and encouraged to report any injuries, swelling or pain.

"Weekend" athletes are often subject to injury. Proper con-

ditioning for total good health requires at least four varied training sessions per week. Vigorous strain on muscle and joints once
or twice a week causes pain and fatigue rather than good health. It
overloads the heart and lungs. We encourage the aerobic conditioning methods.

Conditioning alters all tissues of the body by increasing their
ability to use oxygen, and conditioning takes time. As a general
rule, it takes at least one month of activity for each year of
previous inactivity. That is, in order for an athlete to get in shape
after being out of shape for 10 years, it will take at least 10 months
of training.

Competitive and professional athletes can benefit from our
recommendations. There are many things the athlete can do to
assure proper conditioning, understand potential problems, and
to early recognize and treat injuries. In general, we advise against
oral and injectable medications which mask deeper problems.
Specific examination and evaluation must be done before this
type of treatment should be used.

ATTITUDES TOWARD THE INJURED ATHLETE

There should be an open, helpful relationship among everyone
concerned. We encourage cooperation and respect. There should
be a clear definition of goals and responsibilities. The doctor,
coach and trainer are present to help the athlete, and should not be
there for personal gain. If there is conflict between the doctor and
coach or trainer or even the parents of the younger athlete, the
individuals should meet, away from the athlete, and resolve the
problem.

The self-image of the athlete should be preserved. If injured, the
athlete should be informed fully of the nature of his problem. The
treatment plan and reasons for the plan should be explained fully
to him so that he can participate in rehabilitation without further
injury. In the case of foot injuries, he should be encouraged to
stay in condition through a non-stressing activity for that part
(such as cycling or swimming) while the foot injury heals. He
should be included in all non-stressful team activities.

The sports medicine podiatrist must make firm medical decisions. He will often be asked for medical decisions out of his field of

expertise. At these times, he may give advice on general conditioning and first aid or emergency treatment when necessary. Along with the coach and trainer, his help should be for the welfare of the athlete.

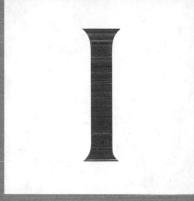

I

FOOT CONSTRUCTION

1

The Normal Foot

The foot and leg establish their basic structure within six years. Beyond that age, the bones continue to develop in size and stabilty, but the foot type is set. Up until this age, certain corrective measures can be taken to prevent future problems. After this age, however, the goals of treatment are to prevent problems through conditioning, to conservatively balance and protect the foot in all functions and environments, to treat acute foot and leg injuries and, finally, to consider correction of severe disabilities and chronic stress syndromes.

The foot is the foundation with our environment, the root between the body and the earth. Any structural, functional or metabolic imbalance within the lower extremity will cause compensation by other body parts, inefficiency, fatigue and overuse. The foot cannot be isolated from other body tissues. The same muscles, tendons and ligaments take part in the integral bone structures which provide support, posture and efficient movement.

Movement of the foot during gait is predictable and synonymous with movement of all the bones of the lower extremity. A small amount of imbalance (even a few degrees of motion) sends shock waves through the ground and up the leg. The foot is a mirror of systemic disease problems, and will reflect problems in all body tissues. The foot is a unique, intricate mechanism which provides a wide variety of services. It cushions the body and adapts to uneven surfaces. It provides traction for movement, awareness of joint and body position for balance, and leverage for propulsion.

The foot is a fascinating structure which is often overlooked because it is so intricate, so non-vital, yet so necessary for normal life. It is forced to function under adverse circumstances, on hard surfaces and in closed shoes. It's often noticed only when it has failed to fulfill these functions. Attention to the feet and legs before they display adverse symptoms will eliminate problems.

Nature produced a magnificent architectural and functional design in the foot, which is designed to work efficiently under excessive loads of unnatural conditions. Throughout the 26 bones, the multitude of muscles, tendons, ligaments, nerves and vessels in each foot, each tissue and structure has a specific function. Each tissue performs this function within its genetic structural ability. Each tissue has a protective mechanism, a warning mechanism, a healing mechanism and the ability to strengthen itself under stress.

What is "normal"? Normal is, according to Dr. Merton Root, "that set of circumstances whereby the lower extremity, and particularly the foot, will function in such a manner that it will create no adverse physical or emotional response to the individual, so long as it is used in an average manner, in an average environment, as dictated by the needs of society at the moment."

When we describe "normal," we talk about ideals, rather than averages. Our goal in corrective treatment is to achieve the ideal normal state, as described by specific structure and function. Most feet do not fit the criteria of the ideal normal foot, yet they function without pain. The goal of diagnosis is to distinguish abnormal from normal. The goal of treatment is to convert the abnormal into the ideal normal condition. This treatment can be in the form of correction or control.

The ideal normal foot in stance is a situation in which:

• The heel bone is in line with the leg and perpendicular to the supporting surface.

• The plane of the forefoot (metatarsal heads) is perpendicular to the rearfoot and parallel to the supporting surface.

•The ankle joint has the ability to dorsiflex 10 degrees.

13

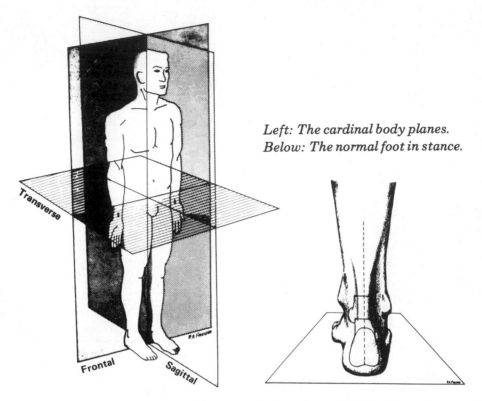

Left: The cardinal body planes.
Below: The normal foot in stance.

• There are no forces on the foot from the leg above in any of the three body planes, causing it to invert or evert, adduct or abduct, dorsiflex or plantarflex.

When describing motions and positions of the parts of the body, we relate them to the three major body planes. Movements of the foot have special definitions, because the foot is at a 90-degree angle to the rest of the body.

• The *sagittal plane* divides the body (from top to bottom) into a right and left side. Motions within this plane are the up and down, forward and backward movements of flexion and extension. Specific movements of the foot are called dorsiflexion (upward movement) and plantarflexion (downward movement).

• The *frontal plane* divides the body (from top to bottom) into a front and back part. Motions within this plane are the up and down, side to side movements of adduction and abduction of the limbs. The motion occurs with inversion and eversion of the foot.

• The *transverse or horizontal plane* divides the body (from side to side) into a top and bottom part. Motions within this plane include the side to side, forward and backward rotational movements of the limbs, as well as the adduction of the foot (where the distal part of the foot moves toward the midline as the leg rotates on its vertical axis) and abduction (where the end of the foot moves away from the midline of the body).

When we describe structure, we describe one part of the foot in relation to another. When we describe movement, we describe the direction of motion of the distal on the proximal part of the foot. The body normally is described in the anatomical stance position (in which the body is erect, the arms extended with the palms facing forward and the feet pointing ahead). "Left" and "right" are the sides of the body being described, not the right or left of the observer. In this position, the center of gravity is supported and stable.

The terms proximal (closer to the center of the body) and distal (away from the center of the body) will be helpful to remember. For example, the ankle is distal to the knee, but the ankle is proximal to the toes.

The term anterior refers to the front, posterior to the back, medial toward the inside and lateral to the outside. For example, the big toe is anterior and medial, the belly button is anterior, and the ears are lateral. The term unilateral refers to one side of the body and bilateral refers to both sides (or both extremities).

INTEGRATED FUNCTION

The human machine is a gloriously smooth and efficient achievement. During rest, stance and activity, all of the tissues of the lower extremity should work with each other. The main tissues of the lower extremity are bone, ligament, muscle, tendon, blood, blood vessels, nerve and skin. Each part of each tissue and all tissues must be coordinated with each other.

When a disruption of this balance occurs through trauma, overuse or imbalance, the injured tissue itself and the other tissues must compensate. Compensation is defined as "an (abnormal) attempt by the body to neutralize an abnormal force." Although usually applied to biomechanical forces, compensation may be applied to any bodily attempt to absorb stress. The goal of

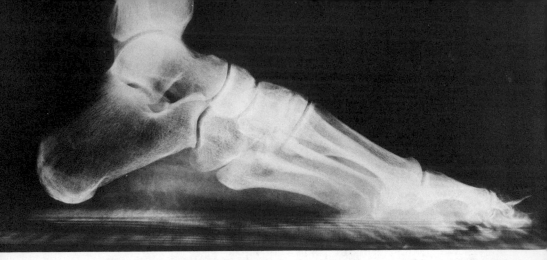

The normal X-ray of the foot shows 26 bones and two sesamoid bones.

treatment is to support the individual (neutral) structure and prevent compensation in order to allow the body to be the best it can be. All body systems work together.

In general terms bones form the skeleton, or basic structure. They serve as attachments of muscles for movement. They articulate (bend at joints) with other bones. The shape of the bone and joint determines the direction and range of motion. The smooth ends where bones contact each other are covered with cartilage and joint fluid, encapsulated, protected and bound down with ligaments. Ligaments maintain joint alignment, provide stability and serve as emergency structures preventing dislocation. They are inelastic, but through flexibility training over time, they will change "position."

Muscles arise from bones and attach to other bones with elastic tendons. When the muscle contracts and thickens, the tendon pulls, producing a shorter distance between the origin (beginning) and insertion (end), resulting in stability or movement of the bones. All muscles of the lower extremity are skeletal voluntary muscles. Each can be conditioned for movement, leverage, balance and accuracy. Each muscle or muscle group has opposing (antagonist) muscles which prevent jerky or excessive movement and stress on bones and joints.

The lower extremity has the elements of strength, endurance and flexibility in the bones, joints and muscles. All the other tissues are necessary for function but should be considered as support systems for these structural tissues. The other tissues providing support to the lower extremity structure are the nerves, the blood vessels, and the skin.

The stimulus for muscle contraction comes through nerves which may work voluntarily, involuntarily or through reflex

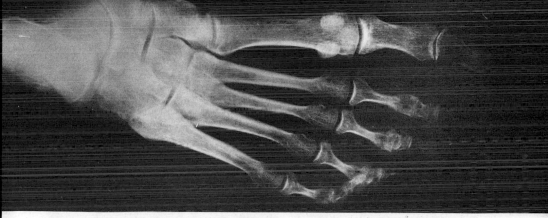

Courtesy of Felton O. Gamble, D.P.M., Applied Foot Roentgenology

action. Nerves are the electrical system of the body. They supply all tissues and control movement and sensations of pain, cold, heat and touch.

The circulating blood in the blood vessels provides nutrition, repair and waste removal. The blood vessels carry cells to and from all tissues. The arteries carry blood from the heart and lungs to the muscles and organs. The veins carry blood back up to the heart and lungs for waste removal and replenishment with the lymph vessels aiding in the process.

The skin itself provides many mechanisms of protection and support. There are many specialized cells in the skin of various parts of the body, including hair and nails, sweat ducts and specialized skin on the palms and soles. The appearance of the skin is a good indicator of general body condition.

This is how all these tissues work together as a unit. Through training, almost all of this integrated system can be improved.

BONES OF THE FEET AND LEGS

Bones make up the skeletal framework of the body. With normal health, nutrition and development, the size and shape of our frame is determined genetically by our ancestors. Bones are living tissues which are firm and yet somewhat flexible. They resist stress and protect vital structures.

At birth, the flexible bones are distorted because of intra-uterine pressure. Newborn babies have inverted feet and bowed legs. From birth to the time the child is "solid enough" to bear body weight for his first step, a dramatic change takes place in body shape. In the lower extremity, the hips, knees, ankles and bones of the feet change so that the feet can be under the body's center of gravity during stance. There are predictable torsions

17

(twists in bone) and changes in joint position (a general "unwinding") during development from the intra-uterine position to the adult's erect stance position. It is not unusual for a young child to moderately toe in or out, to have flat feet or bowed legs which would not be considered normal in an adult. But any abnormality should be evaluated by a professional.

Many of the structural imbalance problems we see in the adult are forms of incomplete development. During development, treatment has the best results with early evaluation and care of the child when the bones and joints are flexible (and have not yet adapted to the abnormal forces). Most normal development of genetically determined structure is complete in the six-year-old child. Beyond this age, it is almost impossible for a doctor to correct a structural abnormality without surgery.

Until the dawning of the age of biomechanics in podiatry, many treatments were empirical. Today, knowledge of normal foot and leg development has been gathered through clear measurement procedures and specific treatment methods. We can predict the compensations that will take place without treatment, prevent compensations with early treatment and control a compensated foot type in an adult.

The bones of the foot and leg work together. We know that as the foot pronates in stance, the leg must internally rotate on the foot. This produces predictable movements of the bones of the foot, the knee and hip joints, and even has an effect on the pelvis and low back. We know that as the foot supinates, the leg must externally rotate with concurrent stress extending up the limb. Problems of overuse, imbalance or shock in the leg are usually related to how well or how poorly the foot pronates and supinates.

There are 26 bones in each foot, and four more bones between the ankle and the hip. These 30 bones on each side, 60 bones in all, comprise the entire lower extremity. It is little wonder that, when the foot is forced to function in non-functional shoes and on unnatural surfaces, it is a source of problems for athletes.

The foot includes the ankle joint and the area below. The foot has two bones in the rear (greater tarsus): the heel bone (calcaneus or os calcis) and the ankle bone (talus or astragulus). The joint between the talus and the calcaneus is called the subtalar joint, and allows complex side-to-side motions of pronation and supination.

All the remaining bones in the foot are part of the forefoot. Those bones include the lesser tarsus, the metatarsus and the phalanges. The forefoot begins at the midtarsal joint which is between the talus (ankle bone), the navicular (a "boat-shaped" bone) and the calcaneus with the cuboid ("cube-shaped") bone. In front of the navicular are the three wedge-shaped cuneiform bones. Consequently, there are five bones in the lesser tarsus.

In front of the lesser tarsus are the five metatarsal bones attached to the tarsus proximally, at their base, and forming the weight-bearing area at the ball of the foot at the distal end or "head" of the metatarsal bones. So each metatarsal bone is long with a base, a shaft and a weight-bearing head. The thickest and most medial of these bones is called the first, and they are numbered laterally to the fifth.

Normally, the plane of the five metatarsal heads is flat. That is, they are all on the same level with no "metatarsal arch." The position of the metatarsals is genetically controlled by the midtarsal joint and should be perpendicular to the weight-bearing direction of the heel bone. Any inward or outward tilt, or differences in the position of one metatarsal relative to the others, is abnormal and may cause symptoms.

Although all the metatarsal heads 1-5 are normally level and on the same plane (parallel with the floor), the first and fifth metatarsals have a range of motion, basically up and down, to adapt to an uneven surface. As the foot pronates and supinates, the first and fifth "rays" tend to "get out of the way" of stress. The second, third and fourth metatarsals are firmly fixed at their base and normally do not move.

Two other bones are in each foot under the first metatarsal head and called sesamoid bones. These are small bones, invested in the tendons which flex the big toe. They serve like the kneecap to protect the larger joint from injury. They move forward as the big toe goes up, and backward as it goes down, so that the front of the joint is protected. They also serve as "pulleys" for the tendons so there is no interference with the joint. The sesamoid bones become a problem if injured or misplaced.

It is possible to describe the ideal normal foot with reference to each of the three body planes. We have described the foot in the frontal plane because this is where most problems arise. We may also describe the normal arches and the normal relative lengths of the weight-bearing bones.

Structural support of the foot is made by the shape of the bones and the aid of the muscles. The ligaments serve as emergency structures only. This means that if a ligament is cut or injured, the arch does not collapse. Shoes are made to support an average arch height. The height of the arch is not as important as its structural integrity. We are concerned about what happens to the shape of the foot when a person stands and moves. If a person has a low arch (pes planus) that is flat before he stands on it, and it stays the same shape in stance and movement, there is no problem. But when an arch collapses in stance, it puts stress on ligaments and muscles, and leads to imbalance and stress.

Osseous, or bony, shape is determined genetically. It can be supported by outside forces, but the basic body shape and size is determined by heredity. This is true for feet, limbs and any other part of the bone structure. The foot then is made of 26 bones and two extra sesamoid bones. Each bone adapts to the supporting surface and gains leverage from it.

Normally, the first and second toes, and the first and second metatarsal heads are the same length, and they get progressively shorter as they go to the fifth. The normal angle between the first and second, and the second and fifth metatarsals is 142.5 degrees. A short first metatarsal (Morton's foot) is biomechanically unstable and the angle is greater, causing pressure on the second metatarsal bone. The relative length of the metatarsal bones is also called the metatarsal parabola and is an important orthopedic consideration in treatment.

The normal angle of gait that each foot makes with the sagittal plane (line of progression) is 5-10 degrees toed outward. This is because of the outward twist in the bones between the ankle and the knee. The ankle bone is held firmly between the tibia and fibula. The bump on the inside of the ankle is the medial malleolus (a bone with a hammer head shape) of the tibia and the bump on the outside is the fibular malleolus. These two bones firmly

20

clamp onto the talus on both sides, so that the ankle joint allows up and down motion. The tibia is also called the shin bone and serves as the attachment for muscles that affect foot movement.

In the anatomical stance position, the center of the hip, knee and ankle joints are in a straight line. In stance, the knee is over the ankle, with no knock knee or bow leg present. This also is true on a side view, so that there is no flexion or hyper-extension (called genu recurvatum) at the knee.

A slight difference between men and women exists in the thigh area, so that there is a slightly greater angulation of the femur into the knee joint in women. This is because of the relative greater width of the pelvis in women. This angulation accounts for specific imbalance problems in women athletes, especially causing stress at the medial knee area.

In the stance position, the pelvis as measured at the top of the iliac crests should be level on the horizontal plane in the front and back views (frontal plane) and the side views (sagittal plane). Any forward tilt of the pelvis, where the front is lower than the back, puts a strain on the low back, causing lordosis (sway back) and postural problems. A backward tilt (kyphosis) limits hip rotation. A side-to-side tilt (scoliosis) produces strain on the spine and/or functional limb length differences.

THE CENTER OF GRAVITY

The center of gravity of the body, where all the major body planes meet at the balancing point of the mass, is located below the umbilicus (navel) and in front of the sacral vertebrae in the normal adult. This varies with each body type and each individual.

Viewed from the side, the center of gravity of the erect body can best be appreciated by imagining dropping a vertical plumb line in front of the face on the chestplate. A continuation of this line will bring it through the front portion of the pelvis, slightly in front of the knees and then in front of the ankles. Viewed from the front, this plumb line courses down the middle, splitting the body into two equal halves.

In order to maintain balance in stance, the center of gravity

21

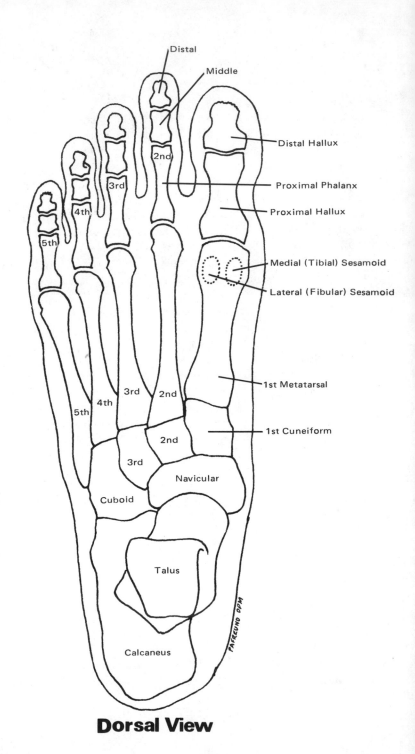

Distal

Middle

Distal Hallux

Proximal Phalanx

Proximal Hallux

Medial (Tibial) Sesamoid

Lateral (Fibular) Sesamoid

1st Metatarsal

1st Cuneiform

2nd

3rd

4th

5th

5th 4th 3rd 2nd

2nd

3rd

Navicular

Cuboid

Talus

Calcaneus

PAFREUND DPM

Dorsal View

22

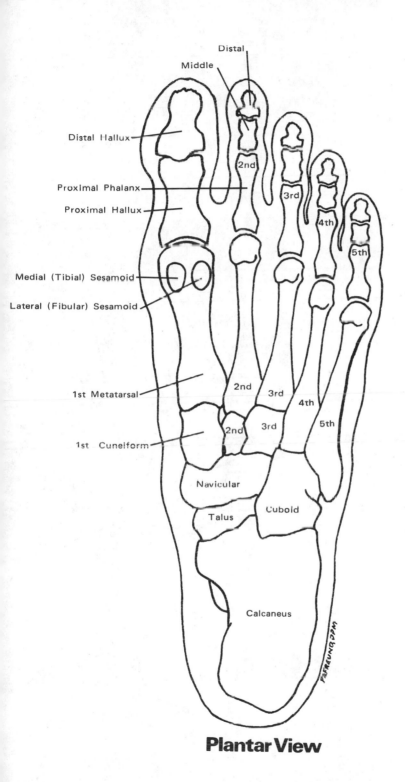

Distal

Middle

Distal Hallux

Proximal Phalanx

Proximal Hallux

Medial (Tibial) Sesamoid

Lateral (Fibular) Sesamoid

2nd

3rd

4th

5th

1st Metatarsal

1st Cuneiform

2nd

3rd

4th

5th

2nd

3rd

Navicular

Talus

Cuboid

Calcaneus

FAFREUNG DPM

Plantar View

Medial View

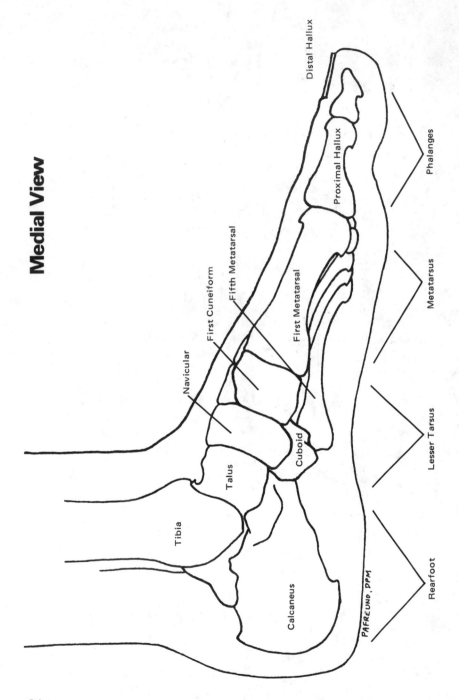

Distal Hallux

Proximal Hallux

Phalanges

First Cuneiform

Fifth Metatarsal

First Metatarsal

Metatarsus

Navicular

Cuboid

Talus

Lesser Tarsus

Tibia

Calcaneus

Rearfoot

PAFREUND, DPM

Lateral View

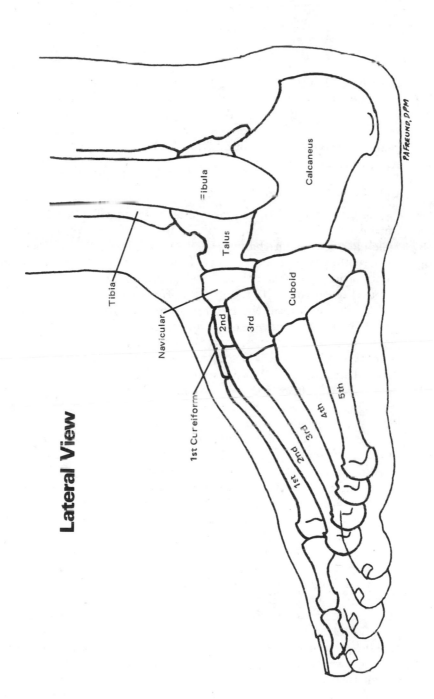

Tibia

Fibula

Talus

Navicular

Calcaneus

Cuboid

1st Cuneiform

2nd

3rd

1st

2nd

3rd

4th

5th

P.A.Freund, DPM

must be within the base of support, and with movement, the base of support (feet and legs) must precede the center of gravity. That is, when momentum is involved, the feet and legs must always be in a position to provide balance and control motion. The lower the center of gravity to the ground, and the wider the base of support, the greater is the stability.

FOOT AND LEG JOINTS

The place where two or more bones meet is called a joint (also known as articulation). The joints are reinforced by ligaments, which are dense white bands of connective tissue. These ligamentous reinforcements aid to provide stability and flexibility or a combination proportional to the nature of the joint and the demand placed on it. It should be noted that the bony structure and the muscles form the main systems of support for the arch and that the ligaments are only called upon as "reserves" such as, when more flexibility or support is required.

Joint surfaces which come into contact with each other are covered with a layer of shiny material called cartilage to protect the bone ends from frictional rubs. Undue frictional forces on these joint surfaces without protection can cause damage to the joint.

A freely movable joint is surrounded by a sac called an articular capsule. The inner surface of the capsule is lined with a thin, shiny synovial membrane, which secretes a clear lubricating fluid called synovial fluid. In some joints, a separate sac of this fluid can be found in places which receive a high proportion of stress (such as the shoulder joint). In this instance, this separate sac is called a bursa and functions like a cushion. The whole joint structure works in a manner rather similar to the shock-absorbing system of a car.

Naturally, not all joints are alike. Some are more freely movable than others, while still others are barely movable. The joints of our body can be roughly divided into several categories. The major joints of the lower extremity are the hip, knee, ankle and the joints of the feet (the subtalar, midtarsal, first and fifth rays, and the toes). Other joints of the foot and leg are firmly bound and allow very little movement.

26

The hip joint is a ball-and-socket-type and can move in all directions. It allows rotation, gliding, angulation and circumduction. In the normal adult, the hip joint allows rotation of the thigh equally internally and externally, so that in the resting position and during the swing phase of walking and running, the knee joint points straight ahead. For normal foot motion, sagittal and frontal plane motions of the hip must be smooth but are not as important as rotation, which controls angle of gait and pronation-supination of the foot.

The *knee joint* is a hinge-type and allows flexion and extension. It allows a small amount of passive rotation and side-to-side motion, greater in young children. Any forces from the foot or leg below, or from the thigh above, which cause rotation or side-to-side motion of the knee are destructive. The knee joint is the largest and most vulnerable in the body.

The *ankle joint* is hinge-type and allows gliding and angulation. Angulation in this joint consists of an upward motion called dorsiflexion (such as bending the foot up towards the leg) and a downward motion called plantarflexion (such as bending the foot toward the ground). In a weight-bearing situation, the gliding motion of this joint compensates for the forward and backward displacements of the body's center of gravity so that the body weight is kept within the normal confines of the supporting surfaces.

Below the ankle joint are the two most important joints of the foot: the subtalar joint (below the ankle) and the midtarsal joint (in the middle of the foot).

The *subtalar joint* is a combination of a gliding and angular joint, allowing motion which continues to form pronation and supination.

The *midtarsal joint* is similar to the subtalar joint, and motion allowed is also pronation and supination. However, the amount of motion available to the midtarsal joint is variable in accordance with the position of the subtalar joint. Like the subtalar joint, the end of motion of the midtarsal joint is dependent on bone-to-bone resistance as well as soft-tissue confinement.

In order to fully appreciate the motion of the subtalar joint and midtarsal joint, we must understand the terms supination and

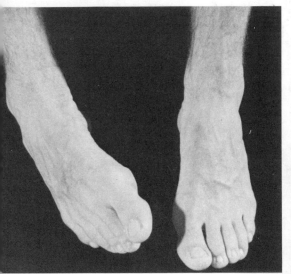

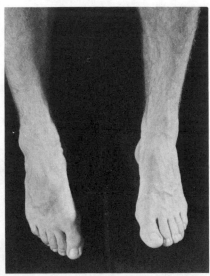

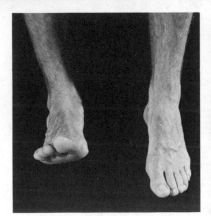

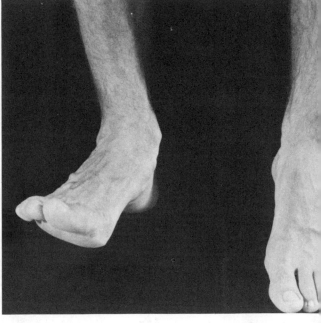

Left: Supination (above) and pronation (below). Right: Plantarflexion (above) and dorsiflexion (below).

28

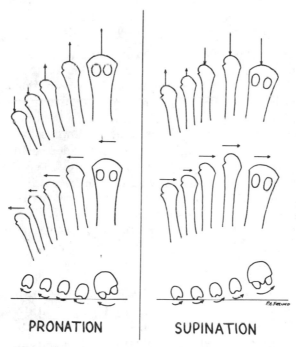

PRONATION | SUPINATION

Motions of the metatarsals with pronation and supination.

pronation. Imagine viewing a person from the front. A line bisecting the body into two equal halves is termed the midline of the body. Supination of the foot is a complex motion involving simultaneous inversion (turning the bottom of the foot towards the midline), adduction (moving the whole foot toward the midline) and plantarflexion (downward motion). A simultaneous combination of these three components will cause the foot to look like this:

Pronation of the foot is also a complex motion consisting of simultaneous eversion (turning the bottom of the foot away from the body's midline), abduction (turning the whole foot away from the midline) and dorsiflexion (up and down motion). A simultaneous combination of these movements will result in the foot looking like this:

Therefore, we can see that supination and pronation are two distinctly opposite movements.

The subtalar joint and midtarsal joint each are capable of performing supination and pronation in the joint itself. When both joints are supinated, they cause supination of the entire foot. Similarly, pronation of both joints will cause pronation of the foot.

As mentioned, the amount of motion available to the midtarsal joint is dependent on the subtalar joint. When the subtalar joint is supinated, it causes a tight bone-to-bone compression in the foot, thereby exerting a "locking" mechanism and decreasing the range of motion in the midtarsal joint. Conversely, when the subtalar joint is pronated, it loosens the bony framework of the foot and thereby "unlocks" it. This unlocking effect causes the midtarsal joint to have more freedom of motion.

Locking and unlocking are essential for gait. When the foot first hits the ground, it is imperative that the foot be unlocked so that it can have more freedom of motion to adapt to the terrain on which it is placed. However, later on, when the foot is about to leave the ground to take the next step, it must get itself ready as a rigid lever in order to propel the leg forward with body weight.

The great toe (hallux) has two bones, and each of the lesser four toes has three bones, which are flexible both where they attach to the metatarsals and at joints where each of these small bones articulate. The toes are also called phalanges, and normally flex up and down as a hinge in the sagittal plane. The toes are normally straight and flat on the ground throughout weight-bearing, and they aid in balance and propulsion.

The position of the toes is maintained by muscle tendons and ligaments. Any imbalance in the rear part of the foot, or pain in the forefoot, will make the toes grip and function abnormally, causing fatigue within the foot or pressure from shoes.

MOTIONS, POSITIONS, ABNORMALITIES

The terms used for motions, positions and abnormalities of the foot and leg are very specific. For each body part in relation to the three major reference planes, there are an infinite number of possibilities. For example, the foot can invert or evert in the frontal plane, dorsiflex or plantarflex in the sagittal plane, and adduct or abduct in the horizontal plane. These are single-plane movements of the foot or part of the foot.

When a joint moves in one plane, we say that it has one degree of freedom of motion (such as the ankle joint); two planes, two degrees (very rare), and three planes, three degrees of freedom of motion (such as the hip joint).

Consistent tri-plane motions of the foot are pronation (in which the distal part of the foot everts, abducts and dorsiflexes), or supination (where the distal part of the foot inverts, adducts and plantarflexes). These are consistent within the foot because the joints, and therefore the axis of motion are inclined to all three body planes.

This is not an example of three degrees of freedom of motion, because it does not allow movement in all directions. Instead, it is a hinge-type which moves in one direction through three body planes. The joints of the foot which allow pronation and supination are the subtalar, midtarsal and fifth-ray joints.

The following table summarizes motions, positions and abnormalities in the various planes. Motion is the act of moving from one place to another. Position is the result of movement. Abnormality is a fixed position (deformed position of the part when it is at rest).

Plane of Motion (reference)	Motion (action)	Position (after movement)	Abnormality (deformed position)
Transverse plane	adduction abduction	adducted abducted	adductus abductus
Frontal plane	inversion eversion	inverted everted	varus valgus
Sagittal plane	dorsiflexion plantarflexion	dorsiflexed plantarflexed	equinus equinus
Three planes	pronation supination	pronated supinated	pronatus supinatus

All motions, positions, and abnormalities in feet may be described in these terms. For example, a subtalar varus is a frontal plane deformity in which everything under the talus (the heel bone) rests in an inverted position, so that the plane of the bottom of the heel bone is directed toward the midline of the body.

All motions, positions, and abnormalities in feet may be described in these terms. For example, a subtalar varus is a frontal plane deformity in which everything under the talus (the heel bone) rests in an inverted position, so that the plane of the bottom of the heel bone is directed toward the midline of the body.

FOOT AND LEG MUSCLES

Almost all muscles of the lower extremity originate proximally from solid large attachments and extend distally via tendons. Muscles produce movement at their insertion into a smaller, lighter part.

The small muscles within the foot are called intrinsic muscles because they arise and end within the foot. They originate proximally and insert distally into the toes for stabilization, and to assist the extrinsic muscles which arise in the leg and produce movement of the parts of the foot.

The main extrinsic muscle groups of the leg are the anterior group (including the anterior tibial which lifts the foot, the extensor muscles which lift the toes and the peroneus tertius which lifts the foot up and out), the lateral muscles (including the peroneal muscles which evert the foot and stabilize the first ray), the posterior muscles of the calf (which form the achilles tendon—the gastrocnemius, the soleus and the plantaris muscles), and the deep posterior muscles (especially the posterior tibial muscle which pulls the foot down and in, and the flexor muscles which pull the toes down).

Four muscles work in balancing the side-to-side position of the foot. Called the "stirrup muscles," they are made up of the anterior and posterior tibial muscles on the medial side, and the peroneus longus and brevis muscles on the lateral side.

In stance, there are "anti-gravity" muscles which help maintain the center of gravity over the base of support in a forward and backward direction. The calf muscles contract to push the ball of the foot down and push the body back as the body pulls forward and the upper attachment muscles pull back on the leg. Conversely, as the center of gravity falls backward, the anterior muscles pull the leg forward so that stress stays in front of the heel bone. Muscles work along the "balancing broomstick" theory in that

32

they pull the body over the base of support, or the base of support moves under the center of gravity.

The main muscles of concern to the athlete which are located around the knee are the hamstring and quadriceps groups. Any muscle of the body can be injured, but those that cross two joints (bi-articular muscles) are especially subject to injury. This is why there is a high incidence of injuries of the hamstring muscles (biceps femoris, semimembranosus, semitendinosus), the quadriceps muscles (especially the vastus medialis, intermedius, lateralis) and the calf muscles (especially the gastrocnemius and the plantaris).

The main function of the knee joint is flexion and extension, a single-plane hinge motion in the sagittal plane. The knee has ligaments on each side for support and limitation of mobility, and muscles in front and back for support and motion with strength.

Throughout the muscle systems of the body, the resting muscles have a moderate tension (tonus) within them, to maintain stability without motion. There is normally a balance of tension in the muscles passing joints so that no inefficient motion or fatigue is encountered at rest, in stance or with activity.

Normal structure allows efficient postural muscle balance. Any inherited structural imbalance, or muscle imbalance acquired through excessive training without total conditioning, will cause strain and fatigue of the imbalanced or overused muscles. That is, if an athlete trains for one specific sport and does not develop strength and flexibility in all muscle groups, then a muscle imbalance will be acquired.

In young athletes, joints are flexible, and greater muscle control is necessary for defined movements. This is why there is a high incidence of muscle problems ("growing pains," sprains) in youngsters and a high incidence of joint problems in adults. Also, this is one of the reasons why children have more difficulty with fine motor skills and movements.

If an athlete develops muscle fatigue repeatedly in one muscle group, it indicates a structural or functional imbalance. For example, muscle pains on the inside of the thigh, in the area of the vastus medialis or sartorius muscles, often are associated with excessive mobility or excessive pronation of the foot, and the reverse is true. Treatment through the use of an artificial support will eliminate this structural or functional imbalance.

Muscle problems of the lower extremity or even around the hips and low back often relate to imbalance which can be corrected with proper foot support. This does not apply to primary traumatic injuries or internal joint derangements, but it is pleasing for podiatrists to be able to help many problems above the foot by balancing foot plant in all phases of activity. This is often done in conjunction with the orthopedist, family doctor, physical therapist and athletic trainer.

TENDONS

Tendons are elastic bands that extend from muscles and attach to bones. When a muscle contracts, the tendon pulls on its attachment (bone) to produce movement. Actually, when the muscle contracts, it pulls equally on both ends, its origin and insertion, producing movement of the lighter or less stable part. For example, the biceps muscle of the arm normally lifts the arm and hand up from the elbow joint, but in doing a chin-up, the body is flexed up on the arm. This is the best way to develop muscle strength through progressive resistance exercise, starting by mildly overloading the muscles and gradually increasing resistance.

Within the foot, long tendons extend from the extrinsic muscles of the leg to produce motion in the foot, or the short tendons of the intrinsic muscles to produce stability and movement within the foot itself.

Tendons are covered with a sheath that allow smooth gliding motion beneath the skin and is free of other attachments. Any injury to this connective tissue can produce adhesions or attachments to other structures which will produce pain with motion or limitation of full joint motion.

Tendons are bound down and held in place by firm connective tissues, fascia, ligaments and bones so that they function effectively. The popping of knuckles or snapping sounds of motion around the foot, ankle or knee often are caused by the movement of tendons over joints.

Tendons are firm bands with a poor blood supply, so they are subject to slow healing and recurrent injuries. In the injuries in which a tendon is ruptured (especially those tendons that do not have an intact sheath) or in areas of excessive motion, professional attention is necessary immediately for immobilization and repair.

BLOOD AND BLOOD VESSELS

Blood is a liquid tissue essential to life. All organs and tissues of the body require nutrition. The blood is constantly being manufactured within the body to transfer required nutrition to the body parts via the red blood cells and to eliminate wastes including carbon dioxide via the white blood cells.

The blood carries hormones, enzymes, antibodies and many other specialized cells to maintain a comfortable internal environment. The blood carries all the elements of healing and repair of injured tissues. Without proper blood supply, healing is incomplete, and excessive scar tissue develops. Those body tissues that have a good blood supply (such as skin and bone) heal well and regenerate completely. Those with poor blood supply (such as tendons, cartilage and ligaments) will never regenerate completely.

In the circulating blood are all the elements of life. The body has other areas of energy storage in muscle and fat that can be converted from storage into usable energy. This ability can be developed through training and conditioning. It is essential to strength during endurance activities.

The major blood vessels of the lower extremity are well protected by bones and large muscle masses. The vessels have muscular walls which expand and contract to increase or decrease blood flow. Blood flow is through an essentially closed system. The heart pumps with its muscular walls through a series of valves so no backward, inefficient flow occurs. Arteries carry blood from the heart to the lungs (where it gets oxygen and releases carbon dioxide), and the muscles, organs, skin and all body parts. The pulse is the heart rate which can be felt along the arteries in various places of the body.

As the blood gets to the body parts, the vessels become smaller (arterioles). Finally, it gets to the microcirculation of the capillaries, where the actual transfer of gases and nutrients passes through the small vessel walls to other cells by osmosis.

After the transfer is complete, the small veins (venioles) begin through muscular milling action to accumulate blood back into the system and enter into the veins. Within the lower extremity, there are two sets of veins, one deep and one superficial. The deep veins run along with the arteries, in opposite directions of blood flow, and so are well protected by the bones and by the muscles and foot. The superficial veins are prominent on most skin surfaces, especially in the extremities, and can be seen as bluish, enlarged lines on the skin.

Veins have a series of valves. In the lower extremity, as the blood moves back up to the heart, the milking action of movement and muscle activity of the major vessels (as well as within the veins themselves) will keep the circulation moving.

The superficial veins drain into the deep veins, also aiding in the movement of blood. This muscular action in the extremities is often called "the peripheral heart" and is essential to normal blood flow. If there is a breakdown in this system, there is pooling of blood fluids in the legs (causing swelling of the ankles). If this pressure continues, or if there is an injury to the vein itself, one of the valves can break, which will apply double pressure and therefore destroy the vein. This pooling of blood causes pain and irritation, along with various types of phlebitis or vein inflammation.

As the pressure increases, more valves break or are separated by the distension. This is the mechanism of varicose veins, and requires medical evaluation and treatment. If all functions as it should, the blood in the veins returns to the heart and continues the cycle.

The blood system is adaptable through conditioning. It is possible to increase blood flow and efficiency through activity, especially through aerobic conditioning programs. Activity exercises vessel muscles. Increased heart rate and pressure with long-term activity will dilate the vessels and help make the vessels more elastic. In this process, the result is increased blood flow to the extremities and the development of collateral circulation in small vessels. Consequently, the heart doesn't have to work as hard to get blood to the tissues, and therefore the resting rate slows down.

In the foot, there are two major arteries: the posterior tibial artery (passing through the tarsal tunnel on the inside and just behind of the medial ankle bone to supply about 75% of the blood to the foot) and the dorsalis pedis artery (which feeds the top of the foot as it passes above and between the first and second metatarsals). Damage to either of these arteries will cause pulsations of blood and damage to surrounding tissues.

If injured, with obvious blood loss or rapid swelling, use direct pressure on the area and seek medical help as soon as possible. If a chronic problem exists in vessels, the person will not be able to participate in athletics.

NERVES

Nerves form the electrical system of the body. The central nervous system is the control center which consists of the brain and spinal column. This has influence over the peripheral nerves which produce motor activity and sensory awareness. The human nervous system is very complex, but all nerves are connected either directly or indirectly to each other.

Parts of this system are automatic, or autonomic, and function independently to support the life processes, such as breathing and the action of the heart. Major abnormalities of the nervous system affect normal activities and negate sports activity.

The main activities of the nervous system in athletes are the motor nerves (which stimulate muscle activity), the sensory nerves (which provide awareness of the internal and external environment) and reflexes (which occur before they are perceived). All of these can be altered through training and conditioning.

Nerve motor function is controlled by the brain and influenced by the emotional or metabolic state of the individual. Motor nerves in the body go from the brain or spinal column to produce action in the muscles. Sensory nerves bring awareness of the environment to the consciousness. Proprioceptive nerves bring awareness of the internal environment, especially balance.

In addition, there are many minute nerves of pain, cold, heat and touch, as well as nerves that supply vessels and specialized structures, such as sweat ducts or hair follicles.

For coordination, it is necessary to have fine hand-eye-brain function. This neuro-muscular control is essential to excellence in sports. Some of this is natural ability, but most is developed through practice.

SKIN

The skin is an organ of the body which provides a selective environment essential to metabolic balance. It absorbs nutrients and rejects waste. It helps in temperature control and fluid balance. It contains sensory organs for touch, temperature, position and pain.

There are basically two divisions of the skin: the epidermis (with four layers of protection and regeneration), and the deeper dermis (which contains the nerves, blood vessels and fat). The epidermis on the palms and soles has an extra layer called the stratum corneum. This layer has the ability to thicken (callous) and increase protection of the deeper, more essential structures.

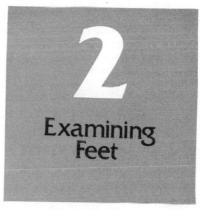

2
Examining Feet

In podiatric medicine, we are concerned with the overall physical condition of the individual, with particular attention to structure, joint ranges of motion, and efficiency of muscles and muscle groups of the foot and leg. There are many specialized methods of evaluation in arriving at a diagnosis and a treatment plan.

In the initial interview, it is important to review all pertinent history which might be related to the athlete's problem. Each doctor follows a diagnostic process through his individual approach, but in each instance he reviews the history, evaluates the symptoms (complaints reported by the patient) and the signs (findings observed by the doctor). He evaluates the present condition through close observation (looking), palpation (touching), percussion (tapping), and auscultation (listening) to the body.

Medical evaluations and examination processes are normally recorded in a standard manner, or SOAP, which refers to Subjective (the complaints of the patient), Objective (the finding of the doctor), Assessment (evaluation of the findings with regard to the patient's needs), Plan (consideration of treatment alternatives, selection of additional diagnostic tests).

The order of recording most examinations of the lower extremity is as follows:

Once a diagnosis is made—that is, the determination of the type and extent of injury to a specific tissue(s)—the appropriate treat-

Areas of Examination

1. Nature of Complaint—a description of the problem in the patient's own words.
    a. total duration—how long it has been noticeable.
    b. acute duration—how long it has been affecting performance.
2. Pain—type of pain; exact location or area.
    a. diseases—present or concurrent.
    b. operations—especially related to location.
    c. injuries or accidents—which might affect lower extremity function.
3. History of Illness or Injury.
    a. present
    b. past
4. Physical and Family History.
5. General Posture—stance evaluation.
6. Gait—normal walking and in activity specific for each sport.
7. Foot Type—general descriptions of high or low arch, wide, narrow, deformed, imbalanced.
8. Visible Deformities—of the feet and legs.
9. Color of Skin—pale, red, cyanotic especially with comparison to the other side or upper extremity.
10. Nails—thickening, splitting or discoloration related to metabolism, nutrition or injury.
11. Skin Lesions—primary or secondary skin changes in response to abnormal internal or external environment.
12. Circulation—pulses, especially the dorsalis pedis and posterior tibial pulses in the foot, the popliteal pulse behind the knee, and the femoral pulse in the upper inner thigh. Also, look for abnormal color changes or problems with the veins, such as varicose veins.
13. Skin Temperature and Texture—related to circulation and nutrition.
14. Edema—specific areas or types of swelling which may indicate local or systemic problems.
15. Reflexes—especially the deep tendon reflexes: the patellar knee jerk, the achilles flexion, and the Babinski test of the foot for hyper- or hypotonicity, indicating problems with the neuromuscular apparatus.

16. Motions of the Foot and Leg—evaluation of the range and quality of motion of the hip, knee and the major joints of the foot: the ankle, subtalar and midtarsal joints. Appraisal of flexibility.

17. Motions and Conditions of Toes.

18. Areas Sensitive to Pressure.

19. Footgear—type, fit and appropriations of casual, training and competition shoes.

20. Conclusion—this may be a diagnosis, differential diagnosis (list of possible diagnoses) or impression, and includes a treatment plan or request for additional tests, such as x-rays, blood tests, special vascular tests or complete biomechanical evaluation.

---

ment may begin. If there is any question as to the specific diagnosis, provide supportive treatment and seek professional consultation.

THE BIOMECHANICAL EXAMINATION

This is a complex process which includes measurements of non-weight bearing positions (seated, lying supine or prone), weight-bearing in stance and in gait. This process is unique to podiatric medicine and has evolved during the past few years. In the past, specific abnormalities were noticed in the resting position, certain things were noticed in the standing foot, and other major neuro-muscular deformities were noticed in gait. Therefore, treatment of these problems was empirical and did not relate to an understanding of function.

This approach is still used by many other professionals who attempt to treat the foot. Podiatrists are concerned with restoration of function and, therefore, try to treat the cause rather than the result of disease processes.

Examination of the foot at rest (non-weight-bearing) is done in order to determine structural and functional ability before compensation occurs. That is, each structural unit is evaluated on a part-to-part basis (such as forefoot to rearfoot, rearfoot to leg, first metatarsal to second metatarsal) in order to determine each individual's neutral position (or position of best function) for each joint.

In this examination, the range of motion (total amount of excursion) is measured, and the quality of motion is assessed. Each moveable joint of the body has an ideal normal position, but the quality of motion is also important.

Normal quality is found whenever a joint can be moved through its full range, in a totally smooth and relaxed manner with an abrupt termination of motion in each direction. There should be no pain, crepitus (grating sound) or restriction of motion. Abnormal quality indicates pain, slowness of motion (created by muscle limitation or swelling), crepitus, unusual laxity or peculiarity of axes of motion.

The quality of motion is the subjective character of a joint, which the examiner or patient feels as the joint is moved through its entire range of motion.

The range of motion is the total available motion of one part to another, as they move around a common joint or joints. All joints of the lower extremity normally demonstrate symmetry of total range between the right and left sides. Unless flexibility exercises are maintained, joint ranges of motion tend to decrease with age. When measured, there may be limitation or laxity compared to the ideal normal range. The major joints of the lower extremity with known normal findings are the hip, the knee and the ankle, and within the foot they are the subtalar joint, the midtarsal joint and the first ray.

When all these measurements are recorded, we then give the patient the stance position examination. This indicates how much the body compensates or does not compensate for structural abnormalities. The stance position of the foot is often different than the appearance of the foot at rest. For example, a foot that is "flat" in stance may actually be a compensated forefoot varus, a normal flatfoot or flat for many other reasons, so it is essential to know the position of the foot in its uncompensated state in order to have a diagnosis of the cause of the foot problem rather than the result.

A review of two specific scientific terms will be helpful here. The neutral position of a joint is the position of best function, from which motions are smooth and predictable. The neutral position must be measured and determined for each individual. In the ideal normal foot, the neutral position is the same as the normal position. Compensation is a change of structure, position or function of one part of the body in an attempt to adjust to, or make up for, the abnormal force of a deviation of structure, position or function of another part. The objective of podiatric biomechanical treatment is to support the neutral position and to prevent compensation.

Normally, the neutral position of the subtalar joint in the frontal plane examination is zero degrees, or in line with the lower leg. From this point, it can invert twice as much as it can evert. If the neutral position is computed to be inverted from zero degrees, it is a subtalar varus which is common; if everted, a subtalar valgus (which is rare).

The midtarsal joint, as represented by the plane of the metatarsal heads, is normally perpendicular to the bisection of the heel bone in the frontal plane. If it is inverted, it is called a forefoot varus; if everted, a forefoot valgus. If the level of metatarsals 2-5 is different than 1-5 it implies that the first ray is either elevated or depressed.

The first ray is normally in line and in the same plane as the second ray. It normally moves equally above and below the second metatarsal head, a total range of approximately two centimeters.

The ankle joint normally allows 10 degrees of dorsiflexion in the sagittal plane with the knee both extended and flexed. If there is adequate dorsiflexion with the knee flexed and limited (less than 10 degrees) with the knee extended, it implies a soft tissue (gastrocnemius muscle) shortage. The measurement of plantarflexion is normally about 45 degrees, but is not important in the average clinical evaluation.

Malleolar torsion is a transverse plane measurement. Normally, the bisection of the medial and lateral malleous is between 13 and 18 degrees. If greater than 18 degrees, it will produce an out-toed angle of gait; if less than 13 degrees, it will produce an intoed position.

Hip joint rotation is a transverse plane measurement. Normally, both with the hip flexed and extended, internal rotation equals external rotation. That is, normally if the hip externally rotates 40 degrees, the neutral position is zero degrees and the knee is directed straight ahead.

The knee joint in stance is normally directly over the ankle joint. If the knees are wider apart than the ankles, and the deformity is within the knee joint, it is termed genu varum. If knock-kneed, it is termed genu valgum. This may be a primary joint problem or secondary to foot malfunction.

Another stance position measurement is the frontal plane of the tibia. Normally, the tibia is straight, but if there is a bowing of the bone in which the distal and is directed toward the midline, it is called tibial varum. If directed away, it is called tibial valgum. Both of these abnormalities have the same effect on the position of the foot as genu varum and valgum, producing rearfoot varus and valgus, respectively.

Normally, the angle of gait is 5-10 degrees out-toed, and is measured as the direction of each foot from the line of progression when walking. When excessively out-toed or intoed, foot function is clumsy and inefficient.

Correlation of the neutral and relaxed calcaneal stance position indicates whether the feet are uncompensated, partially compensated, fully compensated or subluxed. Gait analysis essentially broken up into the contact, midstance, propulsive and swing phases also confirms the diagnosis.

All measurements should be recorded on the Morphological Data Chart as they are observed. If the measurement procedures are correct, all the correlation data will compute to reinforce the diagnosis and treatment plan.

In stance, the foot and leg may or may not compensate for mechanical abnormalities. If enough range of motion is present for compensation to occur, it usually does. But compensation is inefficient in the beginning producing muscle fatigue and later leading to joint pain and possibly arthritis. If compensation reaches the end of the range of motion, it may begin subluxing, which is the term for a slow, forceable dislocation. This produces pain and eventual joint arthritis. If the range of motion is not available for compensation to occur, then with activity there is shock throughout the limb, which also eventually produces imbalance or overuse problems.

The main stance position measurements that are made are postural. In examining posture of the lower extremity in stance,

SUBTALAR JOINT:

Supination	Inversion		20°
Pronation	Eversion		10°
	Total R.O.M.		30°
Neutral Position	Varus		0°
	Valgus		

MIDTARSAL JOINT:

Varus 1-5		0°
Varus 2-5		0°
Valgus 1-5		0°
Valgus 2-5		0°

FIRST RAY:

Dorsiflexion		1 cm.
Plantar Flexion		1 cm.

ANKLE JOINT:

Range of dorsiflexion (knee extended)		10°
Range of dorsiflexion (knee flexed)		15°

ANKLE TO KNEE:

Malleolar Torsion

Internal		13-18°
External		

HIP JOINT:

	Hip Flexed	Hip Extended
Range of Internal Rotation	45°	45°
Range of External Rotation	45°	45°
Total Range of Motion	00°	90°
Neutral Position	0°	0°

KNEE JOINT:

Intermalleolar Distance	6 cm.

Varum	Valgum	Recurvatum
0°	0°	10°

STANCE CORRELATION:

Frontal Plane Tibia

Varum		0°
Valgum		

Angle of Gait

Adduction		5-10°
Abduction		

Calcaneal Position to Floor & Subtalar Joint Neutral

Inverted		0°
Everted		

Calcaneal Stance Position in Static Angle of Gait

Inverted		0°
Everted		

Gait Analysis: See gait evaluation:

Conclusions & Recommendations:

Sample of Morphological Data Chart including normal measurements for one side of the body.

the main measurements are the position of the pelvis, the relationships of the hips to the knees, the knees to the ankles, and the heel bone (calcaneus) to the ground. Rather than forcing the person into the anatomical stance position, we measure the relaxed stance position in the angle and base of gait. (The angle of gait is the direction of each foot from the line of progression when walking, and the base of gait is the width between the feet when walking, so in relaxed stance we duplicate these positions.) The person should stand with equal weight on each limb.

The relaxed stance position of the calcaneus (C.S.P.—calcaneal stance position) should be perpedicular to the floor, vertical and in line with the lower leg. If the calcaneus is tilted inward or outward (inverted or everted), it is abnormal. The lower leg should be vertical to the supporting surface, meaning that the center of the knee should be over the center of the ankle (therefore, there is no knock knee or bow-leg to produce stress). The pelvis should be level, with limbs of equal length. In this position, the knees are pointing straight ahead and the ankles are outwardly rotated about 15 degrees.

Evaluation of the relaxed stance position tells us how much the foot and leg have compensated for structural imbalances. Evaluation of gait then confirms how and when the foot compensates. Various foot and leg abnormalities produce changes at different times during the gait cycle. Since performance in sports is based on efficient function, people with certain foot types will perform better in specific events, specific positions and specific sports.

We do not expect that all athletes, coaches and trainers wish to learn how to evaluate the structure of the lower extremity. Therefore, we will describe a simple field examination, then, for those who are interested, a more detailed clinical evaluation of the lower extremity.

FIELD EXAMINATION

This description is primarily for the trainers, coaches and athletes who wish to check their teams or teammates. Complete examination of the lower extremity is a complex process which involves the history of any sports related symptoms or injuries, examination of structure, function, gait patterns, shoe wear pat-

46

terns, skin callus locations, and often needs x-rays or laboratory tests to confirm a diagnois.

Stance Position Examination: Have the person stand barefoot, wearing short pants, in the angle and base of gait—that is, the angle of the foot from the direction of motion and the distance between the ankles while he is walking. The person should stand relaxed with equal weight on each foot. Normally, the angle each foot makes with the line of progression is 5-10 degrees out-toed, and the width between the ankles is about three inches. In stance, with the body erect, facing straight ahead and the arms at the sides.

• The hips and pelvis should be level, the shoulders level, the spine straight and the head erect.

• The center of the knee joint should be over the center of the ankle joint.

Below: Two views of the one-foot test for balance. Right: Posture chart courtesy of d'Curlin Publishing, P.O. Box 1265, Oceanside, Calif. 92054.

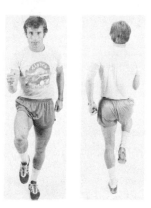

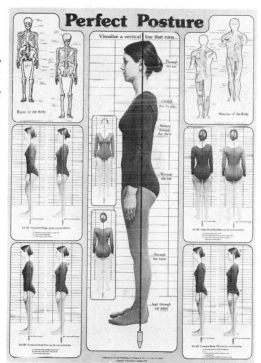

Perfect Posture

- There should be no bow-legs or knock-knees.
- The heel bone should be in line with the lower leg and straight (perpendicular) to the ground.
- The ball of the foot should be flat on the ground, the toes straight and parallel with each other (no bunions, hammertoes or pressure points from shoe irritation).
- The inside arch should form a smooth curve.

The person should be able to stand in this position comfortably with no foot fatigue or low-back strain for at least five minutes. If a structural imbalance exists, muscles try to compensate, with resulting fatigue. The most common problems seen in stance are bowed legs, tilted heel bone, flat feet and contracted tendons to the toes.

The One-Foot Test: The ability to balance on one foot is a good test for structural stability and neuromuscular control. He should be able to balance on one foot for at least three minutes. There should be a balance between the inside muscles (anterior and posterior tibial), outside muscles (peroneus longus and brevis), and between the front muscles (anterior tibial and extensor digitorum longus) and back muscles of the calf. If weight stress constantly falls to the inside, it indicates a mobile, pronated foot type which needs support. If weight stress falls to the outside, causing inversion of the foot, then the range of motion at the joints is not sufficient for normal function, and needs either stretching exercises, external support or both.

This test indicates the general laxity or tightness of joints for the individual and explains how he might function under stress. It also shows the position a foot forms when running, where the support must be under the center of gravity.

Off-Weight-Bearing Examination:

Examine the foot:

- From the bottom: observe any corns, calluses, blisters or skin irritation indicating tissue stress and possible imbalance.
- From the top: observe any tight tendons, crooked, deformed toes, corns or pressure points on toenails, which could become disabling during competition.

48

• With the person seated or lying supine (on his back): The legs should be able to rotate in or out equally, and the resting position from the knee joint should be straight ahead; the legs should extend fully straight with no stress on the hamstring muscles; with the knee straight, the foot should be able to dorsiflex at least 10 degrees at the ankle joint (to form an angle of about 80 degrees with the lower leg).

• With the person lying prone (face down), knees straight, feet hanging at rest: The ball of the foot should be perpendicular or tilted slightly inward (less than five degrees) from the direction of the heel bone; the heel bone should be in line or tilted slightly inward (less than five degrees) from the lower part of the leg.

A small degree of imbalance of the foot or leg will cause compensatory muscle strain, leading to overuse injury during a conditioning program. This overuse may show on the skin, deeper soft structures or even bone (stress fractures). Prevention of overuse injuries is successful with proper examination, training toward flexibility as well as strength and the use of supportive protective footgear. Traumatic injuries need time to heal, but overuse injuries can be evaluated and treated without disability or lost training time. A few minutes of examination early in the conditioning program may prevent a season of nagging injuries.

CLINICAL MEASUREMENT

This description is primarily for the professionals who wish to examine, diagnose, record and treat structural problems of the foot and leg. Some people will find this common sense, others will find this description complex.

Examination is an art. In working with and teaching many individuals, we find that a specific aptitude is helpful, but the process can be learned. An acceptance and understanding of spacial relationships is important. The examiner should have the ability to see things in the three planes. At once, he should be able to relate each part to another in each plane and understand how they function together. Any art requires understanding of certain basic principles, followed by the continued practice of technique. Generally, a greater understanding of basics leads to a more thorough examination and interpretation of findings.

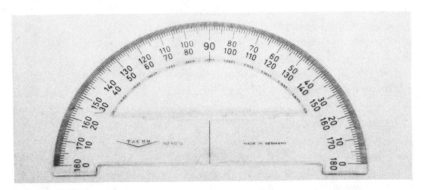

Protractor (above) and tractograph are used in measurement.

Inconsistent technique will lead to false conclusions and treatment failure. Therefore, one should practice these techniques until he is confident and his measurements are reliable.

The purpose of the examination is to confirm normal findings and recognize abnormal structural conditions which affect gait. The examination follows this format:

A. *Major measurements for the thigh and leg.*

1. Hip joint and knee joint: in order to allow normal function in gait, we are concerned mainly with the side-to-side and rotational movement of the hip which allow the knee to function in the sagittal plane around a frontal-transverse axis of motion. Abnor-

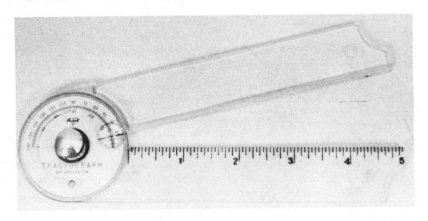

malities of the hip and femur which especially affect this position of the knee joint are: internal and external rotations (whether at the hip, within the femur, or neuromuscular; soft tissue in origin), coxa vara, coxa valga. Major abnormalities within the knee joint are genu varum, genu valgum and genu recurvatum.

Technique of hip joint measurement: All measurements should be made in both the supine and seated positions in order to rule out muscular limitation of motion. If the measurement is the same both ways, it indicates a bone problem; if it's different, it indicates a muscle problem. For normal function, the knee joint axis of motion should allow sagittal plane motion. Internal rotation of the hip should *equal* external rotation.

With the patient supine, support the relaxed, extended limb at the ankle so that there is no friction from the supporting surface. Passively internally rotate the limb to resistance and measure (with either protractor or tractograph) the position of the femoral condyles from the frontal plane of the body. Passively externally rotate the limb to equal resistance at the opposite extent of the

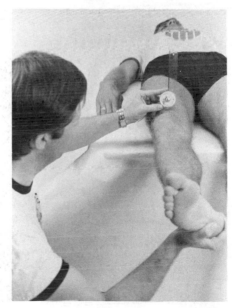

Measuring external rotation of the limb with a tractograph.

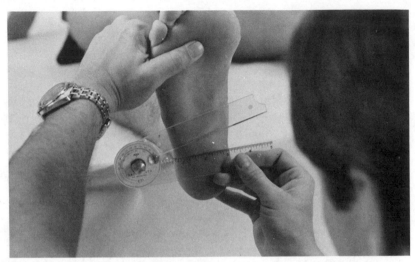

Measurement of outward rotation of ankle bones.

range of motion, and compare the femoral condyles with the frontal plane of the body.

(Do not use the position of the patella as a direct criterion of knee joint position; the patella moves on the femur up to five degrees with internal and external movements, and is under some voluntary control by the patient. The patella may be used as a general impression of femoral position).

Repeat on other limb. Repeat measurement procedure in the seated position for both limbs. Allow *up to* 15 degrees internal or external position of the femoral condyles as the extremes of normal position. The knee joint itself is able to absorb this much variation to allow normal gait (but does not *always* do so!);

Example one: if, internal rotation equals 45 degrees, and, external rotation equals 50 degrees, the total range of motion is 95 degrees; the neutral position of the hip is 2-1/2 degrees externally rotated and within normal limits.

Example two: if, internal rotation equals 65 degrees, and external rotation equals 25 degrees, the total range of motion equals 90 degrees; the neutral position of the hip is 20 degrees internally rotated and will affect the angle of gait by at least five degrees (up to 15 degrees may be absorbed within the knee joint).

In stance, the knee joint should be parallel with the transverse plane and allow the tibia to be vertical (90 degrees) to the transverse plane. The measurement procedure is the same for children (after they begin to walk) and for adults, with minor changes in technique. Consider the fact that there are normal external torsional factors within the limb (femur and tibia) which tend to increase ("abduct") the angle of gait by 8-12 degrees from the time the child first begins to walk, progressing through puberty.

Common sources of error in measurement: (a) position and use of measuring instruments and the patient; (b) patient lifting hip while measuring internal rotation (therefore adding to actual measurement); (c) not rotating limb with equal force to extremes of range of motion.

2. Tibia: For normal function in gait, the tibia must function in the sagittal plane, the plane perpendicular to the transverse and frontal planes. In measurement, consider all three planes:

• Sagittal plane: The tibia should be straight in the sagittal plane. It should be in the sagittal and frontal planes in the anatomical stance position and in the sagittal plane throughout the gait cycle. Abnormalities in the sagittal plane are generally

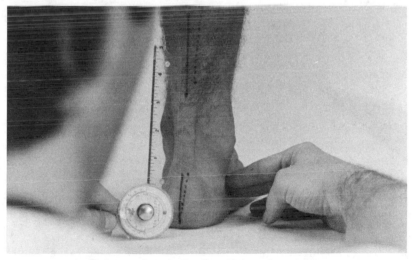

Calcaneal and tibial positions in stance.

seen as an anterior bowing of the shaft of the tibia, as seen in the "sabre shin" deformity of congenital syphilis, Osgood-Schlatter's disease or anterior bowing with rickets and other rare malnutritional states.

Frontal plane: For the adult normal stance position, the tibia is perpendicular and vertical to the transverse plane, and is therefore within the sagittal plane. A frontal plane bowing within the shaft of the tibia places the foot either inverted or everted in relation to the supporting surface, and produces abnormal stresses through the foot when in function during gait. Tibia varum is defined as a frontal plane bowing within the shaft of the tibia, in which the distal end of the tibia is closer to the midline of the body (lateral convexity). Tibia valgum is a frontal plane bowing within the shaft of the tibia, in which the distal end is directed away from the midline of the body (medial convexity). This bowing within the shaft of the tibia will place the ankle joint and therefore the entire foot, in an inverted or everted position, respectively.

False recordings are often made for the young (up to age six) because of the development of the peroneal (lateral) muscle group before the development of the posterior muscle group, altering the appearance of the back of the leg. Rare disease processes may affect the frontal plane relationships of the tibia, such as Blount's disease, rickets or other malnutritional states.

Measurement: (1) body in stance position; (2) foot in normal angle and base of gait; (3) equal weight on each foot; (4) subtalar joint in neutral position; (5) compare posterior inferior one-third of the leg (inferior to the major muscle mass) to the transverse plane; (6) record results in degrees and classify each limb.

Vertical—90 degrees; "inverted" equals X degrees tibia varus; "everted" equals X degrees tibial valgum.

Differentiate tibia varum or valgum (bowing within the shaft of the tibia; a pure osseous structural deformity) from genu varum or valgum (deviation of the tibia from the knee joint itself; a positional or structural deformity).

• Transverse plane: For the adult normal stance position, the ankle joint is externally positioned approximately 15 degrees from the frontal plane of the body. Clinical tibial torsion (malleolar) torsion), as measured by the relationship of the lateral, fibular malleolus and the medial, tibial malleolus to the frontal plane of the body, should not be confused with true tibial torsion, a torsion within the long axis of the tibia itself. *True* tibial torsion is a position of the distal end of the tibia measured in the transverse plane as 18-23 degrees externally deviated from the proximal end of the tibia or frontal plane of the body. This measurement is not possible clinically because the lateral surface of the tibia is not palpable. *Clinical* tibial torsion, or malleolar torsion, in the normal adult ranges from 13-18 degrees externally positional from the frontal plane and is measureable. Measurements of clinical tibial torsion are progressive from approximately zero degrees when the child begins to walk to puberty when the adult normal range of 13-18 degrees external tibial torsion is reached.

Measurement: (1) with the patient seated or supine, support the relaxed extended limb at the mid-foot so there is no friction from the supporting surface; (2) keep the femoral condyles in the frontal plane of the body; (3) subtalar joint in its neutral position; (4) keeping eyes on the level of the shaft of the tibia, look at the foot and ankle from inferior; at this level, palpate and bisect the widths of both the medial malleolus and lateral malleolus; (5) keeping eyes on the level of the tibia, extend the above bisection points to the plantar surface of the foot; (6) placing the upper arm of a tractograph connecting these bisection points, with the axis of the tractograph lateral, and the lower arm of the tractograph parallel with the frontal plane of the body, read angle in degrees; (7) record findings, classify and repeat on opposite limb; (8) findings: 13-18 degrees external tibial torsion for adult, within normal limits; less than 13 degrees, internal tibial (malleolar) torsion; greater than 18 degrees, "excess" tibial (malleolar) torsion.

The measurement procedure is the same for children and adults, but the child yields relatively smaller measurements until the adult normal values are reached near the age of puberty.

In the diagnosis of true tibial torsion, rule out rotational deformities from the knee joint; sometimes called tibial rotations, or "pseudo"-tibial torsion, which has been described similar to tibial rotation, and to a condition in which there is motion available between the tibia and fibula, giving false readings. The subject of "pseudo"-tibial torsion is currently under research.

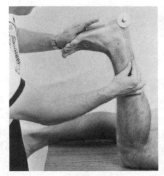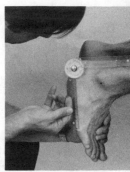

Dorsiflexion of the ankle with the knee extended and flexed.

Common source of error in measurement of clinical tibial torsion: (1) knee not held in frontal plane of body; (2) subtalar joint not held in neutral positions; (3) improper marking of malleoli and extension of those lines to the foot; (4) improper use of measuring device.

B. Structural Measurements for the foot.

1. The ankle joint: The normal ankle joint exhibits at least 10 degrees of dorsiflexion of the foot from 90 degrees with the leg, while the knee is extended. At the end of the midstance phase of gait, the foot must reach an angle of 80 degrees to the tibia. If this is not available, there is stress on the foot to dorsiflex, and this must occur at the subtalar or midtarsal joints, causing excessive pronation.

Technique of ankle joint measurement:

• The patient is either prone or supine with the knee extended; knee parallels frontal plane.

• The posterior surface of the calcaneus is therefore externally rotated from the frontal plane.

• The subtalar joint is placed in its neutral position.

• Passively dorsiflex the foot to resistance, keeping the posterior surface of the calcaneus in a constant neutral position with the leg. This relationship corresponds to the neutral position of the subtalar joint and must not change when the ankle joint is actively dorsiflexed (by contraction of the anterior tibial muscle by the patient).

• When the maximum dorsiflexion is achieved, the angle

between the plantar aspect of the foot and the lateral aspect of the distal one-third of the leg is measured. The plantar aspect of the foot is respresented by an imaginary line from the plantar aspect of the calcaneus to the plantar aspect of the fifth metatarsal head. The lateral aspect of the distal one-third of the leg is represented by a line bisecting the lateral aspect of the leg from the musculo-tendinous junction of the triceps surae to just proximal to the malleoli.

• If midtarsal joint subluxation is present, it is necessary to observe the motion of the plantar surface of the calcaneus throughout the entire range of dorsiflexion. The angle of dorsiflexion is measured at the moment the plantar surface of the calcaneus stops moving. Any further dorsiflexion of the foot on the leg must be a result of midtarsal joint subluxation and not influence the measurement of the ankle joint motion.

Common sources of error: (1) subtalar joint not in neutral position; (2) fifth metatarsal or midtarsal joint subluxed; (3) not using tractograph properly; (4) not positioning yourself properly for the examination.

2. The subtalar joint: This includes the articulations between the talus and calcaneus. The axis of subtalar joint motion is

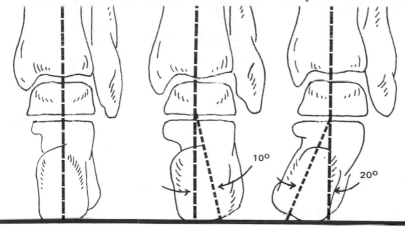

Positions of the subtalar joint: neutral (left), pronated (center), supinated (right).

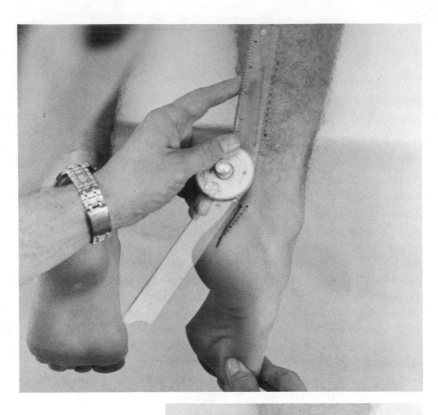

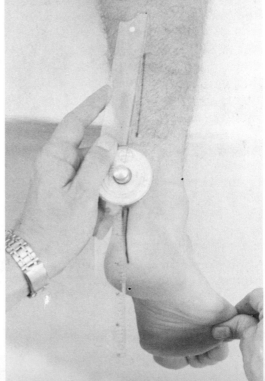

Measurements of supination (above) and pronation (left) indicate neutral position of the individual.

58

inclined to all three body planes and allows the three plane motions of pronation (dorsiflexion, eversion and abduction) and supination (plantarflexion, inversion and adduction), as the talus adducts and plantarflexes in pronation the calcaneus everts. As the talus abducts and dorsiflexes in supination, the calcaneus inverts. Subtalar motion is analyzed by measuring the frontal plane motion of the calcaneus. Normally, the neutral position of the posterior surface of the calcaneus is in line with the tibia, and from this position the calcaneus can invert twice as much as it can evert. Simultaneously, the subtalar joint supinates twice as much as it pronates from the neutral position.

Technique of subtalar joint measurement:

• With the patient prone, place the posterior surface of the calcaneus parallel to the frontal plane. This usually requires internal rotation of the leg.

• Move the subtalar joint to the extreme pronation by holding the foot at the fourth and fifth metatarsal heads and dorsiflexing, everting and abducting the distal part.

• Keeping your head directly over the calcaneus and perpendicular to the frontal plane, bisect the posterior surface of the calcaneus from its most proximal to distal aspect by palpating the medial and lateral edges.

• With your head perpendicular to the frontal plane, bisect the distal one-third of the leg from the musculotendinous junction of the triceps surea (calf muscles) to the proximal aspect of the malleoli.

• Measure the angle of eversion produced by the leg and calcaneal lines with either a protractor or goniometer. Protractor: The base of the protractor is placed in leg line. The apex of the protractor is placed on the most proximal point of the calcaneal line, keeping its base parallel to the leg line. The angle produced by the calcaneal line is then measured, holding the instrument parallel to the frontal plane. Goniometer: One arm of the goniometer is placed on the leg line, and the other arm is placed parallel to the calcaneal line while it is held parallel to the frontal plane.

• The subtalar joint is then moved to the extreme of supination by holding the foot at the fourth and fifth metatarsal heads, and plantarflexing, inverting and adducting the distal on the proximal part.

• The bisection lines of the distal one-third of the leg and the posterior surface of the calcaneus are checked. Usually these lines must be re-established due to movement of the skin over the osseous structures.

• The angle of inversion is measured following the same technique as eversion with pronation.

• Once the range of motion is determined, compute the neutral position of the subtalar joint, according to the formula: neutral position equals maximum eversion minus one-third the total range of motion.

Common sources of error: (1) skin lines too wide or improperly placed; (2) posterior surface of calcaneus not parallel to frontal plane; (3) not positioning yourself properly; (4) not using measuring instruments properly; (5) movement of the skin over the bones; (6) applying unequal pressure at extremes of motion.

3. The midtarsal joint: The midtarsal (transverse tarsal, Chopart's joint) includes the articulations between the talus and navicular, and the calcaneus and the cuboid bones. Like the subtalar joint, midtarsal motion consist of pronation and supination.

In normal stance, the midtarsal joint is locked in the direction of pronation, and the plane of the forefoot is perpendicular to the bisection of the calcaneus. If the forefoot is inverted relative to the rearfoot, there is forefoot varus; if the forefoot is everted relative to the rearfoot, there is forefoot valgus. Frontal plane position of the forefoot is the most important measurement of the midtarsal joint.

Technique of midtarsal joint measurement:

• With the patient kneeling or prone, place the foot in the following position: posterior surface of calcaneus on the frontal plane; subtalar joint in neutral position (which was previously accurately established); ankle joint dorsiflexed to resistance; midtarsal joint pronated; fifth ray pronated.

• This position is maintained by placing digital pressure upward on the distal aspect of the fourth and fifth metatarsal heads.

• Measure the frontal plane angulation which occurs between the forefoot and the rearfoot. The forefoot is represented by a

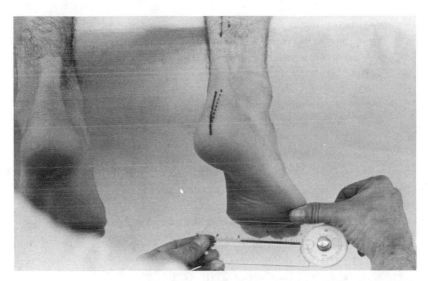

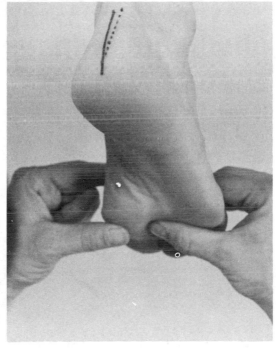

Above: The normal forefoot is perpendicular to the bisection of the heel bone. Right: The normal first metatarsal is level with the second metatarsal.

line from the plantar surface of the fifth to the plantar surface of the first metatarsal head. Since the first and fifth rays are mobile and the 2-4 rays are stable, if there is elevation or plantarflexion of the first or fifth rays, use the next adjacent metatarsal for the measurement. The rearfoot is represented by the bisection of the posterior surface of the calcaneus. It is usually necessary to re-bisect the calcaneus when the subtalar joint is in the neutral position.

Sources of error: (1) calcaneus not on frontal plane or in neutral position; (2) ankle joint not dorsiflexed, mid-tarsal joint not pronated; (3) fifth ray subluxed; (4) lines too wide or improperly placed; (5) pressing the measuring device on the forefoot, depressing soft tissue and distorting the angle.

4. The first ray: This includes the first metatarsal and the first cuneiform which move about a common axis. As the foot pronates in stance, the first ray becomes hypermobile as it dorsiflexes and inverts. As the foot supinates, it may plantarflex and evert. Normally, at rest the first metatarsal head is parallel with the other metatarsal bones. In the abnormal state, the first ray may be elevated or plantarflexed, either flexible or rigid, producing concurrent imbalances of the forefoot. The first ray may function independently of the forefoot and rearfoot. Normally, the range of motion of the first ray is about two centimeters, one above and one below the level of the second metatarsal.

3

The Abnormalities

Throughout Part I, we have stressed that normal is an *ideal* rather than the average. A narrow range of normal that is acceptable for each body tissue, structure or part. In order to function normally, the structure must hold up in an average manner, in an average environment, as dictated by the needs of the activity at the moment, with no adverse physical or emotional response to the individual.

Conditioning enhances the ability of the structure to perform under adverse circumstances. Conditioning allows the structure to perform in a previously limiting enviroment. Those structures that do not respond to conditioning are the weak link in the chain and may need treatment.

An abnormality is that condition that does not fit the criteria for "normal." It may or may not produce pathology, which is the development of symptoms or a disease process in either structure or function. Therefore, "abnormal" refers to a structure or relationship that does not qualify as normal, but does not produce serious symptoms or loss of function. "Pathological" is a morbid or disease process or any abnormality which may disturb the function of all or part of the body, thereby causing symptoms to a greater or lesser degree.

For the most part, congenital (inherited) bone structures dictate the function and performance of the lower extremity. If there is a bone abnormality, joints are at an angle to each other and are inefficient.

Muscles provide movement of bones at joints. There is an intricate balance between the muscle tendons on both sides of a joint. When not moving, there is equal tension on both sides. With movement, one muscle pulls as the other (antagonist) gradually relaxes, so that motion is not allowed to pass beyond the smooth joint surfaces. If muscles function with a mechanical advantage to one side of a joint, the prime-moving muscle becomes stronger than the resisting muscle, leading to an acquired muscle problem which produces fatigue, tendonitis or even muscle pulls. In order for performance to be smooth and predictable, the brain, spinal column and electrical system (nerves) must be coordinated. Sensations, reflexes and motor activities must be specific. Training will help eliminate unwanted actions.

ACQUIRED FOOT AND LEG PROBLEMS

These are the types of problems brought on through injury, disease processes or environmental forces. Injuries disturb the normal function of body parts. If untreated, there may be adhesions, scar tissue and eventual loss of full strength and full function. This will be covered specifically in the later section on the care of injuries.

Disease processes, whether involving the entire body or a local inflammatory area through foreign body irritation, infection or metabolic disturbances, should be evaluated and treated by a professional. Local infection can spread into the bloodstream and cause serious consequences. If an athlete has any ongoing disease process, he should not be allowed to perform or compete without medical approval and supervision.

Acquired foot and leg problems may be brought on by environmental forces, such as faulty equipment or improperly fit shoes and socks. Bad shoes will aggravate minor structural foot imbalances and may actually cause ingrowing toenails, blisters, abrasions, and produce structural and functional problems in the toes. Stretch socks, pointed toe, and high heeled or platform shoes do not allow normal foot motions. They produce problems in the feet through pressure, and in the knees, hips and low back by restricting normal activities. Initially this causes fatigue, and then it produces fixed (bone and joint) structural problems.

64

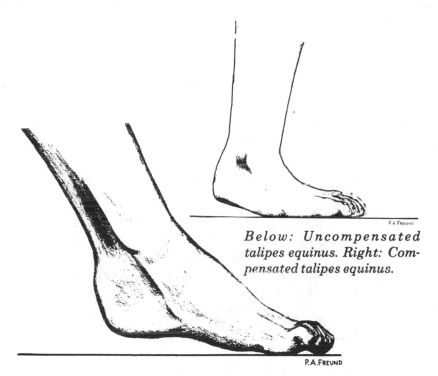

Below: Uncompensated talipes equinus. Right: Compensated talipes equinus.

P.A.FREUND

The human body adapts to its environment. All body tissues to a degree adapt to adverse conditions—bones change, joints change, muscles change and so on. In order to perform to its full capacity, the body must be moderately stressed toward strength, endurance and flexibility under varied conditions. Overtraining of certain muscle groups, produces imbalances that lead to overuse of the underconditioned body structures. Therefore, in order to avoid acquired imbalances, it is necessary to maintain condition in those structures which are not specific to the particular sport.

For example, long-distance runners must work on flexibility of all muscle groups of the legs and low back, as well as moderate upper-body progressive resistance (weight) training to maintain strength and prevent imbalances. The act of long-distance running develops the "go-ahead" muscles, so it is very common to acquire tight, short calf ("runner's equinus") and hamstring muscles, with relatively weak anterior muscles of the leg and quadriceps muscles of the thigh. This same calf muscle imbalance also occurs in the "toes-down" pointed position in swimmers, and in half-point and full-point ballet dancers. When we understand the proper technique necessary for good performance in specific sports, we can then begin to condition those muscles as well as the antagonist (opposite) muscles to prevent acquired imbalances.

NEUROMUSCULAR AND OTHER SOFT TISSUE ABNORMALITIES

Coordination of the body systems is essential to performance. Abnormalities in the neuromuscular system do not allow hand-eye coordination, or fine muscle balance and control. This eliminates many people from certain sports. The so-called "natural athlete" has that rare ability to control his muscle activities, to sense his balance and joint position, and to perform efficiently under varied conditions with less training than most other athletes.

Fortunately, most people can develop coordination through practice. This is why we emphasize learning technique before developing speed. Major neuromuscular physical disorders such as cerebral palsy, poliomyelitis, encephalitis and so on are serious and are beyond the scope of this book. They affect all muscles of the body, even those of speech and general metabolism. Specific muscle spasms or contractures are often an attempt by the body to guard or protect a malfunctioning body part. They should be evaluated professionally.

Some abnormal foot positions are caused by mild neuromuscular imbalances, causing increased tonus (muscle tension) or paralysis (lack of nerve and muscle function) on one side of a joint, and producing abnormal positions at rest and with activity. Since motion occurs around a joint axis, this abnormality affects the quality of motion at the joint, and can be felt during the examination process and observed in gait. Most axes of motion in the body are inclined to the main body planes, so that there may be a "triplane" abnormality. Inherited bone problems are usually classified according to single plane osseous criteria and must be differentiated from the neuromuscular type.

The soft tissues are all those except the bone structures. In general, abnormalities of the soft tissues such as corns and calluses are secondary to structural bone problems or to environmental forces. (They are discussed specifically in the injuries and treatment section.) Soft-tissue problems usually heal quickly and well, as long as the cause of the problem is isolated and eliminated. Many forms of medical treatment such as cortisone injections and pills act on the results of the abnormality rather than the cause. It is essential to understand if one is to cure it.

66

INHERITED ABNORMAL FOOT STRUCTURES
AND COMPENSATIONS

This is the area that is unique to podiatric medicine and the key to many successful treatment plans—first, recognizing abnormal from normal, and then providing rehabilitation, treatment and lasting resolution of the problem.

Minor abnormalities of only a few degrees in the foot or leg will cause compensations of other body parts, with resultant overuse or imbalance. Not all abnormalities produce problems; some are corrected and some are aggravated by other measurable abnormalities. We do not "treat" measurements but use the measurements to help in our treatment. In arriving at a diagnosis and treatment, it is important to understand the nature and demands of the sports, the non-weight-bearing appearance of the foot and leg, the compensations that occur in posture with stance, and the efficiency of motion in the body during gait.

Abnormal foot types are best described in relation to the major body reference planes. Through the measurement and examination process, we are able to record on the morphological data sheet both the normal and abnormal findings. We relate this to the present symptoms of the patient and arrive at a treatment plan.

Since our criteria are in comparision to the ideal normal foot and leg, we must determine the amount of abnormality present, and then decide whether to attempt to correct the structure or attempt to balance it throughout the gait cycle. This accepts the structural abnormality (deformity) that exists and allows the individual to function normally in the presence of the abnormal structure.

Many abnormalities are well absorbed by the body tissues themselves, and those may not produce any problems for the patient. Some abnormalities require corrective procedures, such as corrective casting or surgery, but most structural abnormalities can be controlled on a temporary basis with protective devices such as taping and padding, or balanced on a permanent basis with braces or orthotic devices.

The main single-plane osseous abnormalities of the foot are: equinus, or a neutral position of the ankle joint in the sagittal plane where the foot is plantarflexed on the leg; subtalar varus or subtalar valgus in which the neutral position of the subtalar joint primarily in the frontal plane is inverted or everted on the leg, respectively; forefoot varus or forefoot valgus in which the frontal plane position of the forefoot is inverted or everted on the rearfoot respectively; or metatarsus adductus, a transverse plane abnormality in which the metatarsal bones are angled inward from the rearfoot, causing a convexity to the outside of the foot.

In mild cases, single-plane osseous abnormalities are called positional variations, and in the more severe cases they may be called deformities. Several single-plane osseous abnormalities may be present at one time, causing a grossly distorted appearance of the foot as in clubfoot. The most common types of clubfoot are talipes equino-adducto-varus in which the entire foot is plantar-flexed adducted and inverted, or talipes calcaneo-valgus in which the foot is dorsiflexed, abducted and everted. The term talipes refers to a deformity of the entire foot. Abnormalities are always described as the relative position of the distal on the proximal part.

Abnormalities are first diagnosed through examination of the non-weight-bearing position and motions of the foot on a part-to-part basis. That is, we compare the ankle to the leg, the heel bone to the leg, the forefoot to the rearfoot, the first metatarsal to the second metatarsal and so on. We then compare this to the weight-bearing position to see if and how the body compensates for any abnormality.

Compensation refers to an abnormal, but not necessarily pathological change in one part of the body in an attempt to neutralize an abnormal position or function in another part. With compensation, foot and body parts change posture. The foot has the ability to compensate for abnormal forces coming up from the ground or down through the leg.

Pronation and supination of the foot may compensate for foot and leg deformities. A normal amount of pronation and supination is necessary during gait and in sports activities, and specific sports put specific demands on the foot to adapt. As the foot pronates, the joints of the foot and leg become mobile, causing stress on ligaments, and strain of muscles and tendons. As the foot supinates, the joints of the foot and leg become rigid, causing shock up the leg and impingement on joint surfaces. When pronation or supination are excessive, whether caused by compensation of the body or increased demands of the sport, imbalance and overuse problems occur.

THE PRONATION SYNDROME

As the foot pronates in stance, the talus adducts and plantarflexes as the calcaneus everts. Since the talus is locked in the ankle joint, as it moves inward the leg internally rotates. If excessive, this rotation puts strain on the medial muscles, tendons and ligaments—for example, the posterior tibial muscle and the plantar fascia of the foot. As the talus plantarflexes, the arch flattens, which lengthens the inside border of the foot, stretching all the soft tissues and putting the joint surfaces at an inefficient angle to each other. When joint surfaces are not congruous, motion occurs when those joints should be stable.

Hypermobility is defined as any motion occurring in a joint during weight bearing when that joint should be stable under such load. Hypermobility refers either to excessive motion or motions at a time when there should be none. Hypermobility of the first ray develops whenever the foot is excessively pronated from its neutral position. Therefore, lesions develop under the second metatarsal. Whenever hypermobility is present, hallux abducto-valgus bunions will tend to develop. This occurs with several different compensated foot types.

Whenever the heel bone is everted in stance, it is abnormal and usually means that the foot is excessively pronated from its neutral position. Eversion of the calcaneus produces a medial bowing or convexity of the achilles tendon (called a Helbing's sign) and is present in specific compensated foot types.

As the talus adducts and the leg internally rotates with pronation in stance, there is a stretching force on the medial side of the knee and a pinching force on the lateral side. Normally, the knee joint should function like a hinge in the sagittal plane, forward and backward. When the foot pronates excessively, the knee rotates internally, tending to produce a knock-kneed appearance with medial position of the patella. The kneecap is not attached to any bones but moves along with the muscles of the thigh, the four muscles call the quadriceps femoris.

With pronation, therefore, there is a stress on the medial muscles of the thigh. There is a certain amount of sharp absorption in all directions within the structures of the knee. But as the leg rotates, the thigh rotates, producing a torque within the knee joint as well as excessive motion in the hip joint. This produces a strain around the capsular structures of the sides of the knee, and the front and back of the hip. It comes on with activity and is relieved with rest.

As the thigh internally rotates with force on the front of the pelvis, a forward (anterior) tilting of the pelvis develops, which then begins to limit normal rotations at the hip joint. Anterior tilt of the pelvis, in which the front of the pelvis comes down and the back of the pelvis moves up, produces swayback or lumbar lordosis, a major cause of backache.

Excessive pronation also causes stress fractures in the leg syndromes in the lower extremity. In the feet, it is associated with arch strain and fatigue, plantar fasciitis, the heel spur syndrome, achilles tendonitis, hallux abducto-valgus bunions, contracted or hammertoes, problems with growing bones in children, and stress fractures of the metatarsals, especially the second metatarsal bone.

In the leg, pronation causes stress fractures of the tibia or fibula and acquired muscle imbalances producing shin splints, especially posterior tibial myositis.

At the knee joint, excessive pronation of the foot leads to knock-knee, chondromalcia or softening of the back of the cartilage of the patella, irritation of the medial and lateral menisci and collateral ligaments, and bursitis, especially below the patellar ligament or at the pes anserinus where three muscles of the thigh insert into the medial side of the tibia.

Within the thigh, excessive pronation of the foot causes strains of the vastus medialis, the adductors, the sartorius and other muscles on the medial side, and specifically the tensor fascia lata and the ilio-tibial band on the lateral side. As the thigh internally rotates at the hip, with overuse there may be a "snapping hip" where muscle tendons pop over bone prominences, bursitis or capsular strain.

If posture is affected with an anterior tilt of the pelvis, there may be low lumbar sprains and low-back pains in the area of joints L-5, S-1 or L-4, L-5, or may be painful around the sacroiliac joints secondary to overuse. If pain radiates behind the gluteals and down the lateral thigh, there may be sciatic nerve involvement: sciatica. Biomechanically, all of these problems are associated with excessive pronation of the foot.

As the foot pronates and the arch drops down, there is a functional limb-length difference. With pronation of the foot on one side, that leg is "shorter." With pronation of both feet and internal rotation of both legs, there is an anterior tilt of the pelvis and central low-back strain. With pronation of one foot, there is a drop of one hip and a torque across the pelvis, causing strain on one side. Leg-length discrepancies may be functional (as a result of compensation) or anatomical, where there is a measurable difference in limb length. The objective of treatment is to support the neutral position of joints, which prevents compensation, hypermobility and the overuse syndrome.

THE EFFECT OF ABNORMAL SUPINATION

Supination of the foot in stance, with external rotation of the limb, produces the exact opposite effect of pronation. With pronation, there is increased mobility, a looseness of the joints; with supination, there is a limitation of joint ranges of motion. This eliminates the normal shock-absorbing mechanics of the foot and leg, and produces shock on the skeletal system. As the foot supinates, the talus abducts and dorsiflexes as the calcaneus inverts. This raises the arch and produces a functionally longer limb, with a raising on that side.

Fixed supination or supination in compensation for an abnormality causes the center of gravity to fall to the outside of the base of support, producing lateral instability and inversion sprains. With excessive supination in gait or any condition in which normal pronation is limited, there is a visible shock extending up the leg in gait. A normal amount of supination is necessary for propulsion and proper push-off in activities, but when this is excessive, it is unstable. Excessive supination is a much less common abnormality than excessive pronation.

Both pronation and supination are necessary for performance in

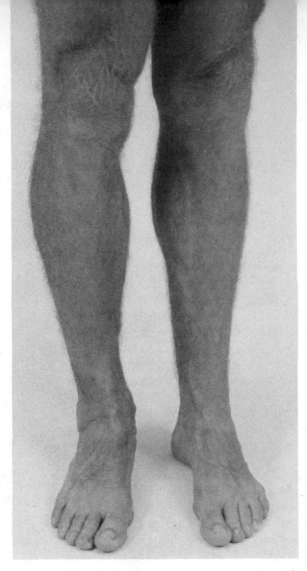

As the upper body rotates to the left, the right foot pronates and the left foot supinates.

sports. Each sport has particular requirements. Running, in which the center of gravity of the body is controlled by one foot, is a part of most sports. Active sports require a greater total range of motion in the joints of the foot. Through training, the athlete learns that point of balance vs. loss of control. He gains a proprioceptive sense, a sense of where his joints are. A trained athelete has greater balance and, therefore, greater confidence in his ability. In a sense, he learns to function in the presence of his abnormalities whether they are compensated or not.

MAJOR ABNORMAL FOOT TYPES

The ideal normal foot has a range of motion available at the ankle joint to dorsiflex 10 degrees; the heel bone is in line with the leg and perpendicular to the supporting surface; the plane of the forefoot is perpendicular to the rearfoot, and there are no forces on the foot from the leg above in any of the three body planes causing it to invert or evert, adduct or abduct, dorsiflex or plantarflex.

Any foot which does not fit these criteria is abnormal, and may or may not produce problems for the athlete. Major classifications of foot types are according to single-plane bone abnormalities. Each foot type has specific predictable appearances, measurements, x-ray findings, skin friction lesions, shoe wear patterns and motions throughout the gait cycle. Each foot type may or may not compensate, but if it does, it is in a predictable manner.

The Ankle Joint. The major osseous abnormalty of the ankle joint is equinus or as commonly called, talipes equinus. Clinically, the defect consists of an inability of the ankle joint to allow 10 degrees or more of dorsiflexion of the foot on the leg at the ankle joint. It affects the midstance phase of gait, when, at the same time the knee is fully extended, the tibia is tilted forward upon the foot so it forms an angle of approximately 80 degrees with the foot. At this moment, the foot should be supinated, and should have passed the neutral subtalar position and be stable for propulsion.

In the talipes equinus deformity, the 10 degrees of dorsiflexion is not present in the ankle joint. The inability of the foot to adequately dorsiflex to this degree, at this moment, results in three possible functional abnormalities, depending upon the range of motion at the subtalar joint and the degree of ankle equinus deformity.

1. If minimal or no motion exists in the subtalar joint and the equinus deformity is much greater than 10 degrees, the heel will never contact the floor, immediately placing the weight on the ball of the foot as would occur in propulsion. Since the foot is not sufficiently supinated to produce complete stability of the forefoot, some shearing of the metatarsal heads occurs, resulting in some element of plantar forefoot callus.

2. If little or no motion is present in the subtalar joint in mild degrees of equinus deformity, the heel contacts the floor normally, but at midstance the heel raises prematurely from the floor.

Again, the foot is not fully supinated in propulsion, and some shearing force occurs to produce plantar callus in the adult foot and has been clinically associated as a major cause of calcaneal apophysitis in the child.

3. If sufficient motion of the subtalar joint is present in mild equinus deformity, the foot will actively pronate at midstance. This pronation occurs at the subtalar joint to allow the small range of dorsiflexion available at this joint to occur. The subtalar pronation unlocks the midtarsal joint so it can pronate excessively at the oblique axis, allowing more dorsiflexion.

Furthermore, since this abnormality is usually present at birth, the abnormal forces at the midtarsal joint gradually sublux this joint about its oblique axis so the forefoot becomes permanently dorsiflexed upon the rearfoot. Such subluxatory change results in retention of the more vertical talus, normally seen only in the infant foot, and a loss of the plantar angle of inclination of the calcaneus, so the arch structure of the foot never develops and a severe pathological flat foot occurs. In cases of major equinus deformity where considerable subtalar joint motion is present, a rocker-bottom foot may develop, and even then the heel may not contact the floor.

Such foot deformity is referred to as compensated talipes equinus since the foot itself develops the needed dorsiflexion by compensatory subtalar and midtarsal joint pronation. The compensated talipes equinus deformity is the most destructive and disabling functional foot problem known. In children, it often produces the symptom of leg fatigue and pain commonly referred to as "growing pains." It is the most common cause of juvenile bunion and hallux abducto-valgus deformity, hammertoes, plantar callosities and juvenile digital corns on toes.

In the adult, this same deformity produces a more severe degree of the same symptoms as seen in the child, plus plantar calcaneal periostitis and heel spurs and severe postural fatigue.

If the patient is undergoing average stance and locomotion, this deformity has been related to an extremely high incidence of low back pain of a disabling degree.

The talipes equinus soon produces a foot that functions throughout the stance and swing phase in a maximum position of pronation. The foot is extremely hypermobile and cannot effectively undergo propulsive-phase function. The individual fails to raise upon his toes, and the foot is lifted from the floor in a nearly flat position in gait. He rolls off his foot rather than pushes off.

The cause of osseous ankle equinus is unknown. This condition is commonly seen in the Negroid foot but rarely in the Caucasian. Conservative treatment has been unsuccessful. In addition, an identical deformity is caused by a short gastrocnemius. Fortunately, most uncompensated and compensated talipes equinus deformities fall into this category, and can be very effectively treated and eliminated in the child.

The Subtalar Joint. The most common osseous abnormality of the foot is subtalar varus. By the time a child has been walking about three months, the torsion of the calcaneus should have developed to the approximate adult level in which the bisection of the heel is perpendicular to the supporting surface and in line with the leg. During early development, calcaneal varus placed the entire foot in an inverted relationship relative to the longitudinal axis of the distal one-third of the leg. The plantar surface of the foot is tilted on the frontal body plane so as to face somewhat toward the midline of the body. As normal valgus torsion progresses, the foot everts until, upon completion of torsion, the plantar surface of the foot lies on the transverse plane and is perpendicular to the longitudinal axis of the distal one-third of the leg. In the older child and adult, the lower leg is vertical to the floor in stance. If torsion of the calcaneus has developed normally, the plantar surface of the foot rests fully upon the floor when the subtalar joint is in its neutral position. The adult structure of the calcaneus on the frontal plane should be approximated at age 15-18 months. At that time, the adult subtalar joint relationship should exist.

Relative to the lower one-third of the leg, the calcaneus should be able to invert twice as far as it will evert during the full range of subtalar joint supination-pronation. In the normal rearfoot, when the vertical bisection of the posterior surfaces of the calcaneus is parallel to the longitudinal axis of the distal one-third of the leg, the subtalar joint rests at its neutral position, and the foot is neither supinated nor pronated. From this neutral position, a foot can supinate twice as far as it can pronate. The neutral position of the subtalar joint is the normal position of the foot in static stance after the age of six.

In a substantial percentage of human feet, the calcaneal valgus torsion is either delayed or fails to ever reach the adult level. In such instances, the residual varus torsion of the calcaneus places the entire foot in an inverted position relative to the talus and leg above. Thus, during stance, if the foot is in its neutral subtalar position as it normally should be, the entire foot is inverted relative to the floor. Weight-bearing occurs along the entire lateral aspect of the sole of the foot, while the medial side fails to contact the floor. Such an inverted position of the foot is rare and requires either very limited subtalar joint range of motion or an extreme degree of calcaneal varus. Such a condition is called uncompensated subtalar varus or talipes varus.

More commonly, there is ample range of subtalar joint pronation to allow the foot to evert until the medial aspect of the sole of the forefoot can make contact with the supporting surface. Such a condition is called compensated subtalar varus. In other words, the foot is no longer in a varus position, but it is abnormally pronated at the subtalar joint whenever weight is borne on the foot. The functional effect of subtalar varus depends upon whether the abnormality is uncompensated or compensated.

Uncompensated subtalar varus is a rigid or semi-rigid foot that develops abnormal distribution of weight in the stance phase of gait. Weight distribution is more lateral than normal at heel contact and continues along the lateral border until lift-off, as evidenced by the characteristic shoe wear pattern in which the entire heel and sole is worn off laterally in a short time. A typical varus gait develops along with plantar callus under the fifth and sometimes fourth metatarsal heads. The fifth metatarsal is short due to early epiphyseal closure related to trauma and is subluxed in a pronatory direction about its axis of motion, resulting in the typical everted and abducted fifth metatarsal called Tailor's bunion. The fifth toe underrides the fourth. The medial plantar aspect of the hallux also develops a large plantar "pinch" callus from the abnormal roll-off in propulsion.

The compensated subtalar varus produces a totally different

76

functional and symptomatic picture. The foot pronates excessively at the contact phase of gait and continues to remain excessively pronated until the heel lifts from the floor. At this time, the foot begins to supinate as the leg externally rotates. But since supination starts very late, the foot never attains a sufficiently supinated position to be stable in propulsion. Shearing forces develop in the forefoot. The first ray is hypermobile, causing callosity to develop under the second, second and third, or the second, third and fourth metatarsal heads, depending upon the structural angle of adductus of the forefoot. A large medial or dorsomedial bunion develops over the first metatarsal head. This type of bunion shows ectopic ossification of bone and a large bursa. Rarely does this foot type produce any major abductory or valgus deformity of the hallux. Hammertoes, minor digital corns and other minor symptoms occur in the forefoot.

The symptoms associated with compensated subtalar varus, while numerous, are seldom acute. The individual rarely seeks professional care unless this deformity is only a part of a more complex deformity. The most disabling effects of subtalar varus are not related to the foot problem by the individual possessing this deformity. Since the abnormal pronation prevents external rotation of the leg until the heel lifts, the result is a temporary jamming of motion at the hip in locomotion with excessive elevation of the pelvis. When unilateral, this condition is often mistakenly regarded as a structural limb shortage on the side opposite the defect. Low-back fatigue and pain of a disabling degree is common, though no relationship is seen between this foot type and sciatica, as is seen in more severe pronatory abnormalities. Lateral instability in gait is synonomous with this foot type, and chronic ankle sprains and ankle joint diastasis are not unusual.

Subtalar Valgus. If any foot merits the designation of "normal flat foot" it would be the subtalar valgus deformity. This is a structurally abnormal foot that functions without excessive pronation. While it is completely flat, it does not produce the typical symptoms associated with flat foot conditions that are related to excessive pronation. Basically, the subtalar valgus foot is one with an everted rearfoot and a supinated forefoot allowing the medial arch to rest upon the supporting surface.

The only structural abnormality which has been identified as a causative factor in this foot type is seen in the talus. In a normal rearfoot, both the ankle joint and subtalar joint lie on the transverse plane parallel to each other. In the talipes valgus abnormality, the talus is more narrow on its lateral side than on its medial, thus tilting the subtalar joint and calcaneus into an everted position. Since the forefoot has a range of supinatory motion at the midtarsal joint, it tends to invert as the forefoot supinates about the longitudinal midtarsal joint axis, and thus the plantar aspect of the forefoot can remain in full contact with the supporting surface while the rearfoot is everted.

The incidence of this abnormality is probably relatively rare. But since it causes no major symptoms there is the possibility of an unrecognized incidence, since the person with this type of abnormality would rarely seek foot care. Concern for the flat-footed appearance, irritation from rigid shank footgear and inability to wear arch supports are the major complaints associated with this abnormality.

Midtarsal Joint. The normal foot, when in the static stance position, exhibits a forefoot that lies fully on the floor at the metatarsal head level. This plantar plane of the metatarsal heads forms a line that is perpendicular to the vertical bisection of the posterior surface of the calcaneus. Stated another way, it can be said that a normal midtarsal joint is one that allows the plantar surface of the forefoot to reach a perpendicular to the sagittal plane of the calcaneus.

At birth, there is about a five degree forefoot varus which resolves by the time the child begins walking. If this development is delayed, it appears to be one of the possible causes of adult forefoot varus. If the torsion develops beyond average limits, it is believed to be a cause of forefoot valgus. This deformity is not fully understood, and the possibility of a contributing developmental abnormality at the calcaneo-cuboid joint is suspected.

While the causative factor in osseous midtarsal joint pathology is still vague, the clinical entities of both forefoot varus and valgus

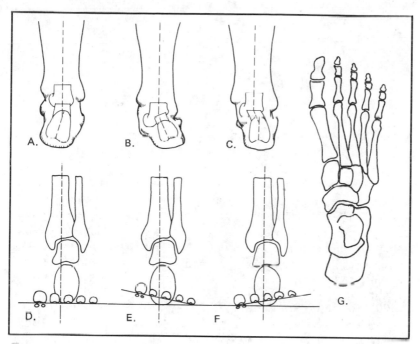

Foot types: a—uncompensated subtalar varus; b—uncompensated subtalar valgus; c—compensated subtalar varus; d—normal forefoot; e—forefoot varus; f—forefoot valgus; g—metatarsus adductus.

can be identified and measured within the limits of practical accuracy.

Forefoot Varus. The forefoot varus deformity places the forefoot in an inverted position when the subtalar joint is in its neutral position during stance. In those rare cases where little or no motion exists at the subtalar joint, the inverted forefoot position is fixed and propulsion occurs at the fourth and fifth metatarsals. This uncompensated defect produces lateral instability of the foot in propulsion and lateral plantar forefoot excrescences.

The presence of subtalar joint motion generally allows the forefoot varus defect to be compensated at the subtalar joint. Eversion of the rearfoot through subtalar pronation allows the forefoot to evert with the rearfoot until the medial plantar aspect of the forefoot comes to rest on the supporting surface. This compensatory subtalar pronation begins to occur as the forefoot makes contact with the supporting surface in the midstance phase of gait. Normally, the leg would begin to externally rotate on the foot at this time, causing a normal foot to supinate and become a rigid lever in propulsion. In the presence of forefoot varus compensatory pronation, the foot remains pronated throughout the stance phase of gait and never develops the stability necessary for adequate propulsive function.

Compensated forefoot varus produces extensive foot and postural symptomatology, and as a cause of foot disability ranks second to the compensated ankle equinus defect. It generally can be said that the symptoms are similar to those of compensated talipes equinus, and as to degree of severity fall somewhere between those of compensated talipes equinus and those of compensated subtalar varus.

Forefoot Valgus. Forefoot valgus places the forefoot in an everted position when the subtalar joint is in its neutral position during stance. With the heel bone vertical to the supporting surface, there is greater pressure on the medial side of the forefoot. Forefoot valgus may be measured in the non-weight-bearing examination as a flat, everted forefoot or as a plantarflexed first ray. Both types may be either rigid or flexible and function differently. If rigid, there is direct pressure under the first metatarsal bone, causing trauma under the medial sesamoid bone. There may be shock extending through the first ray, the mid-tarsal joint and into the subtalar joint, causing supination.

At rest with both types of forefoot valgus, there is a high arch. During gait, rearfoot motion is normal until the medial side of the ball of the foot makes contact, which in the rigid type abruptly stops the pronating foot, causing it to supinate and sending shock up the limb. This often causes lateral instability and may produce an inversion ankle sprain. Rigid forefoot valgus or plantarflexed first ray causes the heel to invert in stance.

Flexible or non-rigid forefoot valgus and plantarflexed first ray are measured in non-weight-bearing examination, but disappear in stance and gait. There is considerable torque within the foot. Although essentially normal in the stance appearance, this foot type has a high incidence of fatigue, postural symptoms, arch strain or fasciitis and lateral instability.

Metatarsus Adductus. Metatarsus adductus is a transverse plane abnormality that affects the angle of gait. It changes the appearance of the foot more than how it functions. Metatarsus adductus is a condition in which the metatarsal bones are adducted or intoed from the direction of the rearfoot, producing a "C" shape or lateral convexity of the foot. Normally, at birth this angle is about 25 degrees and in the adult is less than 15 degrees. The normal foot may be called metatarsus rectus, but if the angle between the front and back of the foot is large, it is considered abnormal. Metatarsus adductus produces no friction lesions because there is no force to compensate. Athletes with this abnormality will tend to toe in and have difficulty getting comfortable shoes, but should perform to full capacity.

Metatarsal Length and Height Abnormalities. The normal metatarsal parabola is 142.5 degrees, with the second metatarsal the longest, then first, then third through fifth in a straight line. When one metatarsal is out of line, it disturbs the flex line of the forefoot. A focal point of pressure develops under the longest metatarsal bone. Pressure is relieved by surgically correcting the problem or by supporting the relatively short metatarsals with padding materials, effectively bringing the ground up to the foot.

Normally, all the metatarsal bones are on the same level. When one metatarsal is lower than others, it acts the same as one which is longer. Depressed metatarsal bones are usually caused through injury of the involved or the neighboring metatarsal bones.

COMPENSATIONS FOR FOOT ABNORMALITIES

The sagittal plane abnormal foot types such as talipes equinus cause vertical forces on the foot. If this force is not resolved with full foot contact and leverage for propulsion, the foot pronates or supinates producing a side to side shearing force which is destructive.

Frontal plane imbalances such as subtalar varus and forefoot varus compensate with pronation of the foot, resulting in the pronation syndrome throughout the limb.

For the most part, transverse plane abnormalities do not need to compensate, because they are already on the supporting surface. They produce angle of gait changes which results in abnormal heel contact and ineffective propulsion. Most transverse plane abnormalities in the foot are osseous and do not respond to treatment; if from above the foot, corrective flexibility exercises may help.

81

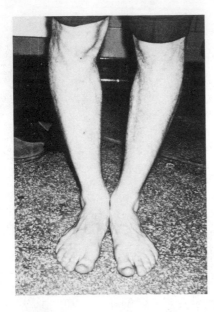

Bowed legs force the feet to pronate to "get to the ground."

ABNORMALITIES ABOVE THE FOOT AFFECTING FOOT STRIDE

Bow Leg. Normally, the tibia is vertical to the supporting surface in stance and during gait. At birth, the tibia is bowed about 15 degrees, but by the time the child walks, most of this resolves. The legs still appear bowed in the early walker because of the development of the lateral muscles for stability rather than the posterior muscles for propulsion. If the bowed leg is still present by age 5-6, it is considered abnormal and called tibia varum.

Tibia varum is a deformity in the shaft of the tibia in which the distal end of the leg is directed toward the midline of the body. The subtalar joint is then inverted from the supporting surface. The effect of tibia varum and subtalar varus on foot function is exactly the same and both are types of rearfoot varus. The movements and function of the subtalar joint are the same with both abnormalities.

Any activity which involves running forces one foot to control the center of gravity. There is an angle from the hip to the point of support which produces of functional runner's varus. Therefore, athletes need a greater range of motion available at the subtalar joint than non-athletes. If this motion is not available, the pronation or supination syndrome will develop, causing imbalance and overuse.

Knock-Knees. Knock-knees may be a primary problem within the knee or secondary to foot imbalance. Knock-knee includes genu valgum, which is a deformity of the knee joint in which the distal end of the tibia is directed away from the midline of the body. The subtalar joint is then everted from the supporting surface, tending to pronate the foot. Pronation of the foot with eversion of the heel puts a force on the leg to tilt further. In most cases, treatment by supporting the neutral position of the foot will prevent pronatory compensation and reverse the knock-knee condition.

Both bow legs and knock-knees affect the base of gait, the distance between the feet with activity, so they affect balance.

Rotational Abnormalities and the Angle of Gait. The normal angle of the foot from the line of progression is 7-10 degrees, or 14-20 degrees between the two feet. Abnormalities in the transverse plane rotations of the thigh or leg will affect this angle. The knee joint, primarily, and the ankle and hip joints all have the ability to absorb these abnormalities. The normal neutral position of hip joint rotations is zero degrees where the knee joint functions straight ahead in the sagittal plane. If the rotation is greater internally than externally, it produces an in-toe; if greater externally than internally, it produces an out-toed position. The same is true of the position of the ankle joint at the distal end of the tibia. Normally, the medial and lateral malleoli are rotated externally 13-18 degrees. If less than 13 degrees, it decreases the angle of gait; if greater than 18 degrees, it increases the angle of gait.

Both in-toeing and out-toeing alter the stress through the foot. Moderate in-toeing helps forward propulsive leverage but if excessive, then stress comes from the inside of the heel out through the lateral side of the forefoot. Out-toeing produces lateral heel wear and stress on the foot, passing medially off through the first and second toes as it should, resulting in an odd appearance and an inefficient non-propulsive gait pattern.

Limb-Length Differences. Leg length differences may be structural, functional, or a combination of the two. Structural differences are actually differences in the length of bones on both

Review of Foot Types and Problems

Foot Types	Non-Weight Bearing Description	With Weight-Bearing the Foot May Compensate by:	Plantar Lesions Usually Develop Under Metatarsal Heads	Descriptive Synonyms
(Sagittal Plane) Ankle Joint:				
Uncompensated Equinus	Measurement shows limited dorsiflexion	(None) (Uncomp.)	Diffuse lesions 2-4	"Toe Walker" (Part of Clubfoot)
Compensated Equinus	Foot is plantarflexed	S.T.Jt. & M.T.Jt. Pronation (Comp.✱) OR M.T.Jt. Subluxation (Comp.)	2, 2-4 ■ ☐ — (Varies)	Pes Planus, P. Valgo Planus ● — "Rocker bottom," "Vertical" Talus
Uncompensated Calcaneus	Limited plantarflexion	(None) (Uncomp.)	(Around heel)	"Heel Walker"
Compensated Calcaneus	Foot is dorsiflexed	S.T.Jt. & M.T.Jt. Supination (Comp.*)	5th–1st	Pes Cavus
(Frontal Plane) Sub-Talar Joint (S.T.Jt.)				
Uncomp. Sub-Talar Varus	Neutral position of the Sub-Talar Joint is inverted from the tibia	(None) (Uncomp.)	5th ☐	Calcaneal Varus, (Part of Clubfoot) — Heel Varus
Comp. Sub-Talar Varus		Sub-talar pronation (Comp.✱)	Nucleated 2nd — 2-5 ■ ☐	Pes Planus, "Weak Foot"
Sub-Talar Valgus	Neutral position of the S.T.Jt. is everted from the tibia	Foot is "flat" No force on Talus to compensate	(Varies)	Pes Valgo Planus ●

Mid-Tarsal Joint (M.T.Jt.)				
Uncomp. Forefoot Varus	Forefoot (plane of the metatarsal heads is inverted from the rearfoot (bisection of the calcaneus)	(None) (Uncomp.)	5th □	Medial imbalance
Comp. Forefoot Varus		Sub-talar and Mid-Tarsal pronation (Comp.★)	Nucleated 2nd; 2 & 5 ■□	Pes Valgo Planus ●
Uncomp. Forefoot Valgus	Forefoot is everted from the rearfoot (as above)	(None) (Uncomp.)	Nucleated 1st (Tibial Sesamoid)	Pes Cavus
Comp. Forefoot Valgus		Sub-Talar Supination (Comp.★)	Nucleated 1st; Diffuse 5th	Pes Cavus; Postero-Lateral Imbalance
(Transverse Plane)				
Mid-Tarsal Joint	Forefoot (anter or to M.T.Jt.) is adducted on the rearfoot	No need to compensate because both the heel and the forefoot are on the supporting surface	None, but tend to aggravate other problems by making foot rigid	Often grouped under: Metatarsus Varus, Met. Adducto-Varus, Met. Adductus (Part of Clubfoot)
Forefoot Adductus	(Differentiated by X-ray)			
Tarso-Metatarsal Joint				
Metatarsus Adductus	Metatarsus is adducted on the lesser Tarsus			

★ Compensation is an abnormal but not necessarily pathological attempt by the body to neutralize an abnormal force from another part. Compensation produces abnormal secondary muscle pulls, affecting joint positions and forefoot abnormalities; in treatment, we attempt to prevent compensation by supporting the abnormality.

■ Hypermobility is defined as either excessive motion or motion at a time when there should be none. Hypermobility of the first ray develops whenever the foot is pronated from its neutral position, therefore lesions develop under the second metatarsal head. Whenever hypermobility is present, hallux abducto-valgus will tend to develop.

□ Pinch callus develops under the medial plantar aspect of the hallux where the upper meets the lower of the shoe.

● Shows "positive" Helbing's sign.

Foot types may be "combined" and have combined signs and symptoms, (e.g., equino-varus, metatarsus adducto-varus).

Foot types may be "partially" compensated if the range of motion in joints is not available for full compensation, and therefore produce gradations of the lesions described.

sides. Functional limb-length differences are the result of excessive pronation which effectively shortens the limb and supination which effectively lengthens the limb. These differences disappear with proper treatment of the foot.

Most people have a moderate limb-length difference which causes them no problems with normal activities. If a limb-length difference is suspected as the cause of problems, it should be treated, but if one is observed and has not produced problems for the athlete, it should be left alone. Dr. Karl Klein has reported that 80% of the knee problems develop on the short side, so it is safe to attempt a heel lift inside the shoe on the suspected short side before seeking professional attention. There are several simple tests that can be done to determine if a limb-length difference exists.

In stance, with the person standing barefoot with equal weight on both feet, observe posture from the front and the back. Look for any hip drop, any curvature of the spine or shoulder tilt.

In one-foot balancing and in gait, the pelvis should remain level. The stride length should be equal on both sides with equal and reciprocal arm swing. If uneven, suspect structural or functional limb-length differences.

Examination in the seated position eliminates most functional or compensatory findings. With the person seated in a straight-backed chair (with nothing in his back pockets), extend the legs out straight by holding the feet. Observe the position of the ankle bones and the level of the bottom of the heels. If the difference is greater than a quarter-inch, suspect a structurally short limb.

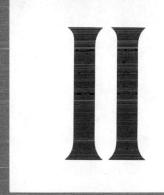

II

FEET
IN MOTION

4

How
Athletes Move

Walking and running are necessary for most sports. With each individual sport, specific phases of the gait cycle are important, since performance, speed, strength and agility are related to how the body handles the center of gravity.

When a person is walking, weight transfers from one foot to the other; there is a side-to-side movement of the center of gravity. In running, the weight is supported on one foot, then both feet are in the air (the double-float phase) and then on the other foot so that each foot must come under the center of gravity of the moving body. Long-distance running is very similar to the walking in its gait cycle. It begins with heel contact, then forefoot contact, then heel-off, then toe-off, and on into the swing phase and the next succeeding weight-bearing cycle.

The stance phase motions and positions of the foot are determined by the genetic structure of the foot and leg, and are treated with external supporting devices, such as strapping and orthotics. The swing phase of gait can be influenced by progressive resistance exercises for strength and yoga-type stretching for flexibility. These conditioning exercises will increase length and strength of stride, as well as balance and controlled reflexes.

The main functions of the foot in gait are to serve as a mobile adaptor upon contact and as a rigid lever during propulsion. Here, we describe the basic gait cycle and stresses in the foot which are essential to all weight-bearing sports, and later we describe specific functions.

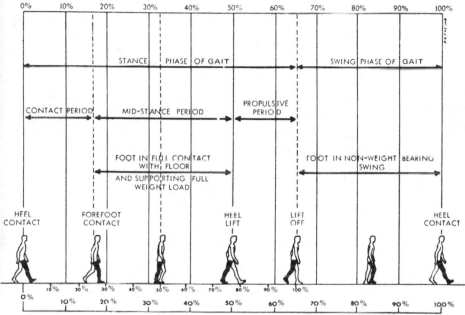

One Complete Walking Gait Cycle of Right Limb

It is important to remember that as the foot pronates, the joints become loose. Pronation of the foot in stance occurs simultaneously with internal rotation of the leg. Supination of the foot, producing rigidity in joints and in stance, occurs simultaneously with external rotation of the leg on the planted foot. In order for normal function to occur in gait, the foot normally pronates a specific amount during the contact phase in order to adapt to the terrain and absorb shock, then supinates during the midstance phase so that it can be rigid for propulsion of body weight.

The exact midpoint in the stance phase of gait should show the foot in its neutral position and be the same as the ideal relaxed stance position. In other words, pronation is normal during the contact phase but not the propulsive phase; supination is normal during the midstance phase but not the contact phase. Compensations for specific foot abnormalities produce changes in predictable phases of the gait cycle.

	Contact phase 25% of stance phase	Mid-stance phase 50% of stance phase	Propulsive phase 25% of stance phase
Phases of Gait	Contact phase 25% of stance phase	Mid-stance phase 50% of stance phase	Propulsive phase 25% of stance phase
Motion of Leg	Internal Rotation of leg	External Rotation of leg	
Motion of Foot At Subtalar Joint	Pronation	Supination \	
Position of Foot At Subtalar Joint	Slight supination / Neutral position	Pronated position / Neutral position	Supinated position

IDEAL MOVEMENTS IN WALKING

As the foot swings through the air before contact, the heel bone and entire foot are tilted inward (inverted) about two degrees. In the normal leg, the tibia is essentially perpendicular to the floor, and therefore the subtalar joint is mildly supinated. The normal contact point is just to the outside of the heel bone. This produces a normal wear pattern on the heels of shoes about one-half inch to the outside of the middle of the shoe. In long-distance running, this wear pattern is slightly more to the lateral side.

After heel contact, the foot begins pronating with eversion of the heel bone (and the entire foot) so that the foot becomes mobile enough to absorb shock and accept uneven surfaces without losing balance. With normal forefoot structure in which the ball of the foot is flat and the metatarsal bones are all on the same level, the forefoot makes contact with the ground. At this point the stress line through the foot is close to the center of the forefoot. With the ground resistance to the forefoot, we reach the end of the contact phase (at approximately 25% of the kinetic stance phase of gait) and enter into the midstance phase, during which the entire foot is on the ground, and the stress line carries on through the ball of the foot.

As the foot pronates into the contact phase, the calcaneus

90

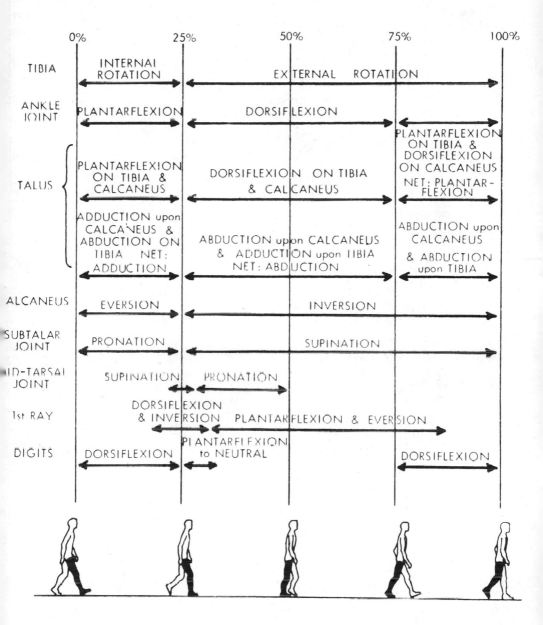

Motions of the foot during the weight-bearing portion of walking.
(Refer also to page 90.)

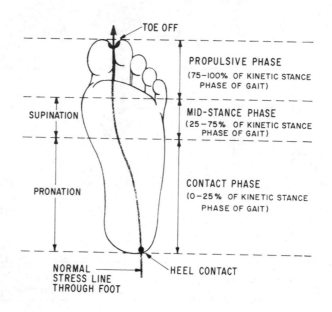

TOE OFF

PROPULSIVE PHASE
(75-100% OF KINETIC STANCE
PHASE OF GAIT)

SUPINATION

MID-STANCE PHASE
(25-75% OF KINETIC STANCE
PHASE OF GAIT)

PRONATION

CONTACT PHASE
(0-25% OF KINETIC STANCE
PHASE OF GAIT)

NORMAL
STRESS LINE
THROUGH FOOT

HEEL CONTACT

KINETIC STANCE PHASE OF GAIT

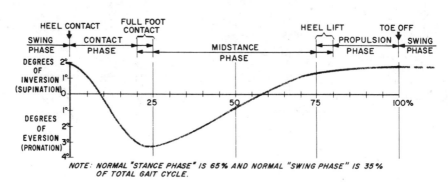

NOTE: NORMAL "STANCE PHASE" IS 65% AND NORMAL "SWING PHASE" IS 35%
OF TOTAL GAIT CYCLE.

everts, so at the end of the contact phase, the heel bone is tilted over about four degrees. As the knee joint comes over the ankle and the leg becomes vertical over the foot, the entire limb begins externally rotating as the foot supinates. When all forces are balanced, the foot and limb are in their neutral position, the best position of function, the one which we would like to see in the normal non-moving stance position.

With ideal normal structure in gait, the position of the foot and leg at 50% of the kinetic stance phase of the gait cycle should be the same as that foot and leg position in the relaxed stance position. Likewise, in the examination process we use the standing position of the heel bone to represent the position of the foot at the midpoint in the gait cycle. This stance position tells us how much the foot and leg have compensated for any imbalance, if present.

For 25% to 75% of the kinetic stance phase of gait, the entire foot is on the ground and the foot is moving from a mobile, pronated adaptor to a rigid, supinated lever in order to propel the body forward. The foot must supinate before the heel lifts off the ground so that stress passes straight out through the first and second toes. If the foot is still pronated as it enters into the propulsive phase, it is unstable and inefficient. The joints are mobile (hypermobile) at a time when they should be stable for propulsion. If the foot is excessively supinated during the propulsive phase, it is unstable laterally and subject to sprains and pressure problems on the soft tissues, especially corns, calluses and blisters.

Normally at about 75% of the weight-bearing gait cycle, the heel raises straight up under force of the achilles tendon (made up of three calf muscles, the gastrocnemius, the soleus and the plantaris) as the center of gravity moves forward over the ball of the foot and out through the toes. When the heel raises, the toes move passively upward. From 75% to toe off (100%), we are in the propulsive phase of the weight-bearing gait cycle. As stress comes off the ball of the foot, the toes move actively downward toward their original resting position. The toes should function straight, with no gripping or twisting motion.

The subtalar joint, with the talus above and the calcaneus below, functions like a universal joint, transferring stresses down-

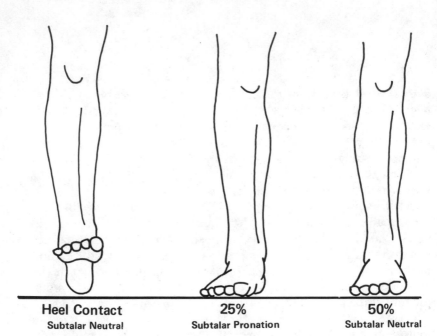

Heel Contact
Subtalar Neutral

25%
Subtalar Pronation

50%
Subtalar Neutral

1

2

3

4

Motions of the feet during the contact, mid-stance and propulsive phases of gait. Note pronation and supination of heel at right.

94

ward from the leg to the foot, and upward from the foot to the leg. The foot is at right angles (90 degrees) to the leg. Motions around the subtalar joint are simultaneous with motion of the limb. They are specific and predictable.

The base line on the accompanying graph represents zero degrees, the position at which the ideal normal foot is vertical to the supporting surface, in direct line with the leg and in its neutral position, the position of best function. Zero degrees represents that position where the subtalar joint is neither pronated nor supinated. Zero degrees, therefore, represents that position where the leg is neither internally nor externally rotated. When the foot pronates with weight-bearing, the limb internally rotates. When the foot supinates, the limb externally rotates. There is a normal amount of pronation and supination that occurs during the gait cycle, and a normal amount of rotation of the limb. But excessive motion is abnormal and may lead to progressive imbalance or overuse injuries.

During the gait cycle with forward momentum and forward leaning, the center of gravity of the body is falling forward. Each step is a combined attempt by the foot and legs to keep up with the center of gravity, an attempt to move the body forward efficiently and an attempt to keep from falling forward. Walking and all movements of the limb depend on the transfer of rotatory movements into straight-line horizontal, vertical or side-to-side activities. The transfer of these many bones, muscles and joint structures, which rotate around fixed structural points to produce movement of the body from one place to another, is a complex process.

Efficiency of motion is essential to good performance in sports. Each activity—walking, sprinting, long-distance running, jumping, kicking and so forth—have specific, definable normal and

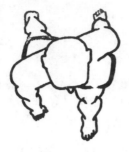

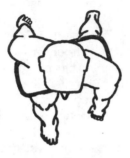

In walking, the upper extremity rotates opposite the lower extremity.

abnormal motions. This is why an understanding of the techniques of the sport and the mechanical abilities and limitations of the foot and leg are essential to a proper conditioning program.

The phases of the gait cycle—contact, midstance, propulsion and swing—each relate to efficient technique in different sports. The contact phase is involved with all sports but is especially important in heel balance, where foot plant, resistance and take-off are necessary, as in running, high jumping and the martial arts. The midstance phase is important for forefoot balance, allowing good lateral movements, as in tennis, squash and soccer. The propulsive phase is especially important to sprinting, pushing off and jumping, as in basketball, hurdles and Nordic skiing. Swing-phase flexibility enhances speed and decreases injuries in all sports. If an athlete is flexible, he gets a greater range of motion from each force, which makes him more efficient.

5

Maintaining Balance

This is a brief discussion describing how an athlete maintains his balance or center of gravity while performing straight-ahead motion, side-to-side motion, ballistics and mixed motions. Generally speaking, the center of gravity is located in the abdominal region. The body parts, primarily the extremities, help the athlete maintain his balance. The lower extremity helps the athlete maintain balance primarily by flexing or extending at the hips or knees. The feet pronate or supinate, lock or unlock to keep the athlete's movement steady and coordinated. Coordination is controlled primarily by the cerebellum of the brain and muscular control is maintained by the cerebrum. Thus, the lower extremity acts only after receiving messages from the brain or through reflexes. If an athlete is losing his balance, he will use his arms to correct himself, and by re-positioning his lower extremity he gains recovery.

In the straight-ahead motions such as running, an athlete may lose his balance and fall forward because his center of gravity was too far forward and/or his arms were too low, thus he could not reposition himself. Usually, decreasing the forward lean or straightening the upper torso is sufficient to regain balance. This puts the center of gravity in direct alignment with the lower extremity. If the athlete cannot perform this repositioning he may catch himself by bouncing off his hands and extended arms.

A football drill is good for balance. The runner uses the hand and arm to maintain balance as he pushes off the ground with his hands while running in a very low-postured position.

In the side-to-side movements as in skiing, the skier maintains his balance by leaning too far forward and bringing his feet and legs under and behind the center of gravity in the opposite direction of the fall. This requires practice, because it is easy to adjust his lower extremity by flexing the knees more or less and creating motion in the feet by locking or unlocking the joints of the feet.

For the most part, if the skiers foot is functioning in or near neutral position, balance is easier to maintain. On the other hand, if your feet are pronated or supinated to a large degree more than five degrees, turning becomes a difficult task because your feet do not have the necessary motion to compensate for the abnormality. The same holds true for torsional problems of the legs or malpositioning at the head of the femur in relation to the shaft of the femur. Thus, in the skier who loses his concentration momentarily and loses his balance, the foot which may have been locked is now unlocked. In order to regain stability, the athlete tries to move the foot back into a locked position with movement in the hips or knees or foot itself. Hence, this rocking or oscillating movement helps maintain balance.

The same kinds of events in the upper and lower extremity occur

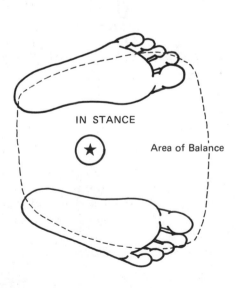

IN STANCE

Area of Balance

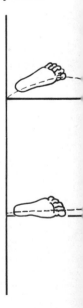

in maintaining balance in ballistic-type movements. In karate, an individual who punches or kicks without control over his body motion finds himself leaning or falling forward or backward. To prevent this, the karate man may slow down his punch or kick, allowing him time to regain correct posture. The kick or punch can be pulled or not completely extended, shortening the movement and thus getting both feet on the ground as in a kick to regain balance. The pulled punch allows the upper extremity and torso to correct itself by leaning back to the correct posture and thus restoring balance.

In the mixed-motions sports such as gymnastics, all these ways of correcting a loss of balance are utilized. Most of the time, the athlete is aware of his bodily reactions as motions and movements are being performed. However, there are many occasions when the athlete is unaware of how his body maintains and regains balance. Basically, practice is the key word, because the athlete is teaching his body to understand its position in relation to the environment. Most specifically, as the athlete gains confidence by practice and competition, he realizes that being calm, relaxed and concentrating without pushing hard will result in the best performances and the most enjoyment.

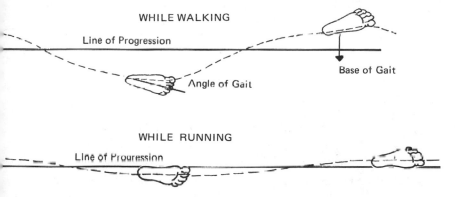

The center of gravity in standing (page 98), walking and running (above).

6

Forward-Motion Sports

The remainder of this section is subdivided into the following categories: (1) primarly "forward" sports—running, swimming; downhill skiing; (2) side-to-side sports—golf, tennis, soccer maneuvers; (3) "ballistic"-type sports—karate, soccer and football kicking; (4) "mixed" sports—football, basketball, gymnastics.

In forward-motion sports, the subject of this chapter, the prime objective is to move the limb and body forward as efficiently as possible.

RUNNING

The biomechanics of running has been discussed previously (Chapter Four). Therefore, only differentiation of the types of running, body posture, dynamic changes of the center of gravity and kinesiology are covered in this section.

The three main types of running are long-distance, middle-distance and sprinting.

On long-distance running, including jogging, the foot goes through all phases of support and recovery. It differs from other forms of running in that at foot strike, the heel usually strikes first. This form of running is similar to the phases of walking with a heel-foot-toe gait during the support phase.

In middle-distance running, for example, the 440 and 880-yard

Steve Prefontaine shows how racing employs the propulsive phase of gait. (Bob Kasper photo)

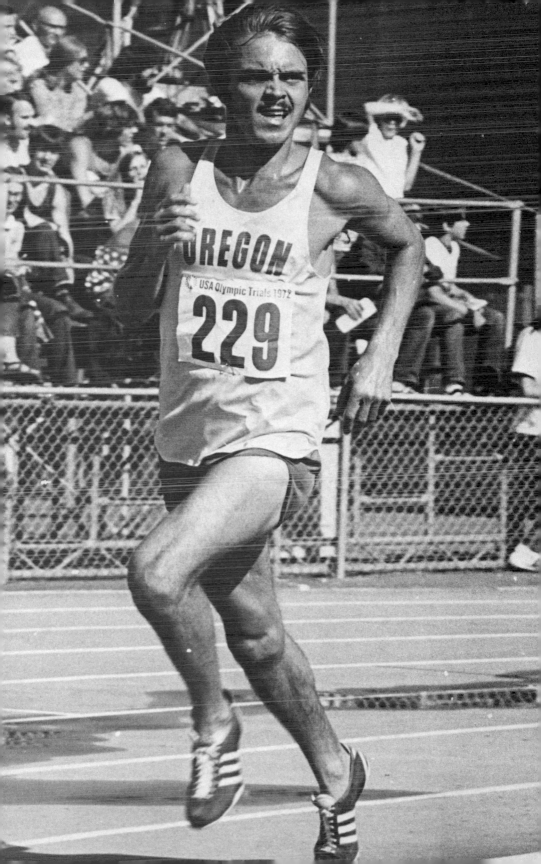

races, the foot and lower extremity go through all phases of swing and support similar to long-distance running. It differs at foot strike because the heel and forefoot may momentarily strike the surface simultaneously, although toward the end of the race, runners may be sprinting.

In sprinting, such as in the 100-yard dash, the foot tends to sag toward the surface during mid-support. Furthermore, foot strike is predominantly on the forefoot or balls of the feet rather than the heels striking first.

The long-distance runner and jogger run basically perpendicular to the running surface with a forward posture. The center of gravity is located within the body planes in the abdominal area.

In the middle-distance running, the runner's body may be leaning forward more than the long-distance runner or jogger. The center of gravity lies within the body planes but more toward the anterior, or front aspect of the runner.

The sprinter, on the other hand, is leaning forward at the start nearly parallel to the ground from the starting blocks, and as he leaves the blocks gradually his body becomes more erect or vertical to the ground. The sprinter may be leaning forward more than the middle-distance runner, although this is not always true. The center of gravity in the sprinter lies outside the body at the start of the race and gradually moves within the body planes.

In calculating the center of gravity in adult males, approximately 56-57% of their total height is the location of the center of gravity in the male. The center of gravity for adult females is at approximately 55% of their total height. These are gross measurements. More specific measurements can be accomplished by photography with planes drawn through the body or by precise mathemathical calculations.

In general, the center of gravity for children and adolescents is higher than adults because of the disproportionate size of the head and thorax, and the relatively small legs. The younger the child, in general, the higher the center of gravity and the lower the stability.

In examining running dynamics, one notices a runner leans forward 20-25 degrees. This tends to decrease the air resistance and keeps the runner's center of gravity ahead of the feet. Furthermore, as the flexion of the knee increases, the speed of the forward swing increases. Increase in speed also occurs with increase in the length of the stride. But any further extension beyond this point reduces speed.

Hip flexibility is important for a full stride. In running, the body falls forward. The muscles then drive the legs, rather than the weight of the body. This means that muscle force and flexibility are necessary for the legs to "catch up" with the center of gravity of the running body.

These principles are true for "straight ahead" running. When a change in direction is necessary, the foot must be planted wider than normal, with the center of gravity low,so that the center of gravity begins to fall in the opposite direction. Then the weight-bearing foot is able to drive behind the direction of motion.

SWIMMING

The primary target sites for injuries to swimmers are the soft tissues. Strained or cramped muscles are frequent, but usually do not end up as serious or complicating problems in the future. Warming up and flexibility exercises (plus a good conditioning program) will alleviate most straining or cramping. So, basically speaking, foot and leg injuries are not common in swimmers.

A swimmer might, however, want to keep a few hints in mind.

1. Develop a style of swimming that suits you.

2. Try out the many variations of a single swimming stroke and see which one suits you the best.

3. Flexibility is important as well as endurance. Stretch and condition yourself gradually, patiently.

4. Learn to do a technique correctly first, then improvise or stylize if necessary. Work on style before speed.

5. There are no taping techniques nor orthoses which can be used meaningfully in swimming. The feet are not as important as the legs in kicking.

6. Follow a balanced strength and flexibility program.

Most swimming events condition the calf muscles to hold the foot in a downward (plantarflexed) position. This is important for swimming itself. But the conditioning causes a "bounce" in gait when walking, and is associated with pain and fatigue in the arches and calves. Therefore, stretching of the calf muscles is important in swimmers.

The faster a swimmer finishes a given distance can be attributed to several factors. The factors associated with speed are dependent on the length of each stroke and the frequency of strokes per given time.

The stroke length is defined as the distance a swimmer travels after one complete stroke cycle. The stroke frequency is dependent on the time it takes to execute one stroke cycle. The stroke length is dependent on the propulsive force generated primarily by the arms and hands, and secondarily by the movement of the legs. Stroke length also is dependent on the resistive forces which oppose the swimmer's movement and the forward motion.

The stroke frequency is dependent on: the time it takes a swimmer to complete the phases of his strokes; time to pull his arms, which produces most of the propulsive force; the recovery phase when the arm no longer is pulling, comes out of the water and is brought forward again to begin the pull phase. How well the swimmer executes these movements is a function of position of the hands, arms, forearms, the range of motion which the limbs move and the torque applied through the shoulders.

Thus, the faster swimmer displays efficient and propulsive movements and decreases the amount of resistive forces acting on his body through proper body positioning. Up and down movements are not desirable because the propulsive force is vertical, not forward. Thus, a swimmer may vary either his stroke length or stroke frequency, as long as he or she does not sigificantly alter the other and decrease speed.

Breathing technique also is an important factor in terms of the swimmer's body position. Usually, swimmers in competition or recreation breathe after one or two strokes as seen in the front crawl. The swimmer must keep his head and face out of the water only briefly to inhale. The longer it takes to inhale, the more legs and lower portion of the trunk sink downward and increase the resistive force. The more horizontal the body is and the lower the profile, the less the resistive force opposing the swimmer's forward motion.

104

Most coaches and athletes regard the arms as the major propulsive force, while attributing very little contribution by the legs. However, in the breaststroke and butterfly, the legs contribute much more to propulsion than in the front crawl and back crawl. The percentage of contribution of the upper versus the lower extremity is widely disputed.

Front Crawl. As the swimmer lifts his arm out of the water and begins to extend forward, the same side or ipsilateral leg is on a downward kick or flutter. The hip on that side is up and out, while the opposite hip is down. The swimmer's head also comes out of the water for inhalation, turning out sidewise on the same side as the arm that is out of the water and being extended. The foot during its downward stroke is plantarflexed, abducted and everted, while the leg is externally rotated. The opposite limb is slightly flexed, while the foot is plantarflexed and abducted.

Researchers have found that swimmers with the best kicks had wide kicks, up to 24 inches apart, and utilized their hips to generate a stronger kick, which in turn used the entire limb rather than just the foot, ankle and lower leg. They also found that the best kickers had better ankle mobility or flexibility than poor kickers. Thus, theoretically any limitation in extension of the leg, as well as the range of motion of the hips, will hinder the swimmer's ability to kick with strength. Any bone block or muscle contracture, at any of the leg and foot joints will thus limit the force of the kick.

Researchers also found that the up-kick was just as important as the downkick in generating propulsion. Also, increased kick frequency without sacrificing width and time of excursion proved to be a better technique than swimming only with the arms, or using a slow-frequency kick.

Back Crawl. The back crawl activity of the legs does not differ from the front crawl except in body position, so this aspect will not be discussed. The swimmer doing this stroke is near a horizontal position on his back with his chin close to his chest. His trunk and legs are loosely extended and his hips just low enough in the water to ensure that the kick will be beneath the surface.

The relationship of his head to his hip also is important. The farther back his head, the more the hips tend to raise out of the water, decreasing the effectiveness of his kick. Breathing is not such a problem here since the face is out of the water.

Breast Stroke. The breast stroke, the slowest of the competitive swimming events allows the swimmer a clear view ahead with minimal output of energy. Breathing is also much easier, although the head is lowered into the water, producing a low profile to decrease the resistive forces against forward motion.

The breast stroke's value also lies outside competition and is useful during life rescue or survival, similar to the value of the sidestroke. The leg action of the breast stroke (frog kick, wedge kick and whip kick) utilizes simultaneous movement of the legs either coming together to propel the swimmer or push with the feet as in the whip kick.

In the wedge kick or frog kick, the width of the internally rotated, abducted legs is wider than the whip kick position. But, this allows for increased resistive force, whereas the whip kick, being narrower, reduces it. As the legs extend and the heels come together, the stroke is ended.

The whip kick, on the other hand, allows the legs to come together quicker, because of less resistive force and distance to travel between the legs, as well as dorsiflex the ankles and push with the soles of the feet. In the frog kick, the post-thrust phase externally rotates the extremities and abducts the feet allowing the heels to come together.

During the pre-thrust phase, both the frog kick and whip kick do not differ. Here, the legs are flexed at the hips, and knees and the ankle is slightly plantarflexed. As the leg flexes completely at the knee, the foot moves from a previously adducted position to an abducted position. The legs begin to internally rotate which allows them to be directed outward.

During this period, the foot is everted, abducted and plantarflexed. As the legs extend completely, they are brought together again for the thrust. Thus, the frog kick (although more powerful) is less efficient than the whip kick. The whip kick can be executed much faster, and the swimmer pushes rather than bringing the legs together to propel forward.

106

DOWNHILL SKIING

In the sport and recreation of skiing, we observe differences and similarities to other sports in terms of biomechanics and kinesiology. We find that the foot gear, and the use of the ski and ski poles accommodate the skier as he traverses down the slope. In review of basic biomechanics of skiing, the main force that edges the ski is the tilt of the leg above the ski. That is, if the leg tilts inward, the inside edge control increases, and if it tilts outward, the outside edge contact increases and often "catches." If the edge catches, the center of gravity is outside the base of support, and in the unconditioned athlete this may cause a fall. If the skier responds quickly, or if his momentum is great enough, he will recover.

The effect of canting a boot or ski is to support the inside of the foot. On a salesroom floor, this tilts the leg outward and feels odd, but on snow, there is more pressure and therefore better control on the inside edge. When the bottoms of the feet are on the same plane and parallel, the inner edge is lower than the outside edge, helping control. Skiers with bowed legs (tibial varum) or an inherited inward (varus) tilt of the foot gain control with canting.

We have seen earlier that internal rotation of the leg causes pronation and excess mobility of the foot. Ski boots are constructed to eliminate inefficient side-to-side motions of the leg within the boot so that all frontal plane motion is transferred to the bottom of the ski. They are constructed to allow some sagittal plane motion through forward tilt at the ankle with dorsiflexion of the foot. But they are unable to control vertical rotation of the leg within the boot, so the foot pronates and supinates as the leg internally and externally rotates.

Most ski boots have little or no arch support. Injected boots form with the shape of the foot in stance, and if the foot is flat, the injection mold comes out flat. Also, if the foot is pronated and hypermobile, the leg must internally rotate to at least that position to begin to get edge control. This is inefficient, ineffective and tiring, so the skier begins to "stem" his turns and "tuck his downhill knee" behind his leading, upper ski.

Therefore, the skier needs inside-the-boot canting or support. This is done with a functional rigid orthotic device with an intrin-

107

sic cant and molded to the foot in the ideal neutral position before it has compensated. There is a need for a commercially available inside-the-boot canting device to control pronation and supination within the boot.

Pronation and supination cause the ski to evert or invert. In the Austrian technique, the skier utilizes a preturn to release the edges prior to a turn. The upper body transverse rotation accentuates the transverse rotation at the knee and finally the foot and the ski. In the French method, the skier utilizes a thrusting motion at the knees which requires a more muscular output and endurance. As the skier goes downhill and crosswise against the slope, the lower limb away from the slope internally rotates and the ski everts. The leg closest to the slope externally rotates, and the ski inverts to hold the uphill edges.

If an individual has difficulty doing these techniques, it may be the result of a lack of practice, not correctly teaching the skier the proper way of doing the technique, or possibly because of one's physical disability or limitations. In skiing, any apparent duration of the perpendicular relationship betweeen the leg, heel and calcaneus and remainder of the foot will affect the ability to perform.

The main problems affecting edge control in skiers are bowed legs (tibia varum) inverted heel bones (subtalar varus) and inverted forefoot (varus) causing pronation of the foot inside the boot. In a soft or loose boot, compensating forces occur at the subtalar joint, resulting in pronation and creating difficulty in controlling the downhill inside edge. If an individual has tibia valgum or knock knee, the area of stress occurs on the inside edges of the ski and supination of the foot within the boot, which results in difficulty with the uphill edge control. Compensating for tibia varum, subtalar varus and forefoot varus occurs when the heel everts to perpendicular or near perpendicular.

One may also see skiers stemming or hopping to begin their turns or tucking their knees when they experience difficulty in controlling their turns. The skier is also flexed at the hips and knees, and is usually leaning forward with his center of gravity down low and forward. The idea of turning corners in the slalom is not to get the center of gravity parallel with the skiing surface or else the individual will fall. Individuals with tight calf muscles or

108

hamstrings may find dorsiflexing their ankles, and flexing knees and hips to be difficult. These individuals will fatigue and tend to lean backward and thus lose their balance more often, especially the beginners.

Skiing Injuries. Sites of injuries are numerous, especially to the lower extremity. Fractures are common occurrences due to tremendous torsional forces acting on the legs. Skiers are prone to falls, and many such accidents produce fractures to any part of the body but primarily to the extremities. The best way to avoid severe injury when falling is to roll in the direction of the fall, and relax and not tighten up or fight the fall. Hitting bodily parts with poles is not infrequent and can produce puncture wounds. Skiing is a contact sport unless you never fall.

Skiing Hints. Make sure the boots fit snugly but not to the point of extreme discomfort or pain. Check to see if the boots allow any motion forward or backward at the lower leg above the ankles. Check to make sure the safety releases are in proper working condition.

Add cants if you have difficulty in turning uphill or downhill. If you have short gastrocnemius (calf) muscles, canting the heels will reduce tension.

7

Side-to-Side Sports

In side-to-side sports, the prime objective is to move the center of gravity, quickly and with control.

TENNIS

In this sport, the motion of the arm swing with the racquet hitting the tennis ball exemplifies ballistic motion. When the player approaches the ball, using the forehand drive technique, the feet are apart approximately shoulder width or more, knee and hips are flexed. As the ball approaches the player, the player steps back or forward, brings the racquet back, and extends and abducts the racquet away from his body, and the shoulder supinates. The arm comes forward during the swing phase, and the ipsilateral or same-side hip turns inward. As the wrist slightly flexes and the arm swing accelerates the racquet, the ball makes contact and is propelled forward while the player follows through with the motion.

Biomechanically, the tennis player uses his back leg and foot for support as the racquet is in the swing phase. The leg begins to turn in, and the foot plantarflexes and everts into the ground, propelling the body forward. The forward limb, at this point in swing phase, begins to flex forward at the hips and knee. As the same-side hip, bearing weight, is adducted forward, the upper extremity moves forward. The opposite limb begins contact with the surface primarily with the ball of the foot in a slightly inverted position. The ipsilateral limb moves forward as the arm is completing the swing phase.

While observing tennis players in action, one immediately sees the fast pace, quick reactions, timing, jumping and stretching used in order to position the body just prior to hitting the tennis ball. Primarily, the tennis player takes a stance position which distributes the weight equally on both legs and feet, and is more on his tiptoes than completely flatfooted. His or her center of gravity is within the body planes and slightly forward, and the player's legs are usually about shoulder width apart. This allows the player the most mobility in left or right, back or forward directions. Hence, in order to prepare for this activity, stretching exercises and knee and ankle strengthening should be used in conjunction with trunk or waist twisting, loosening shoulders and neck, etc. There is running involved, too, so some type of conditioning program with running should be included.

Individuals with flat feet may find problems with foot fatigue, heel cord pain, or foot and ankle instability. Individuals with a relatively high-arched foot may have problems with sprains. These deviances found frequently in the general population can be satisfactorily resolved with orthotic devices or taping. The orthotic is placed in the shoe to control abnormal motion in the joints of the feet.

Injuries in Tennis. Tennis elbow or tendonitis is a common complaint of many tennis enthusiasts. The lower-extremity injuries are primarily restricted to sprains or strains. Since tennis is in a sense a contact sport, injuries may result from direct contact with the tennis ball just being served. Blistering may also occur.

Practical Hints. (1) practice; (2) study yourself—get instruction from the experts; (3) prevent injury by: conditioning, warmup, stretching, proper equipment, properly fitting shoes and taping the ankles if necessary.

GOLF

The golf swing exemplifies ballistic motion, whereby the golfer attempts to hit the ball in such a manner to get the desired distance and accuracy in or near the designated hole. The golfer must know how to correctly grip the golf club, and this can be done by using the overlapping grip, the interlocking vardon grip,

111

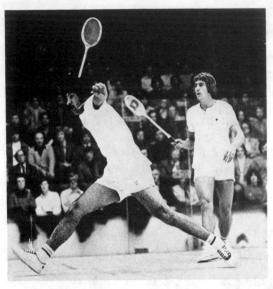

Players use side-to-side motion with quick starts and stops. (Tony Duffy photo)

or the baseball or two-handed grip. It has been found that no one grip was statistically superior to the other in terms of distance and accuracy.

The stance of the golfer relates to the intended direction and distance needed in the shot. For example, the smaller the stance, the more the golfer must be aware of balance during his swing because of less stability. This stance is obviously unstable, and chances of losing one's balance or incorrectly swinging the club might be enhanced. Furthermore, this does not allow the golfer to utilize the maximum force from his swing. On the other hand, a very wide stance also prevents the golfer from using maximum force to hit the ball. Thus, most players utilize an intermediate stance which gives balance, stability and maximum use of the swing.

As the golfer swings the club, the back leg is internally rotating, and the knee is flexed while the foot is everted, abducted and dorsiflexed. The forward leg externally rotates, and the foot is slightly inverted, adducted and plantarflexed. As the golf club is perpendicular to the ground and striking the golf ball, the golfer has to perform the above movement. Prior to that motion, the golf club was brought over the back of the golfer as he "cocked," and the forward leg internally rotated, flexed at the knee, adducted at the hips and dropped, which everted the foot as well as abducting and dorsiflexing it. The back leg was externally rotating, but the foot was neutral to supinated.

112

The follow-through finds the golfer adducting, dropping his hip, internally rotating the leg and flexing at the knee, causing the foot suddenly to evert, abduct and plantarflex into the ground. The forward hip is raised up and out as the forward leg is externally rotated and the foot is neutral to supinated at the subtalar joint. Meanwhile, the golf club is brought forward and over the front shoulder of the golfer as he concentrates on the follow-through.

The critical features for maximum performance during the golf swing:

1. The clubhead is in line with or just behind the hand.

2. The back of the wrist and hand is in a vertical plane perpendicular to the intended direction of the shot.

3. The golfer's center of gravity is forward of a midline between his feet, thus placing a greater proportion of his body weight on his left foot than on his right foot (for a right-handed golfer).

4. The axis of the shoulders-arms-hands lever passing through the golfer's chest is in the same position it has been in throughout the downswing. This is brought about by the golfer's trunk, the lower end of which has been driven forward earlier by leg and hip action, being inclined slightly backward. The golfer's head is inclined forward with his eyes firmly focused on the ball, which ensures that the axis is not lifted and thus tends to eliminate any risk of the ball being topped.

Injuries to Golfers. These usually are strains or sprains. Although injuries are infrequent to most golf enthusiasts, using improper body mechanics and not warming up or being in reasonable physical shape may cause injury or recurrence of old injuries. Besides being traumatized by being walked upon by spiked shoes, the ankle may be sprained due to the exaggerated position of the foot in relation to the lower leg during a golf swing. The usual blistering may result with ill-fitting shoes or worn shoes, especially after 18 or more holes of golf. These sprains and strains apply to the upper torso and extremities as well.

8

Ballistic Sports

Karate is an example of athletic activity that utilizes ballistic movement, as demonstrated by its kicks and punches. The goal of the karate technique is to combine good balance, timing, coordination, power, speed and accuracy into each movement. One of the desired results, then, is the concentrated effort of combining these elements into a single focus of strength and force, enough to break boards and bricks.

Biomechanically, karate instructors emphasize correct posture at all times. The positioning of the lower extremity or hips, legs and feet is essential to produce the "root" or stability of each technique and movement. The feet then are in contact with the ground, and maintain contact until there is movement or kicking. For the most part, the whole foot is on the ground rather than just the balls of the feet.

Since there are many forms or stances in karate, our discussion will be limited to two basic forms. The horse stance or kibadachi, and the front forward-leaning stance or zen-kutsu dachi are basic stances in karatic that demonstrate stability or "root."

In the horse stance, the legs are a little more than a shoulder width apart. The toes are directed straight ahead, and the hips are forward and tucked in to tighten the stomach and protect the groin area. The lower limbs are internally rotated, which allows the center of gravity to reside in the abdominal area. The feet are supinated to neutral as the forefoot is maintained in contact with the ground.

114

In the zen-kutsu dachi or forward-leaning stance, the athlete has one leg and foot two shoulder widths behind the other leg and one shoulder width apart. The forward leg is about one shoulder width apart from the body. The foot is directed forward, whereas the foot of the back leg is pointed at a 45-degree angle or abducted from the midline of the body. The front foot is slightly supinated to neutral, and the back foot is pronated (closed chain kinetics) with the weight distribution primarily 60% on the front leg and foot, and 40% on the back leg and foot.

As the individual moves from a horse stance into a forward-leaning stance, the leg moving forward enters into a swing or non-weight bearing phase. The leg opposite extends at the hip and knee, and the foot plantarflexes, everts and abducts, propelling the body forward. The forward limb re-supinates or internally rotates, and contact is made with both the forefoot and rearfoot. The forward limb is flexed at the hip and knee as the movement is completed.

In the punching techniques, the power, strength and speed begin at the "root" or feet, and the energy is transferred in the motion through the hips as the ipsilateral hip thrusts forward, also bringing the upper extremity forward. The arm is then extended forward and locked at the shoulder, elbow and wrist as the fist is propelled forward, making contact with the first and second knuckles. At that point, the karate-man focuses or locks his motion, extending his energy forward while abruptly ending his own motion.

In the front kick or "mae keri," one leg is thrusted forward with the extension at the knee and flexion at the hip, while the foot plantarflexes, adducts and the toes are dorsiflexed to expose the metatarsal heads which make contact with the target. The opposite limb provides complete weight-bearing support, with the foot locked into place or neutral to supinated position.

In the side kick or "yoko keri," again there is one weight-bearing limb. The thrusted or extended limb is internally rotated, and the foot is dorsiflexed and inverted, with the outside or lateral aspect of the foot used as the point of contact with the target. The thrusted limb is abducted from the body. As the foot approaches the target, the limb bearing weight abducts, ex-

Karate athletes use the rigid foot as a ballistic tool. (Tony Duffy photo)

ternally rotates and supinates or locks the foot in a quick manner, which is coordinated simultaneously with the extension of the thrusted limb.

The kick and punch, when done correctly, utilizes the body structure to transfer the force and energy to a single powerful focus. The techniques are done with speed and smoothness, and with practice are done with great accuracy. Balance in all of these techniques is essential, for not only does the root or stance have to be executed properly, but the arms and legs must be coordinated to further enhance balance as well as produce greater force. As one fist is extended forward, the other arm is flexed rapidly back in the "chamber" or ready position. When done correctly, the effect is a powerful, fast punch. The kicking technique does not differ, for in order to correctly perform a kick, balance is a necessity. This is accomplished in the root or stance as well.

Since karate is a contact sport, sites of injury are numerous. The majority of injuries occur to parts of the body which are used as contact points, the hands or feet. One would find injuries to knuckles, metatarsal heads, wrist, fingers in terms of sprains, fractures and lacerations, just to name the more common injuries. The feet may suffer fractures to any of the bones, as well as frequent ankle sprains. Other injuries occur in areas struck by either hand or feet, such as ribs, nose, hips, knees, back and groin.

The individual punching or kicking injures himself when he does not perform the punch or kick in the correct form. For example, when an individual strikes a board with his knuckles but does not lock his wrist, he will sprain or fracture it. An overzealous individual who is determined to demonstrate his prowess by breaking boards, bricks, etc., may find he has not progressively and patiently conditioned himself to his demise. The individual is on the receiving end of a stray punch or kick and does not have the knowledge to defend himself against a certain technique may become injured. Thus, supervision is needed at all times with proper instruction and emphasis on remaining cool and controlling oneself.

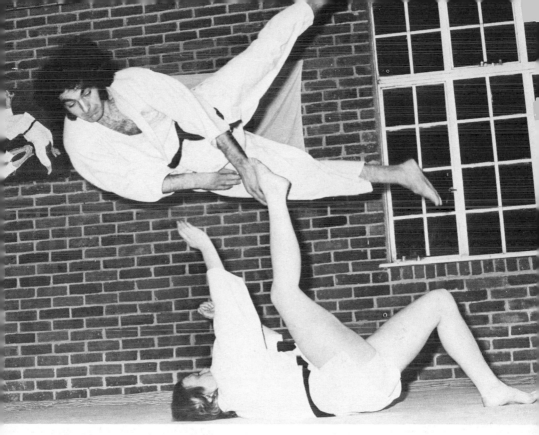

Some hints on karate:

1. Study yourself—practice patience.

2. Maintain proper joint and extremity alignment when making contact. For instance, when you punch with a clenched fist, lock your wrist and keep it in straight alignment with forearm. Contact is made with the first two knuckles (not the thumb). This is to avoid spraining or breaking your wrist. The same is true with your kicks. If you front-kick, make sure your toes are dorsiflexed upwards to expose the metatarsal heads of the bottom of the foot. If the toes are not flexed enough, contact with the toes is not only painful but usually result in sprains, dislocations or fractures.

3. If you find your kicks are weak or you cannot extend completely or high enough, flexibility exercises plus practice plus time will greatly benefit you.

4. When moving from stance to stance, make sure you keep your stances at the same heights. Bobbing up and down during katas when not specifically called for is bad form. Try to find the point where you feel stable and your balance is good with these stances, but always remember to emulate the sensei's instructions and stances as closely as possible.

5. During randori or sparing, try to move smoothly and easily and work on all phases of your instructions. Never lose your control by overdoing it, being overly aggressive or doing techniques for which you are not ready.

6. Concentration is at the end of your punch or kick. Prior to that time, try to be relaxed and flexible, not tight and straining.

Mixed-Motion Sports

FOOTBALL

This sport combines many types of motion. We see ballistic motion in throwing and kicking the football; forward motion in running, rushing the passer, blocking downfield, running a pass pattern; side-to-side motion in running laterally, and a runner avoiding tacklers by suddenly changing directions.

Most of the motion in football is running, which has been discussed in previous chapters. The modification of running in football is called the "cut," or suddenly changing directions while moving forward or backward at or near top speed. The biomechanics of a quick turn, for example, made by a running back at or near top speed, begins where the back decides to turn sharply to the right or to the left, depending on the line of scrimmage.

When the foot is planted, the opposite leg abducts from the leg that is solely supporting the body. The upper extremity turns in the desired direction. At heel contact or heel and forefoot contact, the leg supporting the weight externally rotates, and the foot inverts, plantarflexes and adducts into the ground. At mid-stance, the running back turns his hips outward and abducts his non-weight-bearing limb. The weight-bearing leg internally rotates, and the foot begins to evert, dorsiflex and abduct as the running back propels forward in the new direction.

When the weight-bearing limb is fully extended, the ipsilateral hip is thrust around, allowing the runner to sprint forward toward the line of scrimmage. Hence, a running back with uncompensated torsional problems can't externally rotate or dorsiflex the ankle due to gastroc-soleus or hamstring shortage, or he has a high degree of rearfoot or forefoot varus and will have some difficulty performing this movement in one quick 90-degree turn. In this situation, a running back with any of these problems would have to turn the corner gradually as in an end sweep, but a quick cut back or turning quickly "against the grain" would be difficult for this player. Identification of these characteristics by coach, athlete or trainer can help the player be aware of his particular body and exercise or stretch to improve physical capabilities.

Correct posture is important in order to position the body for maximum stability for contact as well as allowing for flexibility. A running back with a low posture will reduce his target area and place his center of gravity forward, in front of his feet. This individual's momentum is forward, and thus to tackle an individual who persistently runs erect is an easy target for pursuing tacklers.

A low posture and a wide stance allows linemen and linebackers to keep their back straight, body flexed to absorb contact forces and carry movement in any direction. This position also provides the lineman and linebacker with a good leverage system to thrust forward with his upper torso as he simultaneously extends his legs. This low posture provides for good balance and stability while keeping the center of gravity low and forward.

Kicking the football is, of course, also an essential part of the game. We find kicking in the kickoff, field goal and extra point after touchdown, and the punt. The newest innovation to kicking in football has been the soccer style. Studies have shown that the soccer kick produced a greater ball velocity than did the conventional straight approach. It was also found that distances from 20-32 yards from the goalpost, the soccer-style approach proved to have better accuracy. However, using the two-step approach, either soccer style or straight on, produced the same or similar distances kicked.

In the soccer-style approach, the right-footed kicker is off to the left of the ball and moves in an arc as his leg is extended to kick the ball. In the conventional style, the kicker is directly behind and in line with the football. In the soccer-style kick the foot is planted, the leg is slightly externally rotated, which supinates the foot. The right leg now in swing phase is internally rotated, giving the arc affect as the right hip is stabilized and serves as a pivot for the right leg and hip. The foot is slightly plantarflexed, everted and abducted in such a manner that the foot strikes the ball perpendicular or straight forward. As the leg extends from a flexed position, and the lower leg or tibia and fibula is extended, the foot is dorsiflexed upward and forward, and follow-through is achieved.

The kicker's head is forward, and the back is somewhat rounded to allow the eyes to focus on the ball. The arms act to balance the action of the leg—the left forward and the right arm slighly back. Thus, an individual kicker who cannot extend upward beyond 90 degrees or above his waist will have difficulty getting height as well as distance with his kicks. Such players could have hamstring, iliopsoas, gastroc-soleous or calf muscle contractures; quadriceps or thigh muscle weakness, and torsional problems.

The site of injury to football players are numerous. Most injuries occur to the lower extremity—the hip, thigh, knee, ankle and feet. Other common sites of injuries include the head, neck, collarbone, shoulder, elbow, wrists, hands and ribs. These injuries result from contact or great external forces to the body; poor body and joint alignment, and poor equipment and inadequate protection. The knee is the most injured part of the body in football, and muscles, tendons and ligaments are the most frequently damaged tissues. Further research on the common injuries to offensive and defensive members as well as to each specific position would enlighten athletes, coaches and trainers in terms of specific injuries, and the prevention of those injuries by conditioning exercises, improving technique, and adequate taping, orthotics, braces, etc., to maintain proper body and joint alignment.

Practical hints for football players:

1. Study yourself: observe how you make cut, run or pass patterns. Move laterally, and see if you can sight some aspect of your way of posture moving which might be corrected to improve your performance. Have a friend, or coach observe you and ask for his opinion as well.

2. For your foot and ankle: if you have had problems with ankle

sprains, or you feel your ankles are weak or have a tendency to turn in or out on you, tape your ankles and wear properly fitting shoes. If this does not help, padding in the arch or orthotics may control some of the unnecessary motion in your feet which tire you or not allow you to perform as well. Do stretching and strengthening exercises for the muscles around the ankle.

3. For your knee: make sure that your pads in your football pants cover the entire knee while standing and running. If you have a history of knee problems, make sure you give your knee good support such as a knee brace or knee wrap.

4. For your thighs and hips: again make sure the protective equipment adequately protects your hips and thighs so that none of these areas are exposed to external contact.

5. Flexibility is important! Stretch during the warmups and just before you go into the game if called in from the bench. A lot of running is demanded in this sport and flexibility is essential for muscles to work effectively and efficiently. Your warmup routine should be for flexibility, and increased heart rate and blood flow, not to tire you. Therefore, strength and endurance activities, like pushups and situps, should not be done prior to competition.

6. After practice or game: make sure you gradually cool your body. Some stretching exercises or warmup exercises at this time would be very beneficial. Don't expose yourself to extreme temperature changes. Gradually relax yourself with an attitude of feeling good as you slow down.

7. Weights: if you are working with weights to increase bulk and strength of muscles in the lower extremity, make sure you work on the flexors and extensors. Try not to create muscle imbalances, because they cause contractures or shortening of muscles. After working with weights, make sure you stretch the muscles. You don't want the muscle to contract to the point where you can't move as well as before.

BASKETBALL

Basketball is a sport of quick reaction, constant sprinting, running, jumping and endurance. There are numerous skills associated with these activities, such as shooting, dribbling, rebounding

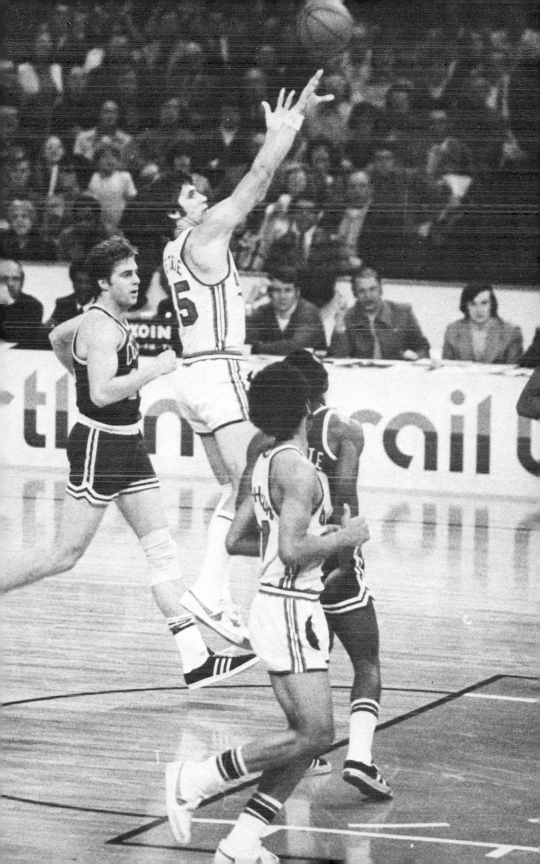

and blocking shots. Our primary attention will, of course, be on the events of the lower extremity during these movements.

In the kinesiology and biomechanics of jumping, the basketball player usually has a wide base or his feet are wide apart (approximately shoulder width). The center of gravity is low and within the body planes as the ankles, knees and hips flex. The arms are usually away from the body part and extended upward during the jump as a part of the accelerating motion upward. The player at this time is on the toes or balls of his feet just prior to jumping upward. When propulsion occurs, the ankles, knees and hip are extended sharply, forcing the foot to plantarflex, evert and abduct into the ground. As the foot lifts off, it has moved from a dorsiflexed position to a plantarflexed, and subsequently moved from an everted position to an inverted and adducted position in the air. It has been observed that taking a few steps or running start before jumping results in higher heights than from a stationary position.

Quickness plays a very important role in the ability of a player, especially the shorter players in order to dribble, pass, shoot and play defense. A player who is shooting must not only jump high enough so his shot is not blocked by the defensive player, but must also aim and shoot with accuracy. Usually, the shot is off just before the player reaches maximum height with his jump, but ideally the shot should be released at the peak of his jump.

There are also many maneuvers one may use before the shot is taken to avoid having the defensive player block his shot or giving the shooter enough defensive pressure to cause the shot to miss the basket. These maneuvers are the "fake" and "pick" and are based on the reaction of the defensive player which allows the shooter to move away from the defensive player, and get his shot off with accuracy and good technique. The offensive player who is "screening" or "picking" usually positions himself to one side of the defensive player. The player has a wide shoulder width or greater stance, and his center of gravity is slightly forward. This allows the offensive player to absorb the force of contact and also block the path of the defender who is attempting to guard the player who is shooting or moving to a position to shoot or pass.

The defender, on the other hand, also utilizes a low posture to get his center of gravity low and slightly forward, and have a wide stance to move laterally, forward and backward quickly. The defender always keeps the offensive player between himself and the basket, and uses his hands to feel for picks or screens coming to his sides even though he is concentrating on the offensive player. Thus, the defenders legs are abducted and internally rotated, and the feet are in neutral to pronated position, allowing the medial aspect of the feet in contact with the floor due to the center of gravity and majority of the weight located midline of the body.

The best position of the body and lower extremity should be with the knees slightly flexed and the weight distributed equally over the feet, completely in contact with the ground as opposed to bearing weight over the balls of the feet. It has been shown that a player on the balls of his feet rocks back onto the heels before propelling forward.

Injuries to the basketball player are predominantly found in the lower extremity or legs, knees, ankles and feet. Most injuries in basketball are a result of tremendous torsional forces on the lower extremity and malalignment of joints. Ankle sprains are probably the most common injury to players in this sport.

Practical hints for basketball players:

1. Study yourself: watch, feel, observe yourself move with and without the ball. Have a fellow basketball player or coach observe you, and ask him his opinion on how you move, shoot, pass, dribble, etc. We're talking about good fundamental basketball techniques. But if you find you can't do something or have difficulty doing something in basketball, assess these difficulties and try to solve them. If you find you're dealing with habits—or the way you taught yourself to move—try to correct them. If the problem is anatomical, specifically the way you're built or the way your bones are structured, strapping the foot, padding the shoes or using orthotic devices may help your feet function better. We're talking about preventing injuries *and* improving performance.

2. Properly fitting foot gear, taping, and orthotic devices may be used to support feet and ankles.

3. Weight training: do not create imbalances. Exercise both agonists and antagonists, and do flexibility or stretching exercises.

GYMNASTICS

Gymnastics requires strength, flexibility, endurance, balance and timing. The gymnasts perform many maneuvers combining many types of motions. In our discussion, the emphasis is on the lower extremity and how it functions and contributes to the total aesthetic beauty of athletes in motion.

Floor exercises: The lower extremity plays a great role in the performance of these floor exercises. Biomechanically speaking, the floor exercises can be classified into motions we have previously discussed. For example, prior to leap or spring with a double twisting somersaults, the gymnast usually runs on the balls of the feet and propels by plantarflexing the foot into the ground, then from a flexed position, extends the knees to obtain the necessary thrust to propel him through his particular movement.

When the gymnast lands, the foot must be in a stable or locked position to help his body halt momentum and unnecessary movement. Again, the knee is usually flexed to help absorb the force of the body weight going through the lower extremity and coming in contact with the floor, as well as stabilizing the center of gravity.

Hence, a gymnast with a large degree of bony deformity or soft-tissue deformity may have difficulty in obtaining the precise coordinated balance that is so necessary in the floor exercises. A foot that does not function at or near neutral position due to the deformities may not give the gymnast the extra lift that is needed to perform a routine perfectly.

This, however, does not necessarily mean a a gymnast is handicapped and therefore should quit. What it means is that the gymnast must recognize his shortcomings and deal with them by working at improving or adjusting a particular movement to suit his body build. If, for example, a gymnast finds his flexibility inadequate, focusing on stretching exercises may help the gymnast improve flexibility and hence that particular routine.

For the static positions, the gymnast is technically and aesthetically required to (1) allow the line of gravity to pass through the mid-point of his base or stance; (2) the area of the stance or base is large as possible; (3) center of gravity is as low as possible.

Front Single-Leg Lever. This hold position can be maneuvered from many different positions, but the simplest way is from the front, erect position. From this position, the gymnast shifts his center of gravity slightly over to one side so that it is directly over the leg which will support the body weight. The head and trunk is then lowered in a forward direction, and the gymnast simultaneously extends their arm forward and upward keeping both legs extended and straight. The supporting limb shifts from a relaxed or pronated position to a more neutral to supinated position to give the gymnast maximum stability from his feet and ankles. The knee is locked and straight ahead. The limb extended backward, up and out is slightly rotated internally, and the foot is in a plantarflexed position. The final position usually reveals a slight vertical arch from the hips and lower back to maintain stability. The gymnast utilizes his neck, wrist and hand flexors to control any forward or backward tendency.

Cartwheel. This is one of the elementary movements generally taught early in gymnastics programs. From a standing position with arms stretched upward and body facing the desired direction, the gymnast steps forward and shifts his weight forward over the front foot. The gymnast then rotates his body sideways, swings the rearleg upward and extended, and lowers his body until his hands on the same side as his front foot has touched the floor. The front leg is slightly flexed at the hip and knee, and the ankle is dorsiflexed. Then with the body weight being partially supported by the front leg and hand, the opposite hand is brought down to the floor as the trunk moves toward the vertical position.

At vertical position of the body, both legs are extended and abducted at the hips, and the foot is plantarflexed. The gymnast then pushes off against the ground and rotates sideways, placing most of the weight on the opposite hand and rearfoot as the body moves away from the vertical. The push-off must be powerful enough to maintain the momentum to enable the gymnast to stand erect again at the completion of the cartwheel. The center of gravity must be aligned directly with the direction of the cartwheel and must not deviate from one side to the other. This would create and imbalance, and the gymnast would fall forward or backward or not complete the cartwheel as desired.

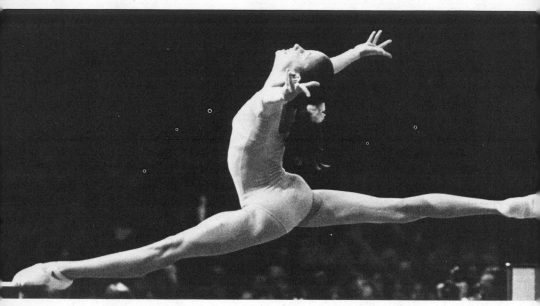

Gymnastics demand all aspects of conditioning. (M.J. Baum photo)

Vaulting. A 5'3" long and 4'5" high horse in gymnastics is used to vault over while doing various movements. In competition judges look for hand placement relative to specific zones painted on the horse, the flight onto and off the horse and form in the execution of the vault. Another basic consideration is the approach, where speed and accuracy in stepping up the the horse are major factors. Running in the approach does not differ from running in any other sport, and biomechanically it is also identical.

The hurdle step or step just prior to takeoff must be done in such a manner as to correctly position the gymnast's body without the loss of speed or accuracy. The legs are flexed at the knees and hips, the feet are together and dorsiflexed at the ankle, and the hands are down by the sides. At takeoff, the hands drive forward onto the horse, and the foot vigorously plantarflexes into the ground. The knees are legs extend, lifting the gymnast upward and forward.

The gymnast, now in flight, must depend on the support of his hands and arms which are extended forward against the horse. This is the phase when the gymnast can control his or her angular direction and momentum. For example, if the gymnast intends to vault forward, the center of gravity is translated straight and forward over the support of the hands and arms as the body also maintains similar position. Momentum is controlled by the duration of support and the angulation of momentum as the gymnasts moves forward. The angulation is similarly dependent on the duration of support, and the longer the support, the sharper the angulation.

During flight, the gymnast changes body position, direction and momentum as a result of the type of support. As the gymnast lands, the body must be positioned in such a way as to allow for adequate reaction to the force of forward momentum and body weight, and does so by moving perpendicular or down to the ground. Any over-compensation or incorrect adjustment results in an awkward landing. As the gymnast comes in contact to the ground, the legs are flexed and dorsiflexed at the ankles and the body is slightly forward with the center of gravity low and forward.

Rings. Two rings are suspended from the ceiling and provide the gymnast with the only means of support during the exercises. These exercises primarily demonstrate upper extremity strength in order to keep the rings still while performing movements like the iron cross and flexibility as seen in the giant swings. The torso is generally perpendicular or parallel to the extremities. The upper and lower extremities are usually extended. The legs are extended most of the time while the feet are plantarflexed and straight ahead, not veering from side to side. The center of gravity is about at the level of the abdomen and is maintained in the body planes, never forward or backward. This is the point of pivot and rotation.

The main objective of gymnast is to perform various movements precisely as well as keeping the rings as still as physically possible. As he performs the iron cross, he gradually extends his arms near full length and turns his body sideways either left or right. At this point, the arms are parallel to the floor and the body is perpendicular to the floor. To keep the rings still, the gymnast must concentrate on equal distribution of strength to the arms. Once the strength weakens through fatigue, the muscles go into spacity and jerky movements are created, moving the rings. The lower extremity is held still, in an extended position. In the giant swings, the upper extremity must maintain the rings still while the lower extremity maintains its extended position and swings the body around the pivot point maintained at the arms.

The lower extremity does not play the major role in balance in this case. The strength in the upper extremity primarily determines the balance and stillness on the rings.

Injuries to gymnasts are usually due to falling. Hence, they can range from strains to lacerations and fractures.

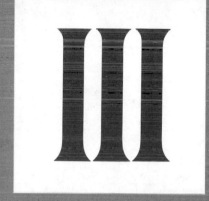

III

FOOT
FAILURE

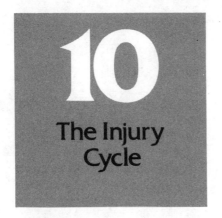

10
The Injury Cycle

Injury is the most feared enemy of the competitive athlete. Nothing can be more frustrating than the knowledge that vigorous activity must come to an end just when personal goals are within reach. In this chapter, injury is defined and its ramifications explored. Traumatic versus overuse injuries are delineated, with special attention being given to overuse syndromes in specific sports. Injuries to specific areas of the lower limb are categorized, as well as the mechanisms involved in each. Clinical evaluation of the injury with diagnostic signs and symptoms most commonly found will be presented, and, where possible, reference is made to a variety of sports where similar injuries occur.

First we must define what an injury is. In its broadest sense, it is any disruption of tissue continuity. This definition is useful because it takes into account all forms of injury from a simple friction blister of skin to a comminuted (fragmented) fracture of bone. This extreme range of injury reminds us that injury can occur to either soft tissue such as skin, muscle, tendon and ligament, or to bone. However, no matter what the tissue involved, certain basic principles must be kept in mind when confronted with an injury, evaluating its severity and determining the best course of treatment.

In all injury, there is an inflammatory response. The degree of the injury will determine the severity of this response. This is nature's way of isolating a specific area and alerting the consciousness to evaluate and treat the problem. Inflammation increases blood flow to the area to bring nutrient blood cells, "flush out" and "wall off" damaged tissue, and begin the deep healing response which proceeds through the blood system and toward the surface. Ideally, this ends when all tissues have returned to their normal condition and function.

Inflammation has five components: pain, redness, heat, swelling and loss of function. The first four are considered "cardinal" signs because they are readily observable by the doctor. The last sign, loss of function, though not considered a cardinal sign, is usually present to some degree. Let us look at these signs and determine the reason for each.

Pain has two components. At the time of the initial injury, pain is more sharp and well defined, especially with motion of the part. During the next 24-48 hours, the pain becomes more throbbing-or pressure-type and noticeable even when the part is not moving. Initial pain is more easily localized than what has been present for a day or two.

Reasons for the difference in pain are that immediately after an injury, especially of a traumatic nature, the torn tissue damage in the immediate area stimulates nerve endings. As the part swells, tissues in the surrounding area are compressed, and thus a more generalized throbbing-type pain is noted. The "throbbing" is actually the resistance to the pulsing of the blood in circulation, so it is the same as the heart rate.

Swelling of an area occurs for several reasons. First, tissue damage results in bleeding because the small blood vessels or capillaries have been torn. Second, fluid between cells and fluid within the cells escapes into the injured area because of this disruption of tissue. Third, special hormones, enzymes and cells within the blood draw more cells into the area to clean up the debris and start the repair processes. Finally, there is a widening of the blood vessels which bring in more blood, carrying the necessary "machinery" for wound healing. All of these contribute to the swelling of an injured area during the first 24-48 hours.

The redness and heat associated with an injury are the result of this last phase of swelling. As the vessels get larger and carry more blood, they make the skin directly over the injured area more red in appearance, because of increased blood flow, and warm to the touch, because the enlarged vessels are closer to the skin surface.

Loss of function is a subjective finding involving a number of factors. Through swelling and muscle spasm, the body attempts to "splint itself," which aids healing. Depending on the severity of the injury, an individual may be totally bedridden or minimally disabled, feeling only mild discomfort with activity. Individual pain thresholds are also a variable; some people can tolerate discomfort better than others. For this reason, following injury, the athlete must be able to demonstrate full function and range of motion before he is allowed to return to competition.

Traumatic injuries to the foot or any part may be caused by a direct blow of short duration, or the result of continuous or intermittent injury (microtrauma) over an extended time period. Cumulative microtrauma "Overuse," will cause tissue destruction. The extent of injury depends on several factors:

1. *Duration:* rapid blow versus continuous or intermittent microtrauma; a rapid injury is more serious because it is not reversible.

2. *Type of injury:* external forces versus internal instability or imbalance; external forces cause greater disability because of the body has no defense against it.

3. *Direction of force:* vertical forces versus twisting forces; twisting (torsional) forces affect more tissues and are therefore more destructive.

4. *Depth of injury:* skin, subcutaneous connective tissue, bone; the deeper the injury, the more destructive.

CYCLE OF OVERUSE INJURY

The inflammatory process includes swelling (edema), redness (erythema), heat, pain and loss of function. It is reversible if irritation stops. Inflammation is the body's method of warning against overuse as well as the beginning of the healing (repair) process.

This is a gradual process progressing from superficial areas of minor skin microtrauma to the deep areas of bone trauma. A severe blow may produce tendon, joint or bone injury before the body has a chance to react. Up to stage 6 (callus), the cycle is reversible if activity (trauma) is stopped.

Foot Injuries, Causes and Cures

(REGION) Depth	Foot Injury	Description	Early Treatment (stop irritation)	Extended Treatment (protect the part)	Expected Disability
(SKIN)	Blister	Separation of superficial layers by fluid	Cool compresses	Sterile drainage and compression dressing	Brief
(SKIN)	Callus, corn	Thickening of upper skin layers for protection	Trimming of excess tissue	Correction by removal of offending irritant	Brief
(SOFT TISSUE)	Contusion (bruise, hematoma)	Damage to the nerve-vessel layer	Cold first 24 hours, then warm; professional help?	Evaluate extent of injury	Varies with depth
(TENDON)	Strain	Tear in the tendon-muscle complex	Evaluate extent, then ice packs; support	Possible immobilization; professional help	4 days to 6 weeks
(NERVE)	Neuritis	Irritation to nerve from pinch or trauma	Evaluate cause; professional help	Relief of impingement	2-3 weeks
(MUSCLE)	Ischemia (cramps)	Loss of blood supply for tissue; fluid imbalance	Evaluate and eliminate cause rapidly; massage	Prevention of overuse	Brief
(TENDON)	Tendinitis	Inflammation of the tendon sheath	Cold first 24 hours, then warm; support; prevent swelling	Prevention of stress; balancing orthotics, professional help	2-6 weeks
(SOFT TISSUE)	Bursitis	Inflamed protective sac or fluid over	Protect or aspirate pressure area, professional help	Correct or relieve irritant; professional help	1 week
(JOINT)	Dislocation	Separation of bones at joint	Immobilization; professional help	Taping, support, orthotics; professional help	2-4 weeks
(BONE)	Periostitis (bone bruise)	Blood between bone and bone covering	Injection, aspiration, support; professional help	Prevention of reinjury	1 week
(BONE)	Stress fracture	Partial crack in skeleton from overuse	Support; compression; professional help	Limited activity	4-6 weeks
(BONE)	Complete fracture	Complete break in skeleton from trauma	Correct alignment of parts; thorough evaluation; professional help	Immobilization of part	4-6 weeks

The body provides several lines of defense against injury. The skin is sensitive to pressure, friction and temperature. Microtrauma to the skin will first produce heat, redness, pain and inflammation, and finally a blister develops to separate the upper from the lower levels of the skin. If microtrauma continues over an extended period of time, a diffuse callus or specific nucleated corn may develop as a protection to the deeper structures.

Beneath the skin is the protective fat layer around the minor nerves and vessels, and surrounding the tendons of muscles. Contusion (bruise) to this area is not disabling unless tendon or nerve damage occurs. Prolonged swelling in this area is destructive in that it produces pressure and ischemia (lack of blood supply) to the deeper, more essential structures.

Strain (a tear in the muscle-tendon complex) may be mild, moderate or complete. The more severe, the more scar tissue (muscles do not regenerate). Rest is essential for healing.

Sprain (a tear in ligaments, fibrous bands that hold bones together at joints) may also be mild, moderate or severe and treatment ranges from two days to six weeks. Pain on pressure and with joint motion is a good indication as to the extent of healing. Ligaments, like muscles, do not regenerate, and occasionally surgical repair is necessary.

Tendonitis (tendon inflammation) is actually inflammation of the tubular sheath, because tendon has no blood supply of its own and therefore heals slowly. The most common cause is a stress tear of the tendon, and it must be treated with adequate rest, or disability is extended.

Neuritis (nerve irritation) can occur through external injury or impingement (pinching) between other structures. This is very painful and disabling. When the cause is found, the treatment is successful.

Bursitis is inflammation of a closed sac of fluid over areas subject to irritation. These are relieved quickly when the area of irritation is found, the inflammation is treated with protection, injection or, on rare occasions, surgical removal of the bursal sac.

Dislocation of bones in joints follows severe trauma and needs professional treatment. Disability varies with the extent of injury.

Periostitis (bone bruise) is a very common injury on the foot because of the many bone prominences. In a bone bruise the perio-steum, or covering of the bone is separated from the bone by a layer of blood. If this is aspirated (drained) and protected, it heals quickly, with a minimum of disability. If it is not treated, it forms an enlargement (exostosis) of bone which produces further fric-tion, irritation and disability.

The most common fracture in the foot is the stress fracture, which is a crack in the shaft of the bone, because of overuse or excessive stress. Bone is a living tissue which must be conditioned for severe stress. When alignment on the fracture bone parts is good, healing is rapid. Most common areas of stress fractures are the metatarsal bones and the heel bone.

HEALING OF INJURIES

How does an injury heal? We have stated that there is an in-creased amount of blood carrying healing elements to the area. These elements have basically two functions: to clear out all dam-aged and non-vital tissues, and to restore tissue continuity by means of regeneration—regeneration of the soft tissue that had been injured or by the laying down of fibrous scar tissue.

These functions will not occur until bleeding into the area has stopped. Once this has occurred, cellular elements are free to clear out damaged tissue and begin laying down new or scar tissue to restore continuity of tissues. It must be remembered that, though the tissue continuity has been restored, complete function may never return to what it was prior to the injury. For example, the sprinter who pulls a hamstring is often subject to re-injury to the same area because the scar that has restored the tissue is not as elastic as the muscle it has replaced.

Some tissues heal or regenerate completely, some heal with scar tissue or "overgrowth" of similar tissue, and unfortunately some tissues do not heal at all. If injury is to the skin, hair or nails on the surface layers, they heal completely with no scar. If the injury gets through the skin to the dermis, which contains blood vessels and fat, they heal with a scar. It is important that there are no attachments (adhesions) between this layer and the layers above or below, or the nerve or tendon structures which pass through it.

Some tendons, especially those with a covering called a para-

Tissue Reaction to Longterm Stress

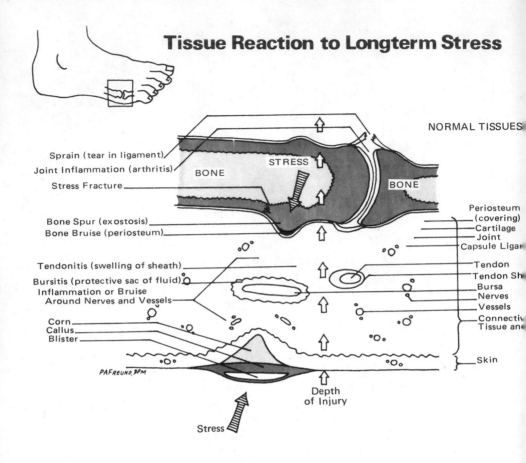

Sprain (tear in ligament)
Joint Inflammation (arthritis)
Stress Fracture

BONE
STRESS
BONE

NORMAL TISSUES

Bone Spur (exostosis)
Bone Bruise (periosteum)

Periosteum (covering)
Cartilage
Joint
Capsule Ligam

Tendonitis (swelling of sheath)
Bursitis (protective sac of fluid)
Inflammation or Bruise
Around Nerves and Vessels

Tendon
Tendon Sh
Bursa
Nerves
Vessels

Corn
Callus
Blister

Connectiv
Tissue an

PAFREUND, DPM

Skin

Depth
of Injury

Stress

tenon, such as tendons on the tops of hands and feet, will regenerate completely. But those without covering, such as deep to the palms and soles, do not heal by themselves and need to be immobilized and often surgically repaired, with resulting scar tissue.

Muscles and visceral (abdominal) organs heal by scarring and never regain full elasticity. Blood vessels are made of muscular walls which expand and contract (pulse), and heal with moderate scar tissue. This is true for the heart muscle as well. The blood itself is a living tissue which is constantly forming and regenerating within the bone marrow, liver and other structures. Transfusions of blood are necessary only when the loss of volume or quality threatens functions of vital organs.

Major nerves such as the brain and spinal cord do not regenerate. They are covered by fluid essential to their function, and loss

138

of spinal fluid or blood flow to the brain for even a few minutes produces permanent damage. Peripheral nerves, such as those in the extremities, are covered with a nutrient-absorbent sheath. If a nerve of this type is injured, it heals completely. A nerve is actually a bundle of small nerve fibers, like electrical wire, so the larger the nerve, the greater the chance of poor healing, entrapment of the nerve in scar tissue, paresthesias (abnormal tingling and shooting sensations), or complete loss of sensation or motor function. Injuries to large peripheral nerves require microscopic surgical repair with gentle handling.

Ligaments are firm, inelastic bands of connective tissue in long fibers. As with tendons, they have poor blood supply. Mild sprains heal with scar tissue, but a complete rupture of a ligament never heals. This is why ankle injuries require a clear diagnosis. If it is not treated properly, the ankle remains unstable (weak) forever. A severe ligament injury must be treated during the first 72 hours following injury.

Periosteum is a covering on bone which provides attachments for other structures and helps supply nutrients to the bone. Periosteum regenerates completely and is essential to healing of bone injuries because it provides the specialized blood cells which organize a bone callus.

Bone is the firm skeletal structure. In the very young, it is flexible and well nourished; in the old, it is brittle and poorly nourished. Children heal more rapidly than adults. For proper bone healing, the parts must be in good position or immobilized so that the thin fibers through the blood clot can form the structural latticework necessary to strength and function of the bone. If this is done, bone regenerates completely.

Each tissue varies with healing time. In general, the more blood supply, the quicker the healing process.

Now that we have some general principles about what occurs with injury, we can use these as guidelines for selecting treatment of an injury. Though specific treatments are discussed more fully in later chapters, here we can outline some of the basic principles regarding injuries and healing.

1. Healing will not occur until bleeding has stopped. Our initial goal is hemostasis (stop the bleeding).

2. Debris in the injured area must be cleared so that new tissue can be laid down. To minimize the amount of debris that accumulates, the swelling must be kept to a minimum.

To minimize swelling, use ICE: I = Ice, C = Compression, E = Elevation.

Ice constricts vessels so that less fluid can infiltrate the area. Compression minimizes the dead space so that there is less area for fluid to accumulate. Elevation allows gravity to assist the body in clearing fluids from the area.

3. Healing will best take place if the part is immobilized. Depending on the tissue involved (bone or soft tissue) healing will best occur if ruptured ends are close to each other and disrupting motion is minimized.

4. Pain is a warning sign and should be monitored. Gone are the days when the choice of treatment was to "run it off." Pain should indicate to the athlete and coaching staff that the injury is still present and that the gradual decrease in pain is a sign that healing is progressing well. However, when returning to activity after pain has ceased, one should progress slowly according to pain tolerance. *Don't expect to be as fit as you were prior to the injury.* Relapses are common when returning from a layoff. Work on conditioning the "good side" as well as the "healing side" when returning to activity. Build a strong foundation that will prevent future injury.

PAIN AND THE ATHLETE

With all tissue injury, comes pain. Pain is a warning signal telling the body that all is not right, that tissue balance and continuity have been upset. In order to diagnose and treat a new injury properly, it is important to have a good understanding of pain and its implications.

Because we have all experienced a variety of injuries, we realize that pain can vary depending on the particular injury. It can vary in two important ways—quantitatively (how much) and qualitatively (what kind). The quantity or intensity of pain a particular injury produces can be misleading. There is no direct relationship between the amount of pain experienced and the seriousness of the injury. A turned ankle, for example, may seem relatively minor.

140

However, serious damage to the supporting structures may have occurred. An athlete who simply "runs it off" may be compounding the problem. Thus, it is important to examine a part before continuing activity, even though the severity of pain is mild in nature.

The qualitative aspect to pain relates to the specific tissue involved. Not all body tissues respond the same way with respect to pain. Each tissue has specialized nerve cells which transfer the message "pain" to the consciousness. By keeping this in mind, a more clear diagnosis can be made. The description of the type of pain experience can guide you to the tissue or tissues involved and thus help determine the possible seriousness of the injury. Warning: self-diagnosis can be dangerous. If there is any doubt, or if you do not respond quickly to first aid treatment, immediately seek professional attention. The different tissues and their most common descriptive type of pain are given. Remember that there may be combined tissue injury with non-specific pain. Try to evaluate these "feelings" as soon after the injury as possible, before swelling occurs. Remember "ICE."

11

Self-Evaluation

It is important to isolate the cause, location and type of pain so you can attempt to make your own "diagnosis" and help your doctor. I find that most athletes go through this process before seeking professional help:

1. *Location and depth:* try to find the point of maximum tenderness.

2. *Type of pain:* "Fatigue" or "aching" pains indicate muscle or tendon problems; "burning" pain indicates inflammation. This can be at various levels—skin or just under the skin (relieved by elimination of friction and pressure); around the tendons and bones (indicating overuse or traumatic injury to tissues, usually relieved by rest), or in joints (indicating a traumatic arthritis, painful with motion and not relieved by rest). "Sharp burning" or "shooting" pains may indicate nerve irritation. "Cramping" is usually associated with muscle injury, but can be related to metabolism and fluid imbalance. "Severe pain" or "loss of function" of any part requires professional evaluation.

3. *Onset:* How did the pain start? Was there any injury or severe change in training or competitive style, such as from long, slow distance to intervals or sprints; from flat to hill running; soft to hard surfaces; hurdles; new events, new shoes? Any change in your conditioning program should be done gradually to allow your body to compensate. Do adequate warmup (stretching) exercises to allow your body to meet new demands. Muscle and joint flexibility are more important than strength.

142

4. *Duration and progression*: How long has the problem been present? Has it been constant, getting worse or better? This will indicate whether the problem is an overuse syndrome or traumatic injury, and whether you have been paying attention to the "cues" of your body.

5. *Treatment:* Has there been any treatment? How do you relieve it? As a general role, ICE—ice, compression and elevation—will be helpful. Heat in any form will increase pain, swelling and inflammation, and probably should not be used for most sports-related injuries. Medications, pills and injections are only temporary, and can mask deeper problems. If pain is not disabling and you continue to perform, can you relieve the pain in any way, such as changing stride, toeing in or out, running on the ball of the foot, on the side of the foot? If so, there is an imbalance causing overuse injury. Orthotics made by a sports-conscious professional will relieve the imbalance.

6. *When:* In activity, when does the pain come on? Pain early in the event may be caused by muscle stiffness or joint arthritis. Pain during the middle of the activity can be caused by a multitude of things, mostly related to conditioning of the various tissues through training. "Overuse = under-conditioning." (To quote Joe Henderson, *Runner's World* editor, "If it hurts, it can't be helping much.") Pain after activity is caused by inflammation of irritated tissues in the body's attempt to bring in healing blood.

7. *Kind of shoes:* What kind of shoes are you wearing? Are they worn down? Good training shoes must cushion the heel on contact, support the arch during full weight-bearing and allow flexibility of motion of the toes during propulsion. Unequal or distorted shoe-wear patterns indicate chronic foot or leg imbalance. If there is a difference in limb length, there are different shoe wear patterns on each foot and greater stress, usually on the shorter limb.

If you can answer these questions about your own performance, you will be close to the resolution of the problem. Never consider an injury lightly. Early treatment will prevent chronic disability. Be patient in allowing nature to heal injuries. When in doubt, get professional help immediately.

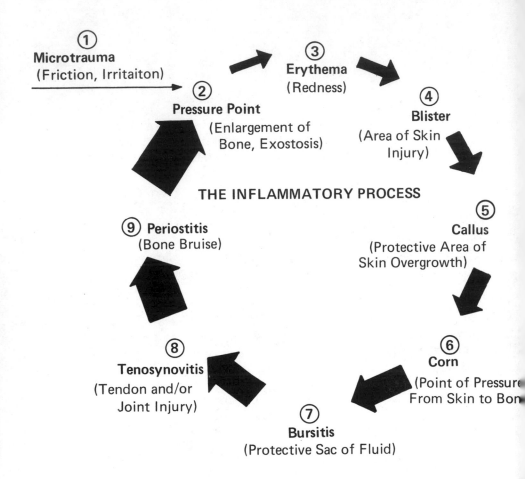

THE INFLAMMATORY PROCESS

① Microtrauma
(Friction, Irritaiton)

② Pressure Point
(Enlargement of
Bone, Exostosis)

③ Erythema
(Redness)

④ Blister
(Area of Skin
Injury)

⑤ Callus
(Protective Area of
Skin Overgrowth)

⑥ Corn
(Point of Pressure
From Skin to Bone)

⑦ Bursitis
(Protective Sac of Fluid)

⑧ Tenosynovitis
(Tendon and/or
Joint Injury)

⑨ Periostitis
(Bone Bruise)

PAIN RESPONSES

Injuries to various tissues of the body transmit different sensations of pain to the brain:

Skin: sharp, focal, brilliant, pinpoint. Hair, nails—no sensations themselves, but injury to their attachments produce skin-type pain. Skin may have referred numbness, tingling, or "pins an needles" pain from deeper nerve injury.

Subcutaneous: connective tissue, fat—less sharp, dispersive.

Blood or blood vessels: no pain in themselves; blood loss leads to shock, fainting (the body's way to get the head to the level of the heart, for circulation to the brain).

Muscle: dull, dispersive, fatigue, cramping, not easily localized; aggravated by movement or pressure.

144

Tendon or deep fascia (covering of muscle): usually sharp or aching, but varies greatly.

Visceral (abdominal organs): dull, sickening, may progress intractable-type pain.

Ligament (bone to bone attachment with fluid capsule at joints): Two types of pain—sharp when ligament is stretched and aching following injury.

Joint: aching, stiffness, painful with motion.

Nerve: shooting, electrical, burning, tingling.

Periosteum (bone covering where soft tissue structures attach): sharp.

Bone: dull, aching, boring, aggravated by movement.

Pain has other characteristics which are helpful in evaluating an injury. It is important to realize, for example, that pain is not summative. That is, an injury to a particular area may involve several structures and specific sites. However, the most severely painful area will obliterate the less painful ones. When this occurs there is a tendency to underestimate the extent of the injury. A careful examination of the total part must be performed to map out the structures involved. As a corollary to this, when the most severely painful area is relieved, minor sites of pain may surface and become paramount.

Pain has a tendency to be more severe at night. This occurs because there is a decrease in external stimuli such as noise, light, movements and intellectual demands. This permits pain to become the dominant sensation. Putting this finding into practical use, it is wise to carry out an examination of an injury in a relatively quiet, calm environment so that subtleties in pain can be brought to attention (immediately before swelling). It is best to get the athlete off the playing field into a quiet room.

With all pain, there are a variety of reflex actions. Most commonly muscle spasm occurs. This spasm usually involves those muscles which either cross over or control motion about an injured area. The purpose of this spasm is to splint the area—that is, immobilize the part so that further injury will not occur. We all have had the experience of turning our ankle, then hobbling around trying to avoid unnecessary motion. It is this motion which exaggerates the pain.

Also, deep, soft tissues (tendons, fascia, muscle and ligaments) usually exhibit pain when under stretch rather than when under compression. Thus, we see that spasm helps prevent stretching of tissue and thus reduces pain. However, a secondary form of pain occurs because of the splinting action of the muscle. In its attempt to prevent motion to damaged tissues, spastic muscle compresses the intramuscular blood vessels, thus reducing or cutting off blood flow. Muscle contraction increases the rate at which nutrients are used thus causing tissue ischemia or lack of oxygen to the muscle. A vicious cycle can occur in which initial injury causes pain which causes muscle spasm which causes pain which causes more spasm, etc. Pain, therefore, can perpetuate itself.

Other reflex activity can occur because of pain. The vessels surrounding a painful area can go into spasm, cutting off blood and nutrients. The result: more pain. Increased sweating can occur in a painful area. This is caused by a stimulation of the autonomic nervous system. This phenomenon can be used clinically to evaluate an injury. Compare the injured side to the non-injured side; the injured side in most cases will be moist.

These simple rules, used in a conscientious manner can be of great benefit when evaluating an injury so that the most appropriate treatment can be used.

TRAUMATIC, OVERUSE AND IMBALANCE INJURIES

We have defined injury as any disruption of tissue continuity. What causes this disruption? Basically injuries can be categorized into two types: traumatic and overuse. A third category, imbalance injury, is related very closely to overuse but involves a slightly different mechanism. All three injuries have different mechanics. They all can be equally disabling.

There is no difference in the result or amount of tissue destruction among traumatic, overuse and imbalance injuries. The location mechanism and rates of injury vary, but the results are the same.

Traumatic injuries happen to everyone, athlete or not. These are the types of injuries that are caused either by some external force

146

applied to a part, as when a football player is "clipped" at the knee, or some abnormal movement which forces a part beyond its normal range of motion, as when an ankle is "turned" when stepping off a curb. Traumatic injuries are acute in nature. That is, they occur suddenly without warning and can cause immediate disability. Because of this sudden onset, the traumatic injury is more easily diagnosed. If the victim can accurately describe the event which led to his injury, and the mechanics of the injury itself, the physician can more easily determine the possible structures affected. Finally, treatment for a traumatic injury is generally specific in nature. When the diagnosis is made, a clear-cut course of action is apparent.

This is not always true with the overuse injury. Overuse injuries occur as a result of longterm, repeated stress on a weak area of the body. The overuse syndrome may be defined as that situation where the functional demands of the sport exceed the physical ability of the individual, resulting in a stress reaction at the weakest point in the structure.

It has only been in the last few years that this entity has been identified with athletes. Before this time, training techniques were such that the athlete tended to "save" himself for the actual competitive event and thus did not push his body to the limits until this time. Training was not as strenuous or as intense as it is today. In today's athletic community, this trend has completely reversed. It is now the training prior to the event which has become the more exhausting. The athlete is forever pushing his body to its limits and beyond. He is constantly working to do more and better than the day before.

This striving to improve is not without cost. People involved in athletics generally are of the opinion that the more exercise one gets, the better conditioned one will be, and thus the more healthy will be the individual. This is only true to a point. Beyond this point there is what is called in economics negative returns on one's investment. There is a disproportion between what is required of a given tissue and what the inherent capacity of the tissue is to receive such stress. In simple terms, the athlete asks more of the body than it is capable of giving. Many authors have written about this:

For instance, Dr. Steven Subotnick, says, "All athletes have one thing in common: the better trained they are, the closer they are to being on the brink of disaster. The brink of disaster is that state between athletic excellence and athletic disaster. Too much training can lead to injury.... Overstress can lead to the symptoms of generalized fatigue and a susceptibility towards contagious diseases such as influenza and colds."

Is there any way to prevent these depressing and incapacitating events? Dr. George Sheehan answers, "Yes, one is to understand and work with GAS. The General Adaptation Syndrome is a three-pound formula of stress and its effects first outlined by Canadian physiologist Hans Selye. It is based on the common and easily observable fact that man exposed to an unaccustomed strenuous task goes through three stages: experiences a hardship, then gets used to it, and finally can't stand it any longer—or as Selye terms the sequence: (1) alarm, (2) resistance, (3) exhaustion. Translated into training, this means increasing amounts of work (Stage 1) with a resultant improvement in performance (Stage 2) but stopping before exhaustion (Stage 3). The coach and his athletes must know that peak ability means exhaustion and staleness are close at hand. The moral is simple: The next time you run out of GAS, fill up your tank with rest."

Three factors contribute to the overuse injury: (1) conditioning (2) training and (3) biomechanical structure of the lower extremity. Each of these three contributes a little to this type of injury, but in combination the results can be disastrous. Poor conditioning or trying to condition too rapidly can cause injury simply because the body is in no way prepared to take the type of punishment that an athlete can give it. It is literally a shock to his system. The "weekend athlete" has a high percentage of injuries. Improper training (that is, doing too much of one thing and not enough of another), poor dieting, not enough rest between workouts, etc., can leave the body unable to sustain this resistance and the final phase of tissue response is reached—breakdown or exhaustion. This, of course, is where injury occurs. Unable to cope with an increasing load the tissue, be it bone or soft tissue, the body finally succumbs to injury.

The main types of overuse syndrome we see in the lower

148

extremity are related to the repeated attempts by the body to neutralize abnormal forces. That is, minor structural imbalances or poor technique require repeated inefficient adjustments for balance and control. Individual structures reach their point of exhaustion. Under normal function, there is no stress, but under the longterm demands of the sport, supportive muscles become fatigued, causing increased stress on joints and bones. The lower extremity is an integral structural entity. Weakness of one part increases stress on another with inefficient compensations. Ideal training methods prepare the body to adapt to stressful situations, but most do not take into account individual structural differences.

There are three stages of overuse syndrome development which may show up anywhere in the body.

Stage I: nagging, bothersome aches and pains after workouts; rapidly reversible with biomechanical evaluation and functional control, causing no permanent disability (for example, an ache in the arch of the foot).

Stage II: pain during as well as after activity, increasing in severity over time, causing concern; slowly reversible with proper treatment and possibly causing permanent damage (knee problem which limits a basketball player from rebounding).

Stage III: pain before, during and after even moderate activity, preventing participation in sports; requires rest and specific rehabilitation, often causing more serious injury or permanent disability.

Structural (bone) imbalances are the main causes of the overuse syndrome, but functional, acquired (soft tissue) imbalances may also produce injury. This type of injury is associated very closely with the overuse injury but has a somewhat different mechanism. We talked about imbalance of structure that may be present in the individual. This imbalance is inherent, and the individual has little control over the situation.

The type of imbalance we speak of now is acquired. For example, sprinters are notorious for their pulled hamstring muscles. If we look closely at possible causes of such disabling problems, we can very easily appreciate the fact that there exists an imbalance between the muscles in the front of the thigh and those in the back of the thigh. Those in the front have a tendency to overpower those in the rear. The result is the hamstrings tend to "give way" when put under the stress of sprinting.

Why has this imbalance come about? As in many sports, certain muscles and joints are more important than other muscles and joints. Each sport requires specialized technique and develops specific muscle groups. There is a tendency to strengthen only those areas that will increase efficiency of performance in a given sport. By strengthening these, other muscles are left unattended, and can be overpowered and susceptible to injury.

The treatment for these imbalance problems is to develop both strength and flexibility. This is stressed elsewhere in the book as essential to proper conditioning. To develop strength, use isometric and isotomic contractions of the weakened muscle groups. To develop flexibility, use gradual stretching exercises on all muscles of the lower extremity. Flexibility exercises are necessary before, when the muscles are tight and inflexible, and especially after workouts when the muscles are warm and easily stretched.

ADVICE TO YOUNG ATHLETES

A few words about young athletes, especially under age 12. Competition and physical conditioning are important to their future personal and interpersonal relationships. Through sports, they can learn much about life, both good and bad. They should be encouraged to develop their full potential, but their motivation must come from within themselves, not from the pressure of "proud" parents and "winning" coaches. In an environment like this, they are afraid to report pains, injuries, or fatigue, which to many of them is a form of failure.

Children are constructed with more protective soft tissue and flexible bones and joints. When they feel pain, it is a greater injury than when an adult feels pain. Injuries to growing structures, especially the ends of long bones (epiphyses) cause permanent imbalance and disability. Youngsters must be allowed to compete in a helpful, open environment where they are at ease to report problems. While healing from injury, they should be encouraged to

150

attend all team functions. Sports competition must be a time of emotional and social, as well as physical development. They should enjoy this phase of their lives.

Proper long term conditioning will prevent injuries. Each individual must understand and respect his ability (and disability) in order to condition himself properly against injury. Each tissue of the body, throught different, reacts to stress in a similar way — there is a time of irritability, during which the tissue is "alarmed," a time of resistance, during which it is at its strongest, and a time of collapse, when it is beyond endurance. The athlete must learn to respect these feelings. In the young athlete who is unable to express these feelings, it is especially important that the coach or trainer make individual contact with the athlete, so that developing problems can be evaluated before they become serious.

Advice on self-evaluation and self treatment is dangerous for us to give. We know that early evaluation and treatment is essential to complete healing. But we also know that during training and in competition, a qualified sports professional is not always present. For that reason, many injuries go overlooked or undertreated. Pain is a signal. It is a necessary and good protective mechanism in which the body clearly tells us what is wrong. It must be respected.

12

Medical Treatment

What makes the team physician and athletic doctor so all-important in the treatment of athletic injuries? This is a question a weekend athlete might ask about the emerging sports-minded physician. One would think that schools of medicine are teaching all that is necessary in each little niche or specialty. This, as many athletes have found, is not necessarily so.

Dr. George Sheehan, medical editor of *Runner's World*, emphasizes in his writings, as we have, that injury prevention is an entirely different specialty of its own. For a doctor to fit adequately into this niche, he must be informed and have a genuine interest in his athletic patients.

This generalization has been stated before, but what does it mean? Is a good rapport with a doctor all that is necessary for a speedy recovery? A direct and closer line of communication probably does come about between athlete and athletic doctor in many instances, but this is secondary. The chief advantage a sports physician has over the regular doctor is the ability to take a meaningful and relevant history of the causative factors leading up to and following the injury itself. A doctor relies heavily on this most important aspect of the patient visit on which to rest his diagnosis. Without some direction or pattern to his questioning, the causation will often be obscured or missed completely.

As you have gathered by now, much of preventive medicine (especially that related to overuse injuries) is based on reversing the factors that cause the injury. If the factors or actions involved in a particular sports participation are not understood, reversing them is impossible.

Take the example of a quarter-miler who continually complained of achilles tendonitis. A careful history in this case reveals that the patient practices daily in training shoes with a substantial heel, but races in an ultra-light, heelless spike. This seemingly minor fact, but one which is all important in this patient's rehabilitation, was missed by the doctor who felt that overdoing it was obviously the cause. This uncertainty in treatment in most cases leads the doctor to prescribe pain medications and withdrawal from participation.

Many athletes wonder if a doctor that advises cutting back from participation is uninformed in sports medicine or in their particular sport? The answer is simply, no. By reading recent articles, you may get the impression that there is an ideal solution to the most injuries and that it is never necessary to take a layoff. But many injuries, especially acute injuries from contact sports, require rest in order to heal and prevent future disability. Other injuries require an easing off merely for diagnostic purposes. The doctor must know what effect a change in routine has on certain obscure injury patterns.

So, again, we state that layoffs from injuries are sometimes necessary and this period of convalescense must be as closely adhered to as a strict training schedule. The athlete must rely on his doctor and follow his instructions to the best of his understanding to ensure the quickest recovery. We often recommend a change in conditioning activity in order to promote healing. That is, if there is a stress fracture in one of the metatarsal bones in a runner, he may substitute cycling, swimming or some other aerobic activity which permits him to stay in shape without trauma to the injured part.

Another common point pondered by athletes is the advantage, if any, of seeking a doctor who actively participates in their particular sporting event. This would be the ideal situation, but such doctors are often hard to find. Dr. George Sheehan quotes Mark Twain as saying, "Anyone who has had a bull by the tail knows five or six things more than someone who hasn't." In other words, a doctor with personal experience has a great advantage.

This set of circumstances, though, is far from mandatory in seeking professional advice or treatment. Usually, look for a doctor who has been involved in some type of sports participation, but many doctors learn other aspects of treatment know-how by keeping up with journals, magazines and in active participation in sports clubs or services as a professional. Doctors, believe it or not, also learn a great deal from their patients.

Sports are often categorized in groups as to their likelihood in causing particular injuries. Being knowledgeable about football injuries, for example, gives the doctor an added advantage when treating a field hockey or lacrosse player. All are contact sports, involve fast running, are played on a similar running surface and require similar shoe gear. This is an example of how the doctor capitalizes on what sports knowledge he has to treat different but similar sports injuries in a competent manner. However, the doctor, in treating injuries from many sports, must realize that treatment and rehabilitation must be specific and directed at that sport only. Having tennis elbow might prevent further participation for a tennis player, but if he was a lineman on a football team he would probably get by with little or no impairment.

One of the biggest questions that affects all athletes and athletic staffs is the problem of differentiation between a mild injury and an injury that requires medical attention. There are several different ways in which to solve this treatment dilemma. The method of resolution, however, is somewhat different when considering a recreational athlete as opposed to an athlete competing on a team or with an organized group.

Let's first consider a daily jogger, as an example, who jogs for enjoyment and betterment of health. One morning, Joe Jogger notices he has a vague ache in one leg. The ache or pain at first is barely noticeable, but in three days Joe finds that even when he is not running there is pain occurring with every step. What will Joe's steps of action most likely be in solving this problem?

Being new at the sport and having had little interaction with other joggers, Joe seeks medical attention at once. Let's now consider some alternatives which Joe might have taken in solving his problem. He might have stopped his running and waited until the pain diminished.

One of the most common first steps an athlete will take in solving an unknown injury is to question fellow athletes to see if this pain is common and what they have done in the past to resolve it. Due to man's nature, this is not surprising, and is often quite valuable in providing many opinions to arrive at a solution. So this action we might call peer advice. If friends speak with confidence, you usually take the most logical advice and plan a self-treatment regimen for yourself that you hope will solve your problem. However, this method may carry a variable risk for a number of reasons.

First, pain seldom feels the same to everyone, and your interpretation of the problem may be different. A common example might be Sam the soccer player who turns his ankle. A friend who had experienced a minor sprain in the past tells Sam that he unfortunately had gone to a doctor who had only put on an Ace wrap and advised taking it easy for a few days. Sam had heard of applying ice to injuries so he goes home, puts an ice bag on his ankle and waits until the next day for his friend to bring him the Ace wrap. Sam goes on for weeks with moderate discomfort and finds months later he has yet to gain the stability and maneuvering power he once had prior to his injury. In this case, Sam obviously had a more serious ankle sprain than his friend and did indeed need medical care that could have allowed him a better future in sports.

How does a lone athlete tell when he should seek medical attention for his injuries? The best method is to get a basic understanding about injury processes and what first aid treatment affords the best recovery. It is, after all, ultimately your decision as to when an injury needs medical attention, so your decision should be made with sound logic. This diagnostic process has been explained in Chapter 11.

The team athlete requires a different approach in medical treatment. A chain of command usually exists by which the athlete is logically screened at time of injury by the coach and trainer to determine the severity of the injury. If the injury is chronic in nature with no acute onset, the athlete usually consults the trainer for advice and treatment.

This chain of command, however, varies greatly depending on

the level of sports competition. High school teams seldom have the benefit of a trainer to coordinate treatment and rehabilitation. Therefore, in high school a much greater responsibility lies on the coach for his unbiased decisions in regard to the "playability" of his athletes. A decision to continue an injured athlete's participation or to allow an over anxious athlete to persuade the coach to allow his continued play can be dangerous. Some basic medical knowledge, common sense and experience are necessary for safer sports programs.

The trainer's responsibility in treating and screening injuries is greater than the coaches. This is part of the trainer's job. He is usually familiar with the athlete's history of injury (or should be), which makes diagnosis and treatment more fluid. A trainer should be a reliable liaison between the doctor or team physician and the athlete. He should record significant injuries of all athletes to facilitate optimum care by the doctor. Trainers should be able to recognize the seriousness of most injuries and be capable of providing first aid until more extensive treatment can be rendered. The optimal condition for athletic treatment is for the team physician to be present at the time of injury for rapid diagnosis and necessary care, or in the case of overuse injuries to be consulted as soon as possible. Coaches and trainers cannot be expected to possess the knowledge of a professional who is trained in medical treatment. It is for this reason that when judgment must be passed by a lay person regarding the continued participation of an athlete, the decision should always side toward conservatism.

MAKING THE DIAGNOSIS

Many of the injuries that occur during sporting events can be adequately diagnosed by the athlete himself. Working with his diagnosis or hunch as to the factors causing the injury, the athlete can then begin a program of rehabilitation specific for that injury and work at preventing future recurrences. We have shown how to assess such injuries and determine their severity. That is the difficult part. Once we have an accurate diagnosis, the treatment plan is clear. We must identify those injuries that require professional attention and those that do not. Identifying this "gray zone" is vital in preventing chronic injuries.

156

Before treatment, take a personal inventory: Keep a clear head, be logical. Write these things down:

1. What factors might have contributed to this disease or injury?

2. Where does it hurt? Identify the boundaries of pain and point to them. Any anatomical "landmarks"?

3. When did it start? Weeks, months, years?

4. How did it happen—suddenly or slowly?

5. Has it changed? Injuries recover in phases; to identify the present phase will affect the way you treat it. For example, you wouldn't put ice on an ankle sprain that happened two months ago.

6. Has the pain been growing worse or is it getting better? To know the progression of pain will give clues to what types of injury you are dealing with. Overuse injuries, for example, usually start with a minor amount of pain and progress with continued use. If the pain is decreasing, the injury may be recovering or healing as you may be "over the hump."

7. Did the injury happen after extreme fatigue?

8. Were you adequately warmed up?

9. Was there any incidence of trauma?

10. Were you hit or did you run into something?

11. Did you trip or stumble?

12. Were you in good shape?

13. Were you using defective equipment or shoes?

Remembering what happened just prior to the injury and re-creating the incident in your mind will clarify the type of injury. For example, if a basketball player jumps at a basket and turns his foot in on landing, he has likely sprained or ruptured the ligaments on the outside of his ankle. Had he heard a snap he may have completely ruptured a ligament or broken a bone.

Now consider any injuries or conditions prior to your current complaint that may have been contributory. Do you have any hereditary abnormalities that you are aware of? Have you had any athletic injuries before this one and how long before did they occur? Any hereditary structural or functional impairment may put undue stress on a vulnerable part of the anatomy. Previous injuries often set off a chain of future injuries. The initial injury may cause you to favor the other leg, therefore putting additional stress on that side. The period of injury rehabilitation, when muscles are weak from disuse, accounts for many secondary injuries.

To recap the previous paragraphs, we see that the history is broken down into relevant questions that provide information on the nature of the injury. Three basic words, what, how and why should all be answered if possible. The why, as you will see in the upcoming pages, is usually the most difficult component to arrive at and without this question answered prevention is hit or miss.

APPROACHING THE DIAGNOSIS

Having taken a good history of the complaint, a physician uses many additional tests and principles in evaluating an injury to arrive at a presumptive diagnosis. Some of these methods of evaluating injuries that have lead to your diagnosis are interpretation of pain, correlation between tissue involvement and anatomical location, and physical tests performed on the body to quantify the degree of impairment.

These tests, however, are by no means all inclusive, for inaccurate interpretation may lead to false security and a serious aggravation of the injury. These have been general guidelines. A physician in an office, hospital or emergency room has many other tests available to him, including x-rays, thermograms, arthrograms, xerographs, blood and urine tests, etc. Used carefully and logically, the guidelines on interpretation will lead to a working diagnosis, which leads to the treatment plan.

TREATMENT PLAN FOR FOOT AND LEG INJURIES

Anatomically, the foot includes all those structures up to and including the ankle joint, the leg is that area between the ankle joint and the knee joint, and the thigh is that area between the knee joint and the hip joint. There is an integral functional relationship between these structures both from the foot up to the low-back area, and from the low back area down to the foot. Acute traumatic tissue injuries require the same treatment plan at

158

whatever level they occur. Overuse and imbalance injuries must be considered with respect for the relationship of one part to the other.

We talk about treatment for major types of tissue injury as well as the structural and functional relationships of one part to the other. The main tissues involved in the lower extremity are the integment (skin and nails), the soft tissues, (muscles, tendons, nerves, ligaments, fat and blood vessels), and the skeleton, (bones and bone covering). This discussion give special attention to treatment of the foot. We then review the areas of injury above the foot related to structural and functional overuse, stress and imbalance injuries. A detailed treatment plan for structures above the foot is beyond the scope of this text.

In this part of the book, we present methods of self treatment for injuries. The specific treatment is precluded by essential signs and symptoms which aid in your selection of the proper treatment. Professional treatments for more serious ailments are presented, although essential signs and symptoms will be included. This approach is intended to allow for a better appreciation of the spectrum of injury without belaboring professional treatment which is beyond the scope of this book. It will be helpful to refer to the Appendix on "over the counter" treatments when considering what to do.

REGIONAL VS. SYSTEMIC APPROACH

There is an ongoing controversy in medical schools as to how to teach anatomy, by regions of the body or by organ systems. If it is taught by regions, the students get a complete understanding of the physiology, or functional relationship of all the various structures and tissues to each other in a given area of the body (foot, ankle, knee, etc.) If it is taught by systems, the student understands the total body function of that system (circulatory system, nervous system, etc.) but finds it difficult to relate these systems to each other on a local anatomical level.

For these reasons, and for the understanding of vital relationships, in most general medical schools, the courses are taught with an emphasis on a systemic basis, and in specialty schools such as podiatric medicine and dentistry, the courses are taught on a regional basis. Interestingly, as general physicians specialize in specific areas (post-graduate internships and residencies), their study procedures are on a regional basis (orthopedics, dermatology, peripheral, vascular disease, etc.), and advanced post-graduate training in the specialty professions such as podiatric medicine will include general hospital experience.

The foot is a specialized regional area that has a direct anatomical and functional relationship with most systems, including bones, ligaments, muscles, tendons, nerves, blood vessels, skin and so forth. We have decided to give a review of the general treatment of organ "systems" in the foot, and in succeeding chapters, to present the treatment of common regional problems extending throughout the lower extremity.

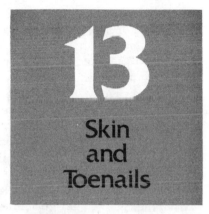

Skin and Toenails

Every athlete is sooner or later confronted with a skin or nail abnormality. It is for this very reason that we put particular emphasis on skin and nail deformities in this section. These ailments are usually easy to differentiate and, barring any complicating circumstances, should respond to basic first aid or self-treatment. If progressing conditions are ignored, however, infection can result and turn a minor condition into a serious incapacitating problem.

LACERATIONS

The severity of a laceration or cut must be evaluated to determine if medical care (usually cleansing and suturing) is necessary. The basic issue to be concerned with is in determining the depth of the injury and if any underlying structures have been disrupted or severed.

A proper evaluation of the wound cannot be carried out until the bleeding has slowed or stopped and the area is cleansed. Direct pressure with a sterile gauze or clean towel will allow for clotting of the small vessels and will slow bleeding. Usually, about two minutes of compression should signficantly slow the blood flow. It is important to use direct pressure and not "blotting" action. If blood continues to pour from the wound, medical attention should be sought. Keep applying moderate pressure.

If you wish to take on the responsibility of treatment, place the injury under cold, running tap water. While immersed in water,

161

lightly but thoroughly scrub the area with a sterile gauze or clean towel using ordinary soap. Hydrogen peroxide (3%), if available, is also very good for irrigation. (Note: 6% hydrogen peroxide is used to "lighten" hair and is too strong to use on the skin.) The depths of the wound must be cleansed, as minute unseen particles or foreign bodies may be trapped within the injured tissue. This irrigating process is often quite uncomfortable, but is necessary for even the cleanest injury has the potential to cause infection. If the interior of the wound cannot be exposed and cleansed, medical help should be sought. It is possible to get tetanus ("lockjaw") if infection is trapped deep.

Once the area is cleansed, look at the wound. If the skin edges are gaping, you should go immediately to your doctor or nearby emergency room for evaluation. A gaping wound usually means the injury has penetrated through the skin and has entered the fatty tissue. Next, make sure you have full function of all parts far from (distal to) the injury and have no numbness distal to the injury. Squeeze the edges together to make sure the skin will approximate well. If a small piece of skin was avulsed or gouged out at the time of injury, the healing process will have to fill this area in. If the edges of the wound will not come together, there is a good chance of having a scar or deep adhesion.

Apply a generous sterile bandage that will keep the injury dry and free from contaminants. Apply the bandage from side to side so that the tension helps hold the wound together. A minor laceration should heal sufficiently in 4-5 days to allow bathing of the part. Complications may arise if the location of injury is near an area of flexion or at a joint level. In this case, normal movement will continue to open the wound and prolong healing, so it may be necessary to immobilize or "splint" the area. If you have any doubts about the severity of the injury, contact your physician immediately.

FOREIGN BODIES

Foreign bodies in the skin, such as slivers, splinters and sand, should first be cleansed, then removed with a sterile instrument. If a deep foreign body is suspected, such as broken glass or a needle, it must be removed professionally.

ABRASIONS

The abrasion occurs secondary to some traumatic force occurring nearly horizontal to the skin surface. The resistance of the surface exceeds the elasticity of the skin. The abrasive nature of this injury is most likely to be seen in a sport where sliding occurs, either intentionally as in baseball or unintentionally as in ice skating or basketball.

Treatment for an abrasion is similar to that of a burn, since a sizeable portion of raw skin in both cases is exposed to the air and can easily become infected. As with the laceration, cleansing is vitally important to remove all foreign particles. Light scrubbing may cause marked pain since a larger portion of skin is exposed, but the bits of dirt and gravel that are frequently embedded in the abrasion must be removed to prevent infection. It helps to do this under cool, running water.

Evaluation of the cleansed wound should reveal only partial loss of the skin layer. If the base does not appear "skin like" the injury is in need of medical care. Sterile bandages should be applied along with a first aid ointment to protect the wound. The bandages should exceed the borders of the injury and be kept dry. Athletic participation is allowable as long as the dressing is reapplied after bathing and no infection is present. Padding should be applied around the injury for protection if reinjury is possible.

BLISTERS

Blisters, undoubtedly the most common of all foot problems, are the separation of layers of epidermis (the superficial layers of the skin) one from another. When the separation occurs, fluid in the area fills the empty space created. This may be blood or a clear serous fluid. The separation of layers occurs because of friction, either linear or twisting, of skin tightly adhered to underlying structures. The two most common causes of blisters to which we direct our treatment approach are improper shoe gear and mechanical disturbances of the feet. Whatever the causative factor, the process of blister formation is that of friction producing epidermal "fatigue" and overuse.

The formation of a blister on the foot begins as a "hot spot" or area of burning, usually on the bottom of the foot or where it contacts with the shoe. If the athlete is not engaged in competition, this is the time to stop and remedy the situation. If the blister has ruptured, pain may be due to raw, tender, immature skin beneath. Take your shoes off, determine the cause of the discomfort and use the appropriate preventive measures as they are described in the following paragraphs.

If the blister has already formed, prompt first aid will hasten an early recovery. Cleanse the blistered areas with alcohol or soap and water, and gently apply pressure on the top of the blister so that the fluid will disperse to the sides. If it is small (less than one-half inch) and there is no pain, leave it alone. But if it is larger or painful or if there is deep bleeding, carefully penetrate the side of the blister with a sterile needle and remove the fluid with continued pressure. The fluid removal will greatly decrease the level of pain. Leave the overlying skin intact. An antiseptic solution or first aid cream can be applied over the entire blister. Apply a bandage or accommodative pad to prevent further irritation. If left intact, the blister should be covered and protected with a bandaid, or it will break and become contaminated.

Blood blisters should be handled in a similar manner, but with greater care than the normal blister filled with serous fluid. Small capillaries have been damaged, causing blood accumulation in the blistered space. A blood blister usually signifies a more traumatic or deeper level of irritation and a greater risk of infection. Again, apply a sterile bandage, accommodate the area with padding for protection, and continue sports participation if the level of pain permits.

In both of these cases, the top layer of skin over the blister will become hardened in a few days. At this time, the bandage may be removed, but continue to leave the dead skin over the blister to provide continued protection for the underlying skin. If there is any infection, the dead skin must be removed.

To prevent blisters, first look to your shoes. If blisters are on the sides or tops of your toes your shoes are either too small in the forefoot or at foot impact your foot is jamming into the toebox of the shoe. For blisters on the bottom of your feet, we recommend that athletes use a cushioning material such as a Spenco insole to absorb friction and shear.

Socks must fit properly. Poorly fitting socks may roll up in wet weather or during vigorous participation. To absorb the maximum amount of perspiration (perspiration increases friction and the likelihood of blister formation), socks should contain natural fabrics like cotton or a blend of cotton and wool. Avoid the "stretch" or tube-type socks. Foot powders also are helpful in decreasing the amount of foot perspiration.

Many runners prefer to go without socks, stating that by eliminating socks you are eliminating a primary causative factor in blister formation. If it works for you, do it. If running without socks, we recommend buying properly fitted shoes with nylon uppers and inserting Spenco insoles. It's usually a good idea to break in new shoes with socks for the first few times and then go without after that time if you prefer.

Many runners use Vaseline to reduce shoe friction. Dr. John Pagliano, podiatrist and marathoner, recommends applying a liberal amount of Vaseline—about a half handful to each foot prior to a long-distance race. He follows this with a comfortable cotton sock and a nylon-top running shoe. He states the Vaseline oozes through the sock and into the nylon to provide a friction-free running base.

If you know your feet well enough to anticipate where you will get blisters (for example, under the big toe is a common location in basketball players), you may wish to put a thin "moleskin" pad or adhesive tape over this area. This method provides another protective barrier between the skin and the shoe.

If your shoes are too narrow for your feet and are causing blisters on your little toes, we recommend buying a brand that offer variable widths. Until that time, you can protect your toes from excessive friction by applying a bandaid or athletic tape over the area. Remove the bandaids between workouts to allow the skin to breathe. If you have buckled (hammer) toes that make blisters inevitable, buy the best accommodating shoe you can find and tape your toes as stated above.

Often, blisters will form under calluses on the foot. Calluses build under areas of stress and irritation. If not treated, a large keratinized plaque forms and gives rise to deeper irritation, which becomes a fluid-filled blister. Again, this can be treated by lancing

165

the blister under sterile conditions. The callus itself should be kept trimmed and smooth. A pumice stone or callus file comes in handy for this. Don't attempt to cut the skin with a razor blade.

If you have tried these blister remedies and find you cannot decrease them, you should consult your podiatrist. This is especially true of blisters occurring on the bottom of the feet. The most common cause of these blisters are mechanical foot imbalances. Most structural or functional deviations stated in previous chapters are those which require abnormal pronation or flattening of the foot to allow for a full foot strike. This causes extra twisting and friction in the skin, and results in blisters and calluses. Orthotic devices are usually corrective. In the case of hammertoes, they usually can be corrected.

INFECTIONS

Infections of the skin may be caused by bacteria, fungus or virus penetration. They may come from the external surface or internal environment. If you have a skin injury from a dirty object or material, or if you have an ongoing infection in your system, such as acne, gum infections or bladder infections, then you are very likely to get an infected wound.

The first and most important treatment is to keep the wound clean, so that it can heal from the bottom up, and not from the top over. If there is pus, drainage, throbbing or red lines (lymphangitis) extending away from the injury, seek medical attention immediately. Any area that has been bleeding and open to the air is likely to become infected. After an injury, it is a good idea to take your temperature daily. Elevated temperature is one of the first signs of infection. This is true for deep injuries as well as skin problems.

CORNS AND CALLUSES

Corns and calluses are local accumulations of keratin or thickened skin in reaction to stress. For clarification, we refer to a corn as occurring on the toes and a callus as occurring on the bottom of the foot, but they are actually the same type of tissue. Corns are usually deeper and show a focal point of pressure. Hard corns are on the tops of toes and at exposed areas.

Calluses and corns occur secondary to the same forces that

cause blisters: those of friction and shear. Superficial (shallow) calluses are very common to the active athlete, and show that the skin has adapted to the increased load and friction placed upon it. It is when skin can no longer tolerate the forces put upon it that the blister forms. The skin of a callus will feel thickened, skin lines will appear exaggerated, and the color will be toward a yellowish hue.

This skin, if not bothersome, can be left alone. A small amount of callus is protective and good, but as it thickens, it impedes circulation, causing a burning sensation. If a slight burning pain exists, use a callus file or pumice stone after bathing to reduce this tissue.

Shearing calluses and corns are a much greater nuisance. They are caused from shear and not just friction. In other words, the skin is stable as the bone moves during activity. The pain from calluses and corns can be sufficient enough to cause a limp or abnormal weight distribution to favor the painful area. This may result in a secondary injury far removed from but directly related to the solitary callus or corn. Early treatment is recommended to avoid this sequence of events.

The shearing callus may look similar to the shallow type but is deeper, and close examination may show a plug or nucleus within which is very much like a corn. It is this hard plug that compresses the surrounding nerves to cause the pain. To temporarily relieve the pressure, the corn must be carefully trimmed down with a sharp instrument and the core removed. We discourage the use of corn plasters for these preparations contain acids which may burn the surrounding normal tissue. The use of corn pads or aperture-type accommodative pads to redistribute the weight and pressure may relieve pain significantly. Pads, if used, must not be placed directly over the corn, for this will only increase the pressure and pain. They must be placed around and behind the lesion. Soft corns may be helped by foam or felt separators.

The cause of corns and calluses are similar to the cause of the blister: pressure and friction. Consider the shoes, first making sure they are the proper size and width. Look for irregularities in the shoe that may be causing abnormal pressure points. If one pair of shoes is the problem, get rid of them.

Most corns on the top of the foot are due to contracted or hammered digits. The contraction, which is the result of a long-standing structural or muscular imbalance, makes the top of the toe more prominent and subject to pressure. With corns, a minor surgical correction is sometimes necessary to straighten the toes in order to provide a permanent relief.

Calluses usually build up on the bottom of the foot under the metatarsal heads. Special types of "pinch" calluses build up where the upper meets the lower of the shoe.

If painful, recurrent calluses are present, medical attention should be sought to determine if the callused tissue is due to a mechanical imbalance. If this is the case, orthoses are helpful in redistributing the weight pattern. Plantar calluses may also be caused by the abnormal position of only one bone in relation to the others. We find that a metatarsal bone can be abnormally depressed, therefore taking a greater than normal amount of stress with each step. A surgical movement in the bone to elevate it is usually curative, or the area can be protected from pressure with a custom orthotic inside the shoe.

WARTS

Warts (verrucae) are caused by a virus infection and are often mistaken as corns or calluses. On close examination, they are very different. Warts on the top of the foot (verruca vulgaris—"common warts") grow like a cauliflower on the surface and are clearly diagnosed, but warts on the bottom of the foot (verruca plantaris—"plantar warts") penetrate deep under the skin like a mushroom because of pressure in standing. (Note: The term "plantar" wart has nothing to do with farmers. The bottom of the foot, or sole, is called the plantar surface.)

Warts may or may not be on pressure and friction areas like corns and calluses, and warts have a very clearly defined border. Unlike corns and calluses, the center encapsulated area usually has dark brown, black or rust-colored sports because the wart has small blood vessels and nerves. For this reason warts are more painful with lateral (side-to-side, pinching) pressure than with direct pressure on top.

Warts are contagious to susceptible people and are usually

found in adolescents. They may be single or multiple (the latter are called "mosaic" warts.) There are many different treatments for warts, some available over the counter. Warts tend to spread and multiply if not treated. They do not respond to mechanical treatment but often respond to chemical treatment or need to be removed professionally. If you are not sure if you have a callus or wart, and it's not going away, see a doctor.

BRUISES OR CONTUSIONS

Bruises occur most frequently in contact sports and are caused by direct blow to the tissues. The injury is usually seen with a crushing- or compression-type injury which causes rupture of the small blood vessels in the area of trauma.

In the evaluation of contusions, two important diagnostic points must be kept in mind: (1) the appearance of the contusion does not necessarily reflect the severity of the injury but rather the vascularity of the area injured; (2) the contusion may not be the only injury sustained; deeper tissue damage may be co-existent.

In treating a moderate-sized contusion, allow 48 hours of ICE compression and elevation. Ice constricts the damaged blood vessels and retards further accumulations of blood and serum. Heating pads and hot packs should not be used during this stage of injury. Compression by means of an overlying pad, held in place by an Ace wrap or an elastic wrap, dimishes swelling. Blood from damaged vessels will flow to the area of least resistence or pressure; by increasing the external pressure, you impede the formation of the bruise or if more severe the hematoma (discussed next). Elevation reduces the pressure within the damaged vessels so clotting will occur faster and blood will have a reduced tendency of escaping into the tissues.

In treating a moderately sized contusion, allow 48 hours of ICE treatment off and on. After that time, the contusion should be well organized and the blood well clotted around the damaged vessels. If any lump or loss of function remains, or if there is any doubt, see a physician. Resolution of the contusion and restoration of the injured part to full function is now of paramount importance.

A large contusion or hematoma left untreated can transform

into scar tissue or calcify, which results in chronic pain and limited function of the adjacent muscle. Warm compresses at this point are helpful in order to dilate the vessels and clean up the localized blood. Stretching exercises should be performed to tolerance at first, and after a suitable range of motion is gained, full athletic participation is allowable. We suggest that a protective bandage be wrapped around the contusion to protect it from damage and maintain moderate continued pressure over the area. As the color of the bruise begins to fade and pain disappears, treatment may be discontinued.

HEMATOMA

A hematoma is a severe contusion that results from marked bleeding into adjacent tissues. On the skin, it may take the form of a blood blister, but deeper in muscle or bone it becomes serious. The pressure by which the blood flows from the damaged vessels is greater, therefore creating a larger accumulation of blood. The hematoma can occur at any tissue depth, and if near the surface of the skin can often be seen and felt as a lump. The blood from a hematoma often gravitates farther down the leg. It is common to see bruising around the achilles tendon when the impact occurred at midcalf onto the toes when the injury was at the ankle.

Hematomas are initially associated with only minor pain, but after the blood is organized a marked inflammatory response sets forth that causes considerable discomfort. This painful stage usually resolves in about three days. Hematomas must be treated vigorously to prevent the complications mentioned for contusions. If the size and mass of the hematoma have not diminished markedly in two days, medical care should be sought. Drainage of the hematoma with a needle, followed by pressure dressings, is sometimes necessary. We recommend seeing an appropriate physician for any hematoma that has readily definable borders on touch or has an egg-type feeling to it.

BONE BRUISE

Bone bruises are caused by direct trauma to bones resulting in inflammation of the bony covering. The most common location for this injury is the heel bone, where it occurs most frequently in the field event athletes who wear track spikes with no cushioning under the heel. The pain is deep, and continued pounding on the heel causes severe pain as the heel is well supplied with nerve endings. Swelling may be minimal or absent.

Bone bruises should be treated with the ICE regimen to reduce the inflammatory process. Residual pain may last for up to a few months and may hamper participation. Padding should be inserted into the heels of the track spike as well as all other shoes. Plastic heel cups are available that will redistribute the weight under the heel. We recommend buying track spikes with slightly elevated midsoles and heels, and using cushioned insoles. This reduces the impact while running and jumping and also plays less havoc with the achilles tendon that has become accustomed to shoes with heels.

ATHLETE'S FOOT

Athletes foot or fungus infections are a familiar companion to most athletes at some time in their lives. The symptoms of fungus infections may vary markedly, depending on the state and type of infection, but characteristically they cause a burning or itching sensation which is made worse by scratching. The most common areas of fungus involvement are the bottom and sides of the feet (particularly the inside arch) the spaces between the toes (particularly between the third, fourth and fifth toes) and the toenails. The appearance is usually that of minor scaling and redness with occasional small vesicles or blisters.

Various types of fungi cause athlete's foot, and some have a "yeasty" odor. On more vigorous and acute stages the infection may present as weeping and inflammed areas with a greater number of vesicles (blisters) seen. The vesicles are easily popped and spread by scratching. Fungus between the toes usually appears as a moist, white tissue with some fissuring. Fungus nails will appear abnormally thickened and flaky with discolorations of the nail ranging from yellow to brown. They make the nail opaque where it is usually transparent.

In evaluating a possible fungal infection, remember that athletes foot seldom will occur on the top of the foot and toes. If this is the case, consider seeing a podiatrist for a more thorough evaluation.

171

Athlete's foot is transmitted by direct contact with the fungus, but some prior injury to the skin is usually necessary for a clinical infection to present. Even more important is host susceptibility. Some patients will contract the infection with miminal exposure, while others seem to have an immunity against the fungus. To prevent the infection, it is essential to keep the feet clean and dry, and to use powder after using public showers.

Diagnosis is often difficult, as other skin disorders may have a similar appearance. Specific treatment depends on the location and severity of involvement. There are many solutions, creams and powders available without a prescription. If there is no improvement in one week, see a doctor.

Treatment of the acutely inflammed fungal infection is best reserved for the podiatrist who can do special tests to clarify the diagnosis. If not cared for properly, these weeping lesions can become infected with bacteria, presenting serious medical problems. Fortunately, for athletes this is not seen often. Self-treatment for the more common chronic scaling and itchy lesion best lies in the condition's prevention, as results of treatment are only fair and recurrences are frequent.

If vesicles and minor inflammation are present, mild acid soaks may be beneficial. We recommend using boric acid powder (one teaspoon to one quart of cool water) or Burow's solution (one tablet to one quart of cool water). This treatment is effective in changing the semi-acute stage into the scaly stage. After the fungus is "dry," use athlete's foot medications available in the drug store. Keep the feet as dry as possible, since fungus thrives in moist environments. This is accomplished by using foot powders, and wearing cotton socks and shoes that breathe. Change socks twice daily if possible.

Results from treatment of fungus nails are poor. Fungus nails are not bothersome but are cosmetically unappealing and may spread to involve all the toenails. If partial involvement is noticed at the sides or end of the nail, keep the nail well trimmed and apply anti-fungal solution daily. With this regimen, it is hoped that the new nail will grow out without the fungus. If the nail is involved all the way to the base, it is sometimes necessary to remove the loose toenail. A prescription oral medication is avail-

172

able for fungus infection of the skin and nails. It is quite effective for skin, but takes nearly a year of use for results in nail infections and recurrences are possible.

Many measures help prevent athlete's foot, and most are centered around good foot hygiene. The two most important measures to remember are to keep your feet as dry as possible and to wear shoes that allow for ventilation. Feet should be dried thoroughly after bathing, and a foot powder should be used routinely. When using powder, treat the shoes as well as the feet, to decrease the chance of re-infection. Synthetic or nylon socks should be avoided. Athletes should wear socks in training shoes (if currently not doing so) and continue wearing them until the infection is cleared. Training without the use of socks can predispose one toward athlete's foot. If possible, wear thongs when using public bathing facilities.

TOENAILS

Normally, toenails are flat plates that sit on top of the toe and protect the sensitive nerve endings from pressure. The original functions of toenails, millions of years ago, were scratching for food, scaling trees and defense. Now they are trapped under constrictive shoes and stretch socks, and forced to function on hard, flat surfaces.

Toenails grow from the nail bed in straight lines. Any injury to the nail bed causes loss or distortion on the nail plate. If the nail is broken or trimmed in the corners, the flesh fills in so that as the new nail grows it goes into the flesh, causing a recurrent pain and pressure cycle. At the first sign of an ingrown nail, it is a good idea to put clean cotton packing under the nail to allow normal growth without pressure.

The vast majority of toenail injuries and ailments involve the big toe exclusively. The big nail is the most prominent one and therefore subject to the greatest amount of extrinsic forces. Forces related to ambulation and shoe pressure can create changes in the nail itself, the skin surrounding the nail or the bone directly beneath the nail. Most athletic nail injuries are caused from the hard nature of the nail embedded or pounding against the surrounding tissues. Most athletic shoes are made over a tapered last, where

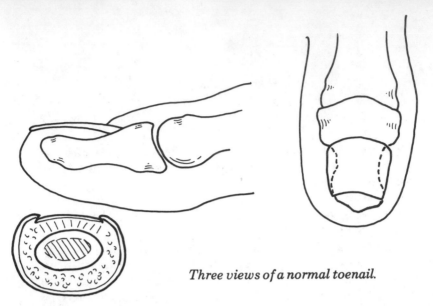

Three views of a normal toenail.

the first toe is assumed to be shorter than the second toe, but this is not always the case.

The ingrown toenail is caused by the sides of the nail embedding into the skin margins surrounding the nail plate. When the nail embeds into the skin, pressure directed at the side of the toe, either for diagnostic purposes or inside the shoe, causes great discomfort. The involved skin may be only tender, but it is often red and swollen. If allowed to continue, the ingrown nail will cause the tissue to puff up on the side in response to the nail acting as a "foreign body." Small corns may form under parts of the nail or within the ingrown border. The corn is a result of continued nail pressure. It is the body's attempt to relieve pressure, but actually causes a greater amount of pain and pressure in the involved area. Unless infected, ingrown nails seldom cause disability, but the chronic pain associated with each step makes the situation unbearable.

Treatment of the ingrown nail involves relieving the pressure or removing the offending border of the nail. This should be done with a steady hand and a pair of nail forceps. The angle at which the involved side is trimmed is critical. Keep the forceps in line with the long axis of the big toe to avoid creating nail spicules that will regrow to produce the same ingrown nail. Nail reduction is often quite painful when unfamiliar with the proper technique. Try not to cause bleeding, which usually produces infection. Pain may be due to pressure under the nail, and not the nail itself. If pain is not diminished 24 hours afer nail trimming podiatric care should be sought. Until the offending nail border is removed, no amount of soaking or medication is going to relieve the pain.

174

Everyone should practice the measures listed to avoid ingrown toe nails:

1. Keep the nails clean. Use a brush, forward and backward to keep the cuticle back and free of irritants.

2. Always trim the toe nails straight across. This helps keep the nail growing out straight.

3. Wear shoes that are the proper width and length. Excessive shoe pressure tends to push the adjacent skin toward the nail, making ingrown nail problems more frequent.

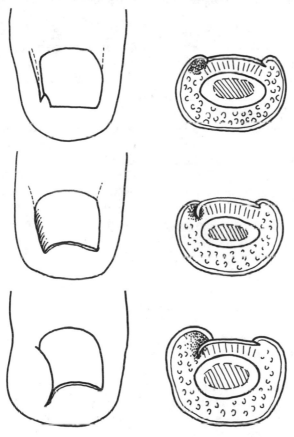

Three stages of an ingrown toenail.

If self-treatment provides only temporary relief and ingrown nails are a recurring problem the offending border of the nail should be permanently removed by your podiatrist. This procedure causes limited disability and minimal discomfort.

"Tennis toe" is any disfigurement of a big toe nail resulting from a jamming process into the end of the shoe. Tennis toe received its name because tennis players are particularly prone to this ailment due to the quick stops involved in the game. Long-distance runners also suffer with this problem more often than they should. In the runner's case, short shoes are more frequently the cause.

Tennis toe is hard to mistake from anything else. The combination of appropriate history and an obnoxious-looking toe nail is enough. The nail is usually lifted up at the end and without treatment will eventually pop off entirely. Under the nail are deposits of dried blood, usually black, blue-black, brownish in color. There may be signs of old blisters around the end of the involved toe. Tennis toe frequently involves the second toe in addition to the first or solely by itself. Athletes with a Morton's-type foot or long second toe are particularly vulnerable to this variance in pathology. Treatment is exactly the same as for the big toe.

Primary treatment for tennis toe is to cut the nail back to the point at which it is lifting from the nail bed. This prevents the lifted nail from acting as a fulcrum when shoe pressure exists and loosening the entire nail.

The most important care is prevention. Check to make sure the shoes are of proper length. If they are short, they should be discarded at once. Often, especially in tennis, the shoe is the correct size. The problem here occurs when the foot is planted on the ground and the foot slides into the end of the shoe. To prevent this, make sure the laces are snug. If the shoe is laced as tight as it can be and still feels loose because of a low instep, put some felt or foam underneath the tongue of the shoe to take up additional space. We also recommend using two small shoe laces for each shoe. Lace the first one up about four eyes and tie it, then lace the other to the top. This provides extra tension on the laces over the forefoot where it is needed. Wear properly fitted cotton socks that will provide some cushioning if the toe does hit the end of the shoe. Trim the nails straight across and short enough so shoe pressure won't pry the nail off.

Subungual hematoma is the accumulation of blood beneath the big toenail, resulting from direct trauma if something smashes the content within the skin through the use of topical creams. If fissuring is involved, the callused area must be eliminated before most creams are effective. Creams are characteristically water soluble and rub well into the skin. Lotions may also be used, although creams have a greater moisturizing effect. Ointments should not be used for dry skin, as they are occlusive and do not penetrate. There are many brands of skin cream on the market today, some of which have special additives that make them more effective. Most skin creams, regardless of brand, should be applied toe nail or from continued jamming as in basketball or with tennis toe. The pressure from the blood makes the involved toe particularly painful, especially the first 24 hours after the injury.

Two methods of treatment exist. One is to ignore it, if it is not too bothersome. If no treatment is rendered, however, the blood will discolor the nail for about a year. Treatment is relatively simple if done within the first 48 hours. Clean the toe and toenail with alcohol. Have a steady-handed friend get a paper clip and straighten one end out. Place the clip over a hot flame and get the clip as hot as possible (red-hot). Without letting the paper clip cool, place it on the nail in the center of the hematoma. This actually melts the nail and allows the blood to be released, relieving the pressure and pain immediately. If you are at all squeamish about the sight of blood, don't try this one! Also, don't do it over a light-colored carpet! This procedure is without pain as long as the clip does not penetrate too deeply under the nail. When the clip has gone through the nail the blood which is under pressure will squirt out. Apply some antiseptic over the hole and apply a band-aid. The nail will be loose in the area where the blood had accumulated. Keep the area covered and clean until it is completely dry. Report any infection to your doctor.

Subungual exostosis is abnormal growth of the small bone beneath the toenail. It grows in response to continuous pressure from the overlying nail or from previous injury. This problem is not visible to the eye, but when pain exists and nothing is visible

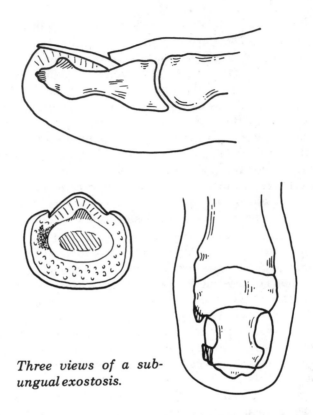

*Three views of a sub-
ungual exostosis.*

consider this possibility. Pain is greatest with pressure straight down on the toenail, while pressure from the sides elicits only minor discomfort. This sign and x-rays are diagnostic. Treatment is done in the doctor's office. Prognosis is very good and lost time is minimal.

DRY AND CRACKED SKIN

Dryness of the skin is caused from a lack of hydration or water in the skin layer. Cracking or fissuring, especially around the bottom of the heel area, is also due to low hydration, although with fissuring you see a build-up of callus around the involved areas. It is aggravated by open-healed or ill-fitting shoes.

Treatment of dry skin is directed at maintaining this water

content within the skin through the use of topical creams. If fissuring is involved, the callused area must be eliminated before most creams are effective. Creams are characteristically water soluble and rub well into the skin. Lotions may also be used, although creams have a greater moisturizing effect. Ointments should not be used for dry skin, as they are occlusive and do not penetrate. There are many brands of skin cream on the market today, some of which have special additives that make them more effective. Most skin creams, regardless of brand, should be applied 1-2 times daily, with one of the applications after bathing when the skin is moist. If this regimen does not prove to be effective use the cream more frequently, up to four times per day.

One particular cream which is effective is Carmol cream. This cream contains a 20% concentration of urea, an excellent moisturizer. It also comes in a lotion which contains 10% urea and is designated for less severe cases. Some other creams available to the public without a prescription are Eucerin cream, Aquacare HP cream and Lubraderm cream.

If cracking and fissuring of the heels is present, first look at the respective area in the shoes to check for irregularities that might be causing irritation to the foot. Carmol 20% can then be used 3-4 times daily. In conjunction with using cream, a pumice stone used after bathing to mechanically remove the callused tissue has proven helpful. If no progress is in sight, your podiatrist has a more complete treatment at his disposal for caring for these problems.

We often see calluses on the heels of athletes wearing rigid appliances. There is usually no cracking, although pressure from the hardened tissue is uncomfortable. A Spenco insole may be put directly over the orthoses in the shoe to remedy this problem. Use a rubber cement, not "contact" cement.

This section on skin and nails is not all inclusive, but should make you more familiar with the care of frequently encountered skin and nail problems. When confronted with a particular problem that raises questions to its cause or treatment, professional care should be instituted.

14

Toes and Metatarsals

Most chronic toe deformities are directly related to hammered, contracted or abnormally shaped digits. As mentioned in the previous chapter on corns and calluses, contracted toes are either hereditary, due to extrinsic forces or secondary to long-standing muscular or neuro-muscular imbalances.

If just the little toe is turned in, consider it to be a hereditary predisposition, but hammered second and third toes are seldom hereditary. By muscular imbalance, we simply mean an imbalanced pull on the toes by the inserting tendons. This abnormal pull over long periods of time results in a buckling effect at the various joint levels in the toes. In children and adolescents, these deformities are often flexible; with increasing age, the joints become fused in this abnormal position. As the top or end of the toes become more prominent, they display areas of redness, blisters, corns or callus formation. The underlying bone often reacts by piling up new bone beneath the pressure point. There may even be an accumulation of fluid, or bursitis between the bone and the skin. Injuries to tendons or spasms in muscles may cause toe deformities.

Treatment of digital deformities should be initiated as soon as the abnormality is detected. When the deformity is not long-standing, self-treatment is often successful in reversing the process of irritation. If the toe is rigid and is not able to straighten out, surgical treatment is often necessary. The first step in the treatment of the hammered toe is to inspect the shoes, making

180

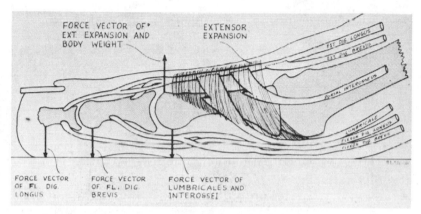

sure they are long enough so the toes don't jam into the end. If one toe in particular seems to be jamming into the end of the shoe because it is abnormally long, as in a Morton's foot, buy shoes to fit the longest toe. Short shoes should be discarded at once. If a corn is forming on the little toe or between the fourth toe and little toe, make sure the shoes are wide enough. Damaged feet are a high price to pay for neglect in buying the proper shoe size. If the shoes have been properly fitted, suspect a biomechanical imbalance of the foot to be the cause of the toe deformity.

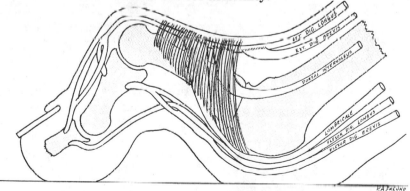

Above: Normal toe. Below: "Hammer" toe.

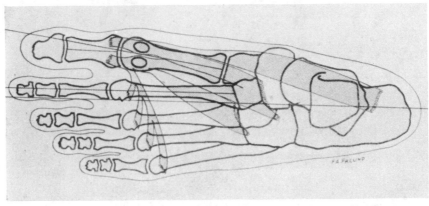

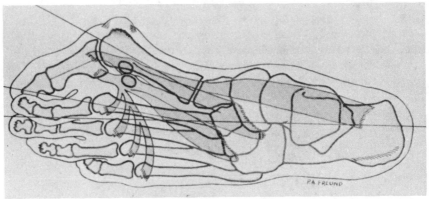

Above: Normal foot. Below: Foot with a bunion.

Primary treatment of the hammertoe involves protecting the irritated tissue or callused area from continued pressure. This can be done with a simple aperture pad. An aperture pad is "donut" shaped and surrounds the point of irritation. (See Chapter 30 for further details.) This reduces the pressure and if worn continually may allow for a complete remission of the pressure point. Aperture pads most commonly have an adhesive backing so they will stick to the toe.

Corns may also form between the toes where there is pressure. These are soft because of increased moisture and must be differentiated from an early fungus infection. If soft corns are occurring between the toes, use lamb's wool, foam or felt to separate the opposing toes. Eighth-inch thickness is usually sufficient for this.

All digital callosities will respond more favorably to conservative treatment if first pared down. This removes pressure from the toe and makes athletic participation more tolerable.

If results of self-treatment are not forthcoming in two months, your podiatrist should be consulted for a mechanical evaluation and treatment. Flexible deformities that have not become rigid and fixed in the contracted position especially in youngsters often respond to tape splinting and rigid orthoses. Intractable (irreversible) corns in the middle-aged athlete often require minor surgical correction to realign the bony structures and alleviate the offending prominences.

BUNIONS

Bunions are bumps on the side of the foot, occurring at the large toe joint. Strictly speaking, a bunion is an area of inflammation over a deformed great toe joint. The severity of a bunion is usually determined by the amount the big toe deviates outward (or laterally) and the size of the bump at the joint level.

Bunions are caused by: (1) pronated feet; (2) longterm use of poorly fitting shoes, and (3) congenital predisposition. Bunions secondary to pronation of the feet are the most frequent, and tend to occur in adolescence and middle age. Pronation causes excessive mobility of the first metatarsal bone, with rubbing of the joint by the shoe, and imbalance of the muscles to the big toe.

Bunions are serious problems if left to progress. Well-developed bunions cause arthritis in the involved joint and create chronic discomfort, besides being asthetically unappealing.

We have seen women distance runners who complain that their big toe is moving outward and a knot is forming at the big toe joint. Apparently, women in general don't have the ligamentous stability in their feet that men do. The extra wear and tear on their feet brings about problems that would normally plague them in their later years. Athletes involved in kicking sports, especially soccer and karate are particularly prone to traumatic arthritis of the first big toe joint that often leads to a stiff joint.

We cannot overemphasize the importance of early treatment for bunions. As soon as a deviation and bump is noticed, even if it is not bothersome, seek professional advice. If there is only redness at the side or on top of the big toe joint and no bony deformity, change shoe gear. The fault may be due to narrow shoes; feet change shape with activity.

The progression of a bunion often can be halted by orthotic devices in the shoes. Orthoses maintain muscular balance and bony stability to the big toe so it won't have a tendency to drift. If the bunion is far advanced, surgical correction to realign the soft tissues and bones is necessary. The convalescent period after surgery is usually 6-8 weeks away from sports participation, although alternative sports such as swimming and bicycling are permitted in approximately 1-2 weeks. We do not consider accommodative padding around a bunion a reasonable alternative to surgery if surgery is indicated. The temporary incapacitation of surgery will greatly outweight the years of chronic progressing discomfort.

Tailor's bunions ("bunionettes") are caused by irritation and pressure of the fifth (outside) metatarsal bone. They originally were described in tailors who sat "Indian style" all day with

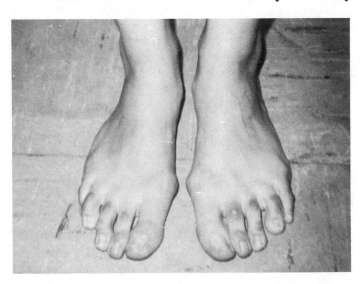

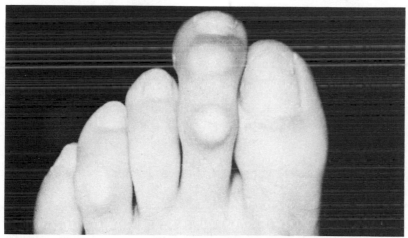

Page 184: Compensated feet show multiple areas of pressure and in-stability. Above: Morton's foot with a long second toe.

pressure on the outsides of the feet. Tailor's bunions are essentially the same as those occurring on the inside of the foot, except there is no severe deviation of the involved toe. The tailor's bunion occurs at the base of the fifth toe where it meets the ball of the foot. The bunion can be on the outside of the foot or on the bottom, and is almost always seen with a prominent callus.

Self-treatment involves using wider shoe gear to accommodate for the bony prominence. Pads in the shape of a half-moon, placed around the prominent callus, often will relieve discomfort temporarily.

Intractable tailor's bunions, not responding to the above care, should be surgically approached. A surgical break is usually made in the bone to move it away from its present position. Tailor's bunions are associated with varus foot types, but orthoses have only limited success in relieving the associated discomfort.

MORTON'S FOOT

The so-called Morton's, Grecian or atavistic foot is a heredity foot type which is very common in athletes and can become disabling with continuous activity. As described earlier, D. J. Morton wrote extensively on foot mechanics. The classic Morton's

185

foot has a short first metatarsal bone. With this condition, normal balance is disturbed and weight stress falls toward the inside arch (pronation). This produces hypermobility of the first ray, displacement of the (protective) sesamoid bones and increased stress on the second metatarsal head, which usually results in a callus in this area.

Initial treatment should support the first metatarsal head, extending from the arch to the sulcus of the great toe. This may be done directly on the foot, on a moveable support or attached to the shoe.

This treatment is temporary. If stress remains on the foot, this padding flattens and loses shape. Usually, a permanent orthotic is necessary.

15

Plantar Fascia and Heel Spur

We often refer to plantar fasciitis and the heel spur syndrome synonymously. It's not completely accurate but does help in keeping the dynamic cause of both conditions in mind. Both conditions involve the long plantar ligament or plantar fascia, and both are aggravated by foot pronation.

Plantar fasciitis is most frequently an acute or semi-acute injury and appears as a strain or partial rupture of the sturdy "ligament" that courses from the heel to the ball of the foot. Pain is in the middle of the heel, extending forward. The plantar fascia is a firm band of connective tissue on the bottom of the foot which is often called a "ligament." It functions in maintaining the inside or medial arch.

The direct cause of injury can be anything that stretches this ligament, such as a lineman in football propelling forcefully from the ball of the foot into an unyielding object. Another cause could be a gymnast jumping off apparatus onto the ball of the foot. With a more gradual onset, the cause is usually pronation, which lengthens the foot and puts a stretch on the fascia.

The plantar fascia is comprised of three slips: the center, the outside (lateral) and the inside (medial) portions. The inside and middle are most frequently involved with injury. The pain from plantar fasciitis usually is in the arch or heel area while standing and running. Direct pressure on the fascia should elicit some tenderness. If you run your fingers along the tender area, you may be able to feel a slight irregularity where the pain is occurring. If

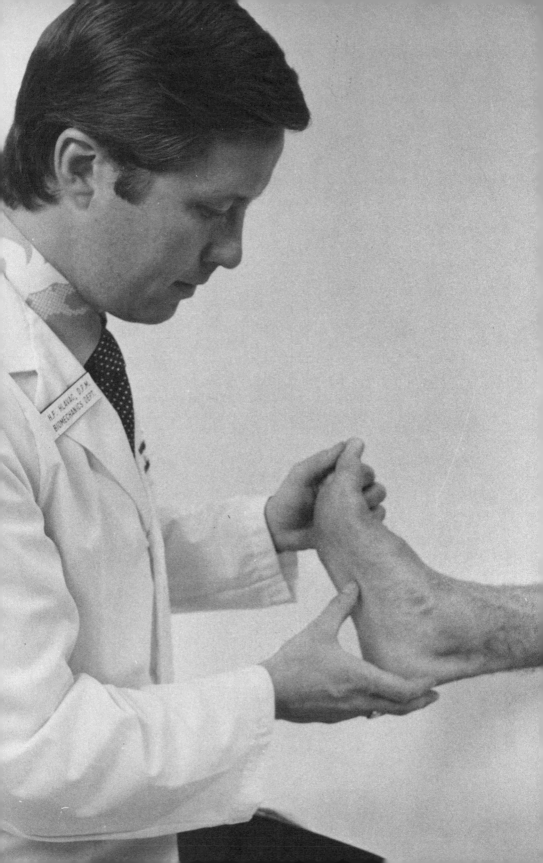

the injury is more acute, swelling can be present and spasm of the ligament often causes this structure to become bow-strung and quite prominent, especially when two toes are bent upward, pain associated with spasm is more severe.

Plantar fasciitis responds fairly well to conservative treatment. If the injury is acute ice should be used immediately to bring down swelling and reduce spasm. During the first 24-48 hours, weight-bearing should be limited, after which further sports participation should be limited to pain tolerance. Felt and tape should both be used to provide additional support and compression over the involved area. A Low-Dye or rest strap (see Chapter 30) should be applied to provide support. In addition, we use a medial arch pad secured with additional tape to provide compression and support. Another treatment is to use a varus heel pad in both shoes to reduce the stretch effect on the ligament. Ice should be used continually after workouts and before bedtime until pain is diminmation. A Sports Wedge, with cupping and tilting of the heel, may be more helpful.

The more chronic plantar fasciitis we see in relation to endurance sports is handled differently. We believe this gradual presentation of pain is most commonly due to abnormal pronation of the foot, and therefore we aim our treatment at this factor. For the first six weeks after injury, the problem is handled the same as acute plantar fasciitis. Ice, again, is all-important to keep inflam-

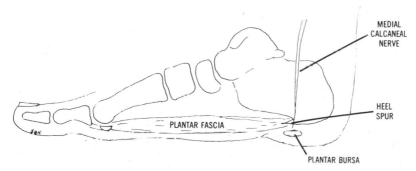

Dorsiflexion of the hallux causes the plantar fascia to be prominent on the arch.

mation at a minimum, and the use of tape and pads provides for additional support and compression.

(Note: Many athletes will adequately cut down training to pain tolerance but continue to compete. This will greatly aggravate the problem. Competition should be prohibited until training is again full scale.)

If pain is near the heel region, x-rays may be necessary to indicate if a heel spur syndrome is taking place. Steroid injections are sometimes indicated to reduce chronic inflammation.

Prevention of plantar fasciitis is best achieved via orthotic devices. By supporting the arch, the devices reduce the strain on the plantar fascia. Our results where orthoses are used in treating plantar fasciitis have been extremely rewarding.

Another type of fasciitis is found in downhill skiers and Nordic skiers who suffer from a "fallen arch"-type pain when they firmly buckle down their ski boots. Pain is relieved by unbuckling the boots but many continue to ski through the pain. This pain is related to the stretching of the plantar fascia and is probably more frequent in skiers with varus-type foot deformities. The abnormal foot, when secured firmly in a ski boot, is functioning maximally pronated in order to maintain inside edge control which in a short period can appear as intolerable arch pain. We suggest trying a rigid or semi-rigid orthotic device or Sports Wedge for this problem.

HEEL SPUR

A heel spur is a bony growth occurring on the underside of the heel bone. This growth appears in response to an abnormal pull from the plantar fascia. Initially, only the bone covering or periosteum is involved. But after years of continued stress and minor inflammation, a bony spur gradually appears. The abnormal stress that causes plantar fasciitis also causes the heel spur, but instead of involving the fascia in the arch area, its involvement is at the ligament's origin on the heel bone. In addition to bone and ligament involvement, we are seeing a large number of cases where a bursitis and nerve entrapment co-exist with the heel spur. The pressure and local irritation cause the bursal sac to form, while the chronic inflammation irritates and binds down the nearby nerve.

Pain is usually greatest in the initial formative stages when

190

only the bone covering is involved. Pain will be present on weight bearing and when pressure is firmly applied over the base of the heel.

Conservative treatment is the same as for plantar fasciitis, although the use of the medial arch pad is not as important here. A pad which has proven effective is one shaped like a horseshoe and placed in the shoe to take the pressure away from the central position of the heel where the tenderness exists. If self-treatment is not progressing satisfactorily, quickly consult a podiatrist. Orthotic devices are again very helpful in cupping the heel and in reducing the pull of the plantar fascia away from the heel bone. When pain is long-standing and unremitting after using all modes of therapy, surgery occasionally is performed with fair to good results.

Looking at plantar fasciitis and the heel spur you see that treatment is directed in two stages. The initial treatment is very similar to that of many overuse injuries, and the extended treatment involves correcting the abnormal forces that initiated the entire injury process.

16

Heel Injuries

HEEL BURSITIS

Bursae are small sacs of fluid located near prominent bones or around moving body parts, and they function as shock absorbers. Occasionally, after chronic trauma or overuse, these sacs become enlarged and inflammed. Bursitis often occurs with the heel spur syndrome, but is more frequently seen in back of the heel between the achilles tendon and the heel bone.

This particular presentation, called retrocalcaneal bursitis in medical terminology, is brought about by abnormal pressure from the shoe counter which creates a shearing force within the bursal sac. Athletes with high-arched feet are particularly prone to this ailment as their heel bone is more prominent in the back of the shoes. The condition usually starts as an area of redness or blister formation at the back of the heel. The heel movement that causes this bursitis is predominantly a side-to-side motion, or inversion and eversion of the heel.

If your heels are not moving up and down within the shoes, but you notice an area of continuing irritation, take heed. This is the stage in which conservative treatment is most beneficial. If blisters are your only problem, first check the counter of your shoes, making sure there are no points of irritation. If the area is reddened and the pain is deeper when pressure is applied, suspect a bursal irritation. A bursa has a "spongy" feeling. Heel bursitis should be distinguished from achilles tendonitis. If no pain is associated with jumping barefoot, suspect bursistis.

192

Treatment of the heel irritation should involve some type of accommodative padding. Anything that encircles the irritated area will do fine. Pads for the back of the heel need not be thick, as they must fit into the shoe; one-sixteenth- to one-eighth-inch felt is usually adequate. If swelling is evident and does not respond to ice applications, you should consider seeing your podiatrist. Professional care may involve a steriod injection to calm down the bursal irritation.

The best prevention is again through orthotic devices. As stated, it appears to be the excessive side to side motion of the calcaneus that aggravates the condition. A rigid orthoses with a heel stabilizing post limit this motion and decrease the shear within the involved soft tissues. In addition to soft tissue involve-

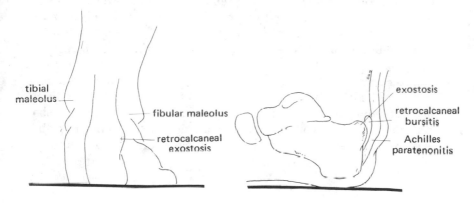

tibial maleolus

fibular maleolus

retrocalcaneal exostosis

exostosis

retrocalcaneal bursitis

Achilles paratenonitis

Two views of the development of rectocalcaneal bursitis and exostosis.

ment, long-standing shear and pressure also can result in bone deposits in the back of the heel. This bony deposition makes the back of the heel more prominent and subject to greater irritation.

APOPHYSITIS

Apophysitis is inflammation of the growth area of the heel bone, which develops in two parts. Apophysitis also appears with pain in the heel, although this condition is restricted to youngsters between the ages of 10 and 15 years. The associated pain from apophysitis is directly in back of the heel and therefore somewhat lower than that of achilles tendonitis and bursitis. The cause of apophysitis is thought to be hampered circulation to the developing heel bone. It is associated with certain foot types (equinus) and is aggravated by sports.

Pain is greatest whenever vigorous activity such as running and especially jumping are involved. The symptoms are usually seen in the physically active child. Many times, the apophysitis comes on with new shoes, especially baseball spikes that have a metal heel plate at the point of irritation.

Treatment is relatively simple and in nearly all cases provides relief of symptoms. When this condition is suspected, felt heel lifts of about a half-inch thickness should be placed in all shoes. This reduces the pull from the achilles tendon inserting into the painful portion of the heel. In addition to using pads, some limitation of sports participation is mandatory for relief of pain, especially fast-running sports and sports such as basketball which require jumping.

After a period of three weeks to a month, allow sports participation to pain tolerance, cutting back if symptoms recur. Pain usually diminishes in 1-2 months. With further development of the heel bone, the symptoms of apophysitis disappear. If no treatment is given, the area still heals, but it may take six months or more.

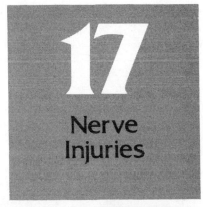

Nerve Injuries

CUTANEOUS NERVE ENTRAPMENT AND COMPRESSION

Cutaneous nerves are those occurring just below the skin. Their superficial location makes them particularly vulnerable to entrapment and compression. Nerve entrapment usually results after some previous inflammatory process or after surgery. The nerves involved become entrapped in the fibrous tissue. Professional treatment is necessary to break up the scar tissue with injections or by a surgical procedure. Nerve compression usually results after wearing tight-fitting or irritating shoes.

This condition is extremely common with snow skiers and ice skaters. In both sports, a high degree of foot support is needed so shoe gear is bound down very tightly. The cold environment lessens the pain that would otherwise warn you that the shoes are a little tight. The skin numbness that results may last from one week up to two months. Little can be done except wait for skin sensation to return. If it is necessary to lace shoes to the point you are bordering discomfort, consider putting sponge rubber or felt pads under the tongue of the shoe to better distribute the pressure on the underlying nerves.

GANGLIONS

Ganglions or ganglionic cysts are herniating outpockets from joint sacs or tendon sheaths, and are filled with fluid. Trauma is felt to be the cause that weakens the lining of the joint or tendon. Ganglions grow at a fairly slow rate. They feel rather firm and are

195

filled with a gelatinous substance. They are not freely movable because they are attached (and move along with) tendons and joints.

A podiatrist should be consulted in the first stages of presentation. He can rule out other more serious conditions and coordinate your treatment. If ganglions are not particularly bothersome, they can be left alone. Conservative treatment is to see that the ganglion is not subjected to unusual pressure or friction. If the ganglion is in a prominent area, an accommodative pad might serve well as a protective device. If the cyst is believed to have come from the tarsal joints, orthoses may be helpful in reducing abnormal tarsal joint motion. For the same reason, it is wise to use orthoses after surgery is performed.

Some doctors attempt to inject and drain ganglions and have reported fair results. If the ganglion is bothersome, we recommend having surgery. Surgery probably should be done under general anesthesia as meticulous attention is necessary to excise the entire ganglion to help safeguard against recurrences.

NEUROMA

A neuroma is a benign nerve tumor. It is fairly common in the feet where there is friction and trauma, or with mechanical imbalance on hard flat surfaces. Normally, the major nerves pass deep inside of the ankle bone through the bottom of the foot, extending between the metatarsal heads and out to the sides of the toes.

A neuroma can occur anywhere there is irritation to the nerve sheath. Nature actually made an anatomical "mistake," so there is pressure from the bones on the nerve. This causes a thickening of the nerve sheath or covering, producing scar tissue and causing nerve pains. The most common location is between the third and fourth metatarsal heads. This neuroma was first described by Dr. T. E. Morton (not the same D. J. Morton who described foot imbalance) and is often called Morton's neuroma or Morton's metatarsalgia.

Neuromas also can occur between other metatarsal spaces or under the heel when associated with the heel spur syndrome. Neuromas produce needle-like shooting, electric or tingling pains

196

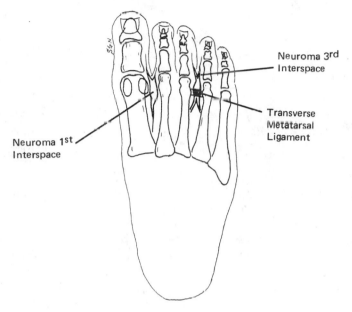

Interdigital neuromas.

with certain standing positions. As they advance, they can produce numbness or muscle cramping in the affected toes.

About 50% of all neuromas can be relieved with conservative treatment. First, the person must wear a shoe that does not cramp the feet. Sometimes, they must change the heel heights in order to change the weight-bearing point on the foot. Often cushioned insoles or pads to separate the metatarsal heads will do. If not, professional help is needed. The neuroma may respond to local injections or orthotics, or it may require surgical removal. This is a soft tissue procedure (no bone surgery) so disability is minimal and the person is able to bear weight immediately after surgery.

18

Tendon Injuries

Tendons are the means by which muscles attach to bones and produce movement. Tendonitis (or tenosynovitis) refers to inflammation of the tendon (or tendon covering). The inflammation is caused by a single process, irritation arising either from overuse or from direct trauma. Such things as a blow to the tendon, a rapid change in workout routine, shoes or surface all can contribute to the inflammation.

Essentially, any tendon of the lower extremity that is subject to continual trauma, overuse due to excessive pronation of the foot, or a muscle imbalance can develop tendonitis. Tendonitis can be prevented with extensive warmups and flexibility training. The athlete should never attempt to "run through" possible tendonitis.

Tendonitis shows up as localized pain and tenderness when the involved muscle tendon is put to use. Depending on the severity of injury, pain may be present at rest or only after vigorous exercise. There may be evidence of local swelling, but this is not always true. The most common areas of tendonitis are the achilles tendon, the top of the foot, and the front, back or sides of the knee and ankle joints. These areas are most commonly affected because of their great mobility.

When the first pains of a possible tendonitis occur, effort should be made to limit the motion of the involved part. If the pain is minor, a decrease in activity may be sufficient. Check your foot gear and make sure they are not badly worn.

198

If you are a skier, ice skater or involved in any sport that requires wearing a tight boot, be suspicious of a compression tendonitis over the top (dorsum) of the ankle. This problem is caused by having the shoes or boots laced too tightly. A compression of adjacent nerves is also common in these areas.

If the tendonitis is on either (medial or lateral) side of the ankle, suspect a mechanical foot abnormality. If tendonitis occurs at the attachment of the achilles tendon, suspect a muscle imbalance, improper training techniques or a mechanical foot imbalance.

Initial treatment for achilles tendonitis is elevation of the heel with a quarter-inch pad in the shoe. This relaxes the tendon and promotes healing. Tendonitis on either side of the knee, if from overuse, is again usually caused by abnormal foot mechanics. Tendonitis over or under the kneecap (patella) can be attributed to a multitude of factors, again including poor foot structure (see knee injuries).

In treatment, reduce the primary cause of excess motion. This can be done by reducing activity. But if this is not enough and pain continues, tape should be applied to restrict joint motion. Caution must be taken to avoid improperly applied tape that could further compress the tendon and aggravate the tendonitis. Tape should be used primarily for joint restriction. If taping fails and pain is sufficient, plaster casting is necessary to eliminate totally the use of the involved muscle. This technique should allow healing within three weeks' time. In addition to restricting motion, ice and elevation are helpful both in the acute and chronic stages of injury to reduce inflammation.

Ice massage is recommended for almost all acute sports injuries. In the case of chronic tendonitis with soft tissue crepitus (a rough crackling sensation with movement) and fluid surrounding the tendon, moist heat applications may be necessary to mobilize the fluid. This is one major exception to the ICE rule. Never use heat during the first 48 hours after injury, but if a chronic condition is present, try moist heat.

Once an episode of tendonitis has occurred, the athlete will have a greater tendency toward recurrences. This is true because the inflammation often leaves a small amount of scar tissue behind, which hinders the gliding motion of the tendon within its sheath.

The result can be recurrent episodes of inflammation. The tendon sheath, if damaged enough, can cause continuous pain on motion. Local injections of anti-inflammatory medications may be sufficient, but surgical removal of the scar tissue may be necessary.

A biomechanical evaluation should be performed to see if abnormal foot mechanics is resulting in abnormal stress to a particular tendon group. If this is the case, rigid appliances should be prescribed to correct his unwanted motion. As in other overuse injuries, the athlete can attempt to reduce foot motion with soft appliances, taping or pads as described in Chapter 30. Stretching exercises are very important to maintain strength and elasticity in the leg and foot muscles. The muscles in the front of the leg and thigh, if prone toward tendon inflammation, should be strengthened to reduce muscular imbalances that occur naturally with running sports.

19

Joint Injuries

Within the foot, there are many joints. They have different sizes and shapes which govern the amount and direction of motion of each bone on another. Where one bone articulates on another, there is the covering of the bone (periosteum) which flows into the capsules and ligaments which cover the fluid-filled joint spaces. The fluid provides smooth gliding motion between the cartilagerous ends of the opposing bones. With normal function, stress is absorbed within this "hydraulic" system.

Injury to the joint can occur at various structures. Basically, when there is joint injury, there is stiffness and pain with motion. Because of the variety of structures in and around a joint, many different things can happen with a traumatic, overuse or imbalance injury, but the important thing to remember is that because of their intrinsic poor blood supply, joints heal very slowly.

The most common types of joint problems are: arthritis (inflammation of the joint); capsulitis (inflammation of the covering of the joint); ligament injuries (sprains); cartilage damage; dislocation; crepitus (roughness within a joint giving a "grating" sound and sensation with motion in certain positions).

Arthritis is a general term which refers to any inflammation of a joint. It can be caused by injury (traumatic arthritis), disease processes (rheumatoid arthritis), osteoarthritis, psoriatic arthritis, tubercular arthritis, gonorrheal arthritis, metabolism (gouty arthritis), drug or chemical reactions, or infection.

The main type of arthritis seen in athletes is the traumatic type, where the stress through the joint exceeds the range of motion allowed by the structure. When this happens very suddenly, there is a stretch of the ligaments (which are inelastic). This pulls on the attachments. If it is severe, the ligament breaks and may permit joint dislocation, with or without bone injury. This demands immediate professional attention. Don't attempt to manipulate a dislocated joint! If the injury is less severe, there may be rupture or partial tear in the joint capsule or ligament.

There are four classes of sprains, from mild to severe, depending on bone and joint damage. If there is any disfigurement, it indicates dislocation. If there is any grating or roughness in the joint, it indicates a fragment interfering with motion. If there is deep bleeding with rapid swelling, it indicates broken vessels in the area. All of these require immediate professional attention. While waiting for help to arrive, use ICE.

Less severe joint injuries often go unnoticed during competition, when the body is warm and moving. As the body cools down after competition, one joint remains swollen and stiff. It is important at this point to use ICE. Heat application will increase pain, swelling and disability. Often, this joint pain will not show until well after the activity, even until the next morning, when mild joint inflammation goes on during the night. Upon arising in the morning, the injured joint feels stiff and motions are slow, "like a car with cold oil." Sudden movements are painful. If swelling is evident, use ice. Do not attempt to return to activity without an excessive warmup and complete relief of joint pain.

If untreated, joint arthritis is progressive. With the inflammatory process, the healing blood cells bring in scar tissue around the joint and thickening of the bone. The inflammatory process must be stopped as soon as possible to prevent permanent disability.

Any joint which is injured can become arthritic. The most common lower-extremity joint injury in sports is the inversion ankle sprain which is described in the chapter on ankle and leg injuries. Within the foot, certain entities are so common as to have special names:

"Turf-toe" is a football injury which occurs when there is forced dorsiflexion (upward extension) of the first toe as the leg comes

202

forward on the planted foot. This is especially common on relatively hard surfaces, such as artificial turf, with a flexible shoe. Therefore, we recommend a multiple-cleated (up to 22) football shoe with a rigid shank when playing on artificial surfaces. Natural turf does not produce this injury (but results in others). "Turf-toe" is one form of capsulitis where the stress on the joint exceeds its normal functional range of motion.

If there is imbalance, leading to overuse stress on joints, arthritis can develop. Any structured imbalance which causes the joints of the foot to compensate and function at the end of their normal range of motion will produce progressive joint strain and inflammation, sending "shock waves" through the foot and up the leg. Ligaments and capsules around joints are meant as "emergency" structures and should not be under stress with normal activities. Well-conditioned muscles maintain normal joint alignment. With muscle imbalance or weakness, or with hereditary functional imbalance, the joints are forced to function under stress. These are the points of injury in sports. The injury may be rapid or cumulative.

Young, growing athletes are especially susceptible to joint injuries. Their joints are often especially loose, so it is difficult for them to gain stability for contact sports. In other sports, because of this laxity, many of their movements are less efficient than an adult's. Their coaches and trainers must emphasize strength and flexibility exercises for the normal function of joints.

For example, never use a side stretch or "lotus position" on the knees, especially in youngsters. The knee is a hinge-type joint, and is most efficient with flexion-extension strength and stability exercises—never with a lateral force on the joint, which only increases susceptibility to injury.

Injuries to joints in youngsters are especially serious. If there is damage to the growth area of the bone, there is a progressive deformity with permanent disability. Therefore, all suspected joint injuries in children must be examined professionally.

Other types of arthritis, through disease processes, faults in metabolism, and exposure to specific drugs and chemicals are not within the scope of this book. However, athletes, coaches, and trainers should be aware that any puncture wound or injury to the skin near a joint can produce an infection inside the joint (pyogenic arthritis). Also, if there is an injury to a joint while an athlete has an infection elsewhere in his body, it is possible to get the infection in that injured joint. The most common symptom with this is pain and stiffness of the joint, with fever and chills. This demands immediate medical evaluation.

Joint problems in athletes are very common. Most are mild, transient and self-limiting, with no disability. In any case, the situation must be evaluated carefully and treated promptly. Immediate treatment for joint problems anywhere in the body is ICE.

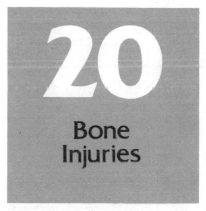

20

Bone Injuries

An injury which is serious enough to damage bone requires professional evaluation as soon as possible. The most common bone injuries in the feet are bone bruises, fractures, stress fractures and injuries to the growth plate in youngsters.

Bones are hard but flexible tissues of live cells which are well supplied with blood, and are constantly fortifying and replenishing themselves in the healthy body. Most bones in the feet and legs are long bonds with ends ("head" and "base"), hard sides (cortical bone), soft insides (cancellous bone, marrow or matrix) and a covering (the periosteum). The shaft of a long bone is called the epiphysis and the area between is the diaphysis; the area of bone growth in youngsters is called the metaphysis. The periosteum helps support the blood and nerve supply to the bone, and serves as the attachment of tendons to muscles and ligaments to bones.

A bone bruise ("stone bruise") occurs from a sharp blow on a bone prominance. This causes an immediate sharp pain and damage to the periosteum, which stimulates the inflammatory process. If the damage is minor, there is soft-tissue swelling around the area which resolves quickly. If there is a break in the periosteum itself, there is healing activity which brings in new blood and periosteal cells, often resulting in a bone spur formation.

Early treatment with ICE will prevent the inflammatory process. If the injury is greater, there can be a hematoma, or blood bruise between the periosteum and the bone. (This is a frequent cause of heel spurs). If untreated, the blood blister fills in with bone cells. Therefore, within 24 hours after an injury, if there is a lump in the area of the bone bruise, there is probably a hematoma which requires professional treatment.

A fracture involves a break in the cortex of the bone. There are many descriptions of types of fractures: simple (crack in cortex, no displacement); transverse, oblique or spiral (the direction of the break through the bone); comminuted (multiple, fragmental); compression (one part pushed into another); compound (a fracture breaking through the skin); "green-stick" (half-broken and bent); intra-articular (into a joint); epiphyseal (through a growth area); displaced (movement of the fractured part from its normal position).

When a fracture occurs, there is usually a sudden move or acute trauma. The victim often hears or feels a distinct crack. There is usually a numb, "shocky" or unstable feeling distal to (away from or beneath) the area of injury. Weight-bearing and motion of the part are painful. Pain increases with motion, rather than decreases as with many other injuries. Usually, a bruise follows, but this takes several hours.

The earlier a professional sees the injured athlete, the better. He should be examined away from the noisy area of competition, before swelling has started. Initial treatment for a suspected fracture again includes ICE. Professional treatment includes setting and immobilization if necessary.

Stress fractures are very common in the military, where they are called "march" fractures. They usually occur with a poorly trained recruit who must endure physical stress with a heavy pack. In fact, Dr. Richard Gilbert, who has served as a military podiatrist and is now in private practice in San Diego, California has treated more than 25,000 stress fractures. He reports that they usually occur on the left foot on the day the drill instructor known to have said, "let me hear your left . . . your left . . . ."

Since bone is a living tissue, it adapts to stress. This structural change takes time, and again shows the need for long-term conditioning, with moderate training year-round. Stress fractures in the foot occur most commonly in the metatarsal bones of the calcaneus. Usually, there is no point of acute injury, but with activity

206

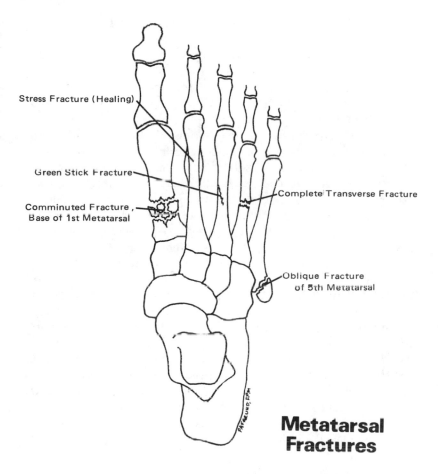

Stress Fracture (Healing)

Green Stick Fracture

Comminuted Fracture,
Base of 1st Metatarsal

Complete Transverse Fracture

Oblique Fracture
of 5th Metatarsal

FAFREUND, F/M

Metatarsal Fractures

the top of the foot or the sides of the heel bone become swollen and painful. This often is mistaken for a tendonitis and treated as such, but it doesn't respond to treatment like a tendonitis.

Often, the stress fracture will not show on x-rays for up to three weeks in the metatarsals and up to 4-5 weeks in the heel bone. Stress fractures usually do not require casting but some form of immobilization. While the foot is swollen and painful, you must limit weight-bearing activity. We often recommend substitute activity, such as cycling or swimming, or some non-weight-bearing aerobic activity. This way, the athlete maintains good condition while the injured part heals.

Returning to training from an injury must be very gradual; recurrences and other tissue injuries are common. Never begin activity until the swelling and pain are gone. A suspected stress fracture or "tendonitis" that doesn't respond to treatment should be examined by a professional.

Epiphyseal injuries can be very serious. If there is a suspected fracture at the growth line of the bone or injury into a joint in the growing athlete (up to age 20), it must have medical attention. With epiphyseal injuries, it is possible to have distorted growth patterns and increasing deformity with age. The name orthopedics means "straight child." The symbol of orthopedics is a growing tree. The old adage, "As the twig is bent, so grows the tree," has a great deal of truth and should not be taken lightly.

A baby has a thick soft, spongy foot. As he grows older, the tissues form to muscle and bone with less fat, and less protection. Throughout the 26 bones of each foot, there are many bone growth centers. These growth centers must be protected with good sports equipment. Many of the less expensive athletic shoes causes irritation from the placement of rivets, plastic stitching or the misplacement of spikes. Most children don't complain unless a problem is quite serious, yet "growth pains" are not normal. They indicate increased stress, overuse or muscle imbalance. The cause of that imbalance must be understood and treated, or the body will compensate, causing other problems.

With increased emphasis on competitive sports in younger age groups, there has been a phenomenal increase in injuries in young athletes. Parents and coaches must respect the fact that all parts of the growing child are in the formative stages. Any suspected injury must be treated immediately.

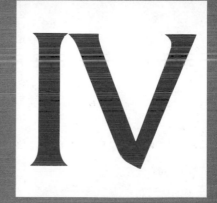

IV

RELATED
AILMENTS

21

Ankle
Injuries

This chapter concerning ankle injuries includes ankle sprains and a condition called the tarsal tunnel syndrome. In addition, we discuss fascia problems of the ankle and leg.

In many ways, the ankle joint functionally resembles the knee joint. Both joints bear the entire body's weight, allow motion predominately in the same direction, are supported by strong ligaments on either side, and frequently are injured and later re-injured. They are both parallel to the supporting surface, and allow the hinge motion of flexion and extension.

Let's consider the anatomy of the ankle and see how and what parts are responsible for its stability. The ankle is made up of three bones, the tibia, fibula and talus. The tibia and fibula bones end in two easily felt prominances on either side of the ankle called malleoli. The talus is a bone of the foot and has a flat surface that lies between the two leg bones. The ankle is often described as a saddle-type joint; the talus resembles the saddle with the body pivoting over it. The upper nature of the ankle joint is supported by three means: (1) gravity and joint congruity; (2) strong ligaments; (3) muscle tendons.

As with the knee, body weight helps maintain ankle joint alignment as long as there are no postural or structural defects which may favor joint malalignment. Bones and ligaments are the ankle's mainstay of stability. Every aspect of the ankle is supported by a maze of ligaments arranged to offer maximum support with maximum mobility. The strongest sets of ligaments are on

210

the medial and lateral sides of the ankle. These ligaments restrict excess foot inversion and eversion. When the ligaments are damaged, so is the ability to maintain proper ankle stability, and recurrent sprains are the result. Muscle tendons which cross the ankle on either side also aid in stabilization. On the medial side, the posterior tibial tendon offers ankle support, while on the lateral side the peroneal tendons exert their force. One set pulls the foot into inversion and the other into eversion. It is through their antagonistic effort that the neutral position is achieved.

ANKLE SPRAINS

There are two basic types of ankle sprains. The first, called an inversion sprain, accounts for more than 75% of ankle injuries. This sprain occurs when the foot severely inverts or turns in with relation to the leg. The force of body weight stretches the soft tissue on the lateral side of the ankle. This injury is most common in a normal or high-arched foot type; it usually occurs when walking or running or jumping.

The other sprain, called an eversion sprain, occurs when the foot is severely everted or turned out in relation to the leg. This force tears soft tissue on the medial side of the ankle and is most frequent in the flat foot type; it usually occurs with falling or jumping.

The severity of an ankle injury is classified in three degrees. The first-degree sprain results in swelling and prolonged pain, although no frank rupture or ankle instability is noted. The second-degree sprain involves a partial rupture of the supporting ligaments, and mild instability is noted on examination. The third-degree sprain causes marked instability and involves a total rupture of the supporting ligaments. All sprains fitting into one of these categories require immediate medical attention.

Doctors frequently are blamed for the mismanagement of ankle sprains, although much of the blame should be placed on the victim who attempts self-treatment on an ankle that clearly requires medical attention. If moderate to severe sprains were properly treated, starting the minute after injury instead of 1-2 weeks following the injury, the end result would be much better.

Unfortunately, the familiarity with ankle sprains is probably the greatest reason why people avoid medical treatment. There seems to be a universal misconception that all ankle sprains are alike and will respond favorably to ice, then heat, then an Ace bandage. We hope to clear up this feeling by defining which ankle injuries require medical attention. Also, we suggest first-aid measures to be used until medical help arrives.

We use one simple criterion to determine if an ankle requires medical attention: If a person who sustains either an inversion or eversion ankle sprain cannot walk it off in a period of five minutes so he can return to daily activities with no impairment other than minimal pain for a few hours, he should seek medical attention. Prolonged pain usually signifies bleeding around the ankle from either vessel or ligament damage. This type of injury requires strict medical care to assure quick recovery with maximum flexibility and stability.

If you sustain an ankle injury that requires medical attention, stay off it until it can be examined. This is especially important if you hear a snap or tear during the injury process. A signal such as this could mean a fracture or serious tear in the ligament. Call for an emergency appointment or go directly to an emergency room. .

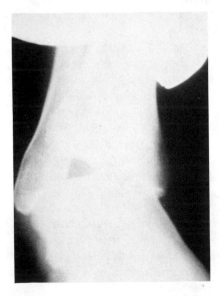

X-ray of an out-of-joint ankle.

Immediately after the injury, place compression and ice around the ankle region. If participating with a team, see that ice is readily available in case of emergencies. Keep a wet ankle wrap in the ice box, and immediately after injury firmly place the wrap around the ankle. Over this wrap, place ice packs. This treatment serves a threefold purpose: (1) compression keeps swelling down mechanically, and the ice constricts the blood vessels to retard swelling; (2) the ice also works as an anesthetic to reduce pain; (3) keeping the extremity elevated except during necessary ambulation holds down swelling by reducing the force of gravity.

Because of the high incidence of recurrent sprains and inadequate treatment, we feel there are few ankle sprains that should be handled by a lay person. Professional treatment varies with each individual's point of view, although there are certain guidelines that must be followed with any ankle sprain.

1. Classify the severity of the ankle sprain through digital palpation, by means of x-ray to rule out fractures, stress x-rays to determine abnormal ankle motion and arthrogram, if indicated, to quantitate ligament damage.

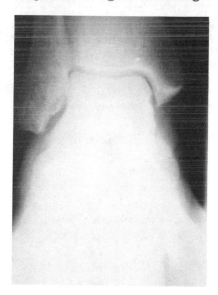

X-ray of a normal ankle.

2. Strictly immobilize, apply ice, compression and elevation until the acute phase of injury has subsided.

3. Immobilization to allow for soft tissue healing.

4. After soft tissue repair has occurred to regain strength and mobility in the ankle joint.

Specific ankle sprain treatment may be beyond the scope of this book, but prevention is not. A good percentage of ankle sprains in every sport could be avoided by applying a few basic principles regarding training and technique. There are four reasons why ankle sprains occur: (1) uneven terrain; (2) unnatural activity requiring unnatural body movement; (3) poor foot gear; (4) inherent structural weakness or imbalance.

The surface on which a sport is played is a significant determinant of ankle injuries. It stands to reason that if you play on a field of grass, there will be uneven surfaces involved (not to mention sunken water sprinklers!). These surfaces are often unseen since the grass makes the entire surface appear consistent. If you anticipate playing on grass, take special precautions by checking for small holes and marking them prior to a game.

Runners often ask whether to jog on grass surfaces or on the roads. For injury rehabilitation, we usually advocate running on grass. The softer surface absorbs a great deal of shock and dissipates the sudden trauma going through the body with each step. Another consideration, however, is the more serious runner who logs more than 50 miles per week at a faster speed. For this individual, it is unrealistic to find grass or soft surfaces everywhere he goes.

The point we find most significant is that this runner must weigh the chances of sustaining an ankle sprain while running on grass against a more probable overuse syndrome on concrete. We are faced with the "choice" of the overuse syndrome or the ankle sprain. The point to be made is that athletes should condition themselves slowly for new surfaces and new events. They must develop balance from movement. They must develop a propriceptive sense through practice.

Cause two refers to nearly all sports that use some sort of ball— football, basketball, soccer, etc. In these sports, repeated changes in direction put a great deal of stress on the ankle, especially the lateral ligaments. These are also the sports that report the greatest frequency of ankle injuries. This point is the only one of the four that cannot be manipulated. The player with weak ankles either compensates by working with the other factors or switches to another sport that requires less ankle strength.

Cause three refers not only to worn shoes but new shoes as well. Manufacturers of training flats for distance runners began modifying their shoes 4-5 years ago by widening the heels. Many of the multi-layered heel models at that time were so narrow that a runner took his life in his hands if he had to run down a gravel road. Recently, however, "flared" heel seems to have caught on widely. This type of heel gives maximum ankle stability. The athlete with weak ankles should make sure that his shoes are of good quality and have a solid heel counter; we recommend the flared laminated heel for those runners with ankle instability.

There are two areas of shoe wear that should tell you when to purchase new shoes. Look from behind at the heel counter. If it is badly sloped over to one side, it can't be repaired. If the heel is badly worn, either repair it with a glue gun or similar device, get the heel resoled or buy new shoes. This is vitally important, since severely worn heels can throw off your entire gait.

In considering the causative nature between skeletal abnormalities and ankle sprains, it must be remembered that the ankle is a weight-bearing joint. The heel bone directly below the ankle supports it and determines the stability of the ankle, depending on its position. If the heel is turned in, body weight is shifted to the outside and a stretch is placed on the lateral ligaments. Conversely, if the heel is turned out or everted excessively, force is placed on the medial ligaments. Therefore, it is the upright nature of the heel bone that maintains ankle stability.

Any structural foot or leg deformity which causes the heel bone to shift form its vertical position will most likely favor ankle sprains. Deformities such as forefoot valgus and rearfoot varus especially favor sprains, because they shift the heel bone in an inverted position. Inversion sprains are more predominant, because the foot moves more freely and to a greater degree in this direction and because the medial ligaments are said to be stronger.

215

Evaluation of Ankle Sprains

An athlete has an ankle painfully swollen due to a recent injury. Do not allow him to bear weight on the injured ankle.

Place the foot in plantar flexion and invert *gently*. Move the foot into dorsiflexion and invert again.

Is there point tenderness lateral or medial to the malleolus?

↓ YES

Suspect a fracture rather than a sprain. Obtain X-rays. *Get a doctor.*

Have the athlete describe the accident—whether he twisted the ankle or fell on it, how far he fell, whether the foot turned in or out, whether he felt or heard a snap—and estimate the degree of rotation.

Feel from the lateral malleolus to the anterolateral aspect and from the front of the lateral malleolus across the interosseous ligament. Palpate the sinus tarsi and the lateral aspect of the forefoot. Tap both malleoli. Note athlete's response.

Now examine both feet with the athlete standing. Look for abnormalities and signs of weakened ligamentous structures.

Examine both feet with the patient lying down. Note the location of the swelling.

Is the sprain moderate with a suspected tearing and capsular damage?

↓ YES

Choose between early weight-bearing (EWB) or nonweight-bearing (NWB) management.

↓ EWB

Have the athlete keep his ankle elevated and on ice for 24-48 hours.

NWB

If the sprain is mild, choose between early weight-bearing (EWB) or nonweight-bearing (NWB) management.

Have the athlete keep the ankle elevated and on ice for 24-48 hours. After 48 hours apply a walking cast to be worn two to three weeks.

Wrap the ankle in figure-eight style with a 3-inch-wide elastic bandage, to be rewound and tightened three times a day until the swelling has receded. Apply in a direction that *supports* the injured area.

↓ EWB

Instruct the athlete to keep the ankle elevated and on ice for 24-48 hours. Wrap the ankle with an elastic bandage over a compression dressing.

When the cast is removed, apply an elastic bandage.

On the third or fourth day following injury, have the patient begin soaking his ankle in warm water for 20 minutes 3-4 times a day, following each soaking with dorsiflexion, plantar flexion, inversion, and eversion exercises with leg elevated.

Have the athlete walk with fitted crutches for at least a week. Instruct him to touch the heel of the injured foot to the floor and push off gently with the forefoot while bearing his weight on his hands and arms.

Have the athlete begin simple exercises—raising up on the toes, rocking back on the heels, and finally rolling the injured foot sideways and bearing his body weight on the lateral aspect. He may begin nonweight-bearing sports, such as cycling and swimming.

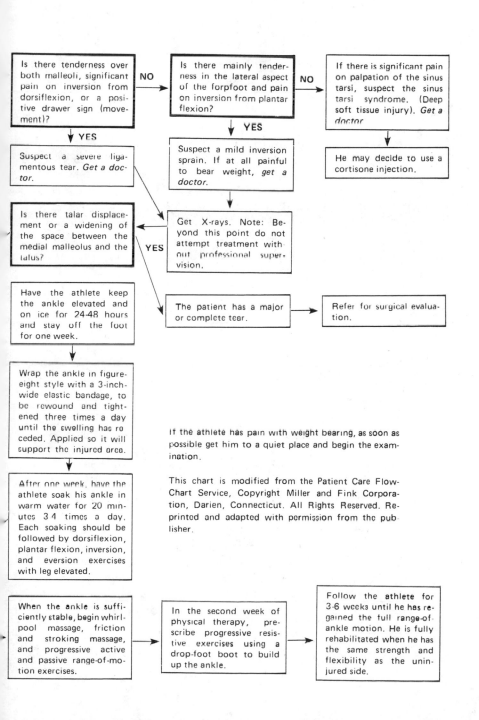

Is there tenderness over both malleoli, significant pain on inversion from dorsiflexion, or a positive drawer sign (movement)?

NO →

Is there mainly tenderness in the lateral aspect of the forefoot and pain on inversion from plantar flexion?

NO →

If there is significant pain on palpation of the sinus tarsi, suspect the sinus tarsi syndrome. (Deep soft tissue injury). *Get a doctor.*

↓ **YES**

Suspect a severe ligamentous tear. *Get a doctor.*

↓ **YES**

Suspect a mild inversion sprain. If at all painful to bear weight, *get a doctor.*

He may decide to use a cortisone injection.

Is there talar displacement or a widening of the space between the medial malleolus and the talus?

YES ←

Get X-rays. Note: Beyond this point do not attempt treatment without professional supervision.

Have the athlete keep the ankle elevated and on ice for 24-48 hours and stay off the foot for one week.

The patient has a major or complete tear. →

Refer for surgical evaluation.

Wrap the ankle in figure-eight style with a 3-inch-wide elastic bandage, to be rewound and tightened three times a day until the swelling has receded. Applied so it will support the injured area.

If the athlete has pain with weight bearing, as soon as possible get him to a quiet place and begin the examination.

After one week, have the athlete soak his ankle in warm water for 20 minutes 3-4 times a day. Each soaking should be followed by dorsiflexion, plantar flexion, inversion, and eversion exercises with leg elevated.

This chart is modified from the Patient Care Flow-Chart Service, Copyright Miller and Fink Corporation, Darien, Connecticut. All Rights Reserved. Reprinted and adapted with permission from the publisher.

When the ankle is sufficiently stable, begin whirlpool massage, friction and stroking massage, and progressive active and passive range-of-motion exercises.

In the second week of physical therapy, prescribe progressive resistive exercises using a drop-foot boot to build up the ankle.

Follow the athlete for 3-6 weeks until he has regained the full range-of-ankle motion. He is fully rehabilitated when he has the same strength and flexibility as the uninjured side.

A thorough biomechanical workup is necessary to determine if there are any deformities contributing to the frequency of sprains. If the answer is yes, correcting the deforming force with the use of orthotic devices with a rearfoot post to properly balance the foot should reduce the chance of future sprains.

Patients that have extremely flexible and elastic joints also have a greater tendency toward ankle sprains. In these cases, the ligaments are so able to stretch that even moderate forces can cause the ankles to give way. Once an ankle is sprained it is never as strong as before the injury. The once-healthy ligaments are replaced with scar tissue which possesses a lesser ability to withstand the forces of body weight. The result is a greater tendency toward future sprains. If measures are not taken to obtain stability through ankle taping, orthotic use or surgery, recurrent sprains will plague the athlete throughout his active life.

Surgery for the acute ankle sprain requires tying the disrupted ligaments back together. The procedure itself is not difficult, but the rehabilitation time required to achieve adequate ankle motion is quite lengthly. On the other hand, if the plaster casting technique is used, there is a chance that stability will not be adequate for the damage put to the ankle. There are pros and cons to each medical opinion, but the most important factor is the individual under consideration.

If the athlete is young and has a bright future in sports, he probably deserves the more aggressive repair to achieve maximum stability. If the patient is not extremely active, plaster casting usually will suffice. Surgery for the "chronic" ankle involves rerouting adjacent tendons to support the ankle joint. This procedure is indicated for the patient who has recurrent swelling and pain with sports activity.

Dr. Hirata does not recommend surgery for the athlete with instability associated with an increased range of motion but no associated pain. He prefers to tape the athlete before each practice or game. In this way, the athlete functions quite normally and avoids the convalescent period involved with surgery.

So, generally speaking, surgery is reserved for the more severe acute ankle injuries of the young athlete, or those athletes troubled with chronic pain and aggravation following a history of

218

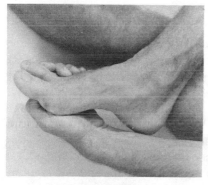
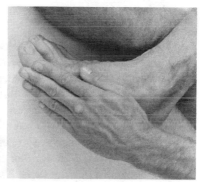
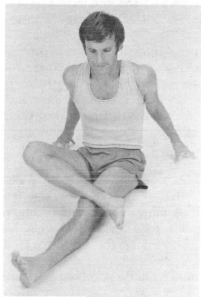

To help rehabilitate an injured ankle, exercise it through the full range of motion.

severe ankle trauma. If surgery is a last-ditch effort for weak ankles, what then are the alternatives?

Ankle taping is a very good way to achieve additional support for the weak ankle ligaments. The tape functions as an external ligament and restricts extreme ranges of motion. The tape is placed in a special manner around the ankle so as to prevent the heel from maximally inverting. Taping is usually best done by a physician or trainer who has a good working knowledge of the anatomy. However, the athlete can learn basic pre-game taping if these personnel are not available.

When taping the foot or ankle, the foot should be in an over-corrected position to allow for the normal "give" that occurs with all types of tape. For example, if you wish to prevent inversion sprains or hold the foot in a neutral position with a Low-Dye Strap, don't tape in the relaxed foot attitude, but hold the foot at a right angle to the leg and invert the heel a little so when the tape loosens a moderate amount of restriction will still be maintained.

Whenever taping, remember not to pull or cinch up on the tape and to avoid folds in the tape. Tape should be applied with a minimal amount of tension. If tape is applied too snuggly, this will cause pain on motion from the binding effect, and can compress nerves and blood vessels.

There are a few drawbacks to using tape for pre-game prevention. It takes someone trained in taping to apply it, and treatment requires a few minutes of time. The greatest physical drawback to taping for injuries is the fact that stretching and loss of adherence decreases its ability to properly support the involved part. Good functional control from taping is said to diminish after only 10-15 minutes of active use. Therefore, it is important to moderately over-correct with your tape.

Taping for ankles has proven to be effective over extended periods of time by the mere fact that it restricts the last few degrees of motion at the ankle that might have caused injury. Also, the pull of the tape on the skin tells the athlete when his ankle is starting to "go."

Plastic orthotic devices have been beneficial in reducing ankle sprains in a number of athletes. Ankle stability is gained by reducing abnormal torques in the foot that may be twisting the foot toward a potential sprain and by using a wide rearfoot post that prevents the heel bone from turning in or out.

Semi-rigid or soft leather appliances do not effectively work to prevent inversion ankle sprains as there is no firm platform to prevent heel twisting.

TARSAL TUNNEL SYNDROME

Tarsal tunnel syndrome in the ankle is similar to the carpal tunnel syndrome in the wrist, where many structures pass through a small space. This puts pressure on the nerve.

The classical tarsal syndrome is not an overuse injury. It occurs on the inside of the ankle where abnormally tight ligaments or possibly scar tissue from a previous injury binds down the underlying nerve. The compressed nerve relays a tingling or needles-and-pins sensation either locally or into the foot along the inside of the arch. This ailment usually requires surgery if pain persists after conservative attempts to relieve localized swelling or pressure have failed.

The tarsal tunnel syndrome that occurs in conjunction with athletic participation (usually endurance sports) is clearly overuse in nature and more apt to occur with a pronated foot type. Other causes may be localized trauma or tendonitis around the inside of the ankle. The nerve compression, therefore, results from either external or internal pressures. If an athlete has a foot type requiring a large amount of heel eversion motion, such as a rearfoot varus, forefoot varus or an equinus, the movement stretches the attaching ligament with every step. This action irritates and compresses the underlying nerve. If swelling occurs around the ankle for any reason, the pressure in this closed space will rise with a similar consequence.

Symptoms of this condition are numbness, burning or tingling sensations on the inside of the arch and bottom of the foot. Tenderness may be present over the tarsal tunnel region, just below and behind the ankle joint. Tapping the invoved area may elicit a similar sensation either locally or in the foot. This is called Tinel's sign, where there are nerve sensations from the point of compression along the course of the nerve.

Treatment begins by determining the causative factor. An athlete's history might bring forth a past incident which may have initiated the current injury. More important with athletes is a thorough biomechanical evaluation to rule out any foot abnormality.

If an abnormality is present, rigid orthoses are necessary to prevent the heel from everting, thereby reducing the stretching or tightness of the tarsal tunnel. The orthotic device grasps the heel bone and, with the addition of a rear platform or post, only allows the heel to move to the amount necessary for normal function. This heel control is necessary in preventing the foot from prona-

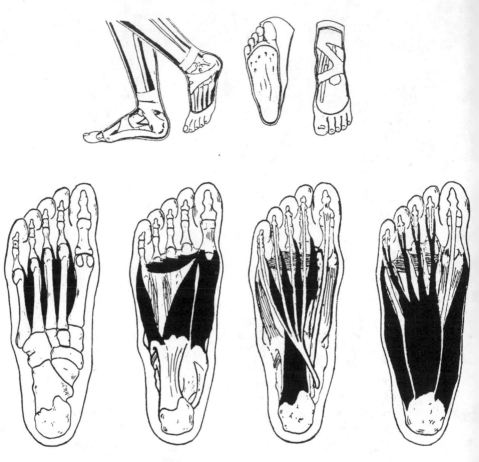

Fascia and muscles of the foot.

ting, and is the main difference between an orthoses and an arch support which attempts to hold up the arch farther out on the foot. Initial attempts should be made with tape strapping or varus heel pads in the shoes to see if any benefit is gained. Consider using a Sports Wedge. Reversal of symptoms may take weeks.

FASCIA PROBLEMS

Fascia is a specialized connective tissue that protects, separates structures and keeps things in place. Superficial fascia is soft and flexibile and it makes up most of the connective tissue and fat in the protective layers of the body. Scar tissue disturbs the normal function of superficial fascia. Deep fascia has several forms, and serves as a protective and separating material between muscles and muscle groups, and may form firm specialized bands like ligaments.

Problems can arise when fascia is too tight or too loose. Not much is known about these conditions, but they are playing an increased part in our understanding of athletic injuries. Fascia is distributed throughout the body, but the areas of concern for us are around the bottom of the foot, the ankle and the leg.

Recognition of a problem is the first step toward treatment. Problems of fascia are often mistaken for other things. For example, a disturbance of the plantar fascia is often mistaken as the heel spur syndrome; problems of the Y-shaped "ligament" around the ankle are often mistaken for tendonitis or stress fracture; problems of fascia around the leg are often called shin splints, and problems of fascia behind the knee are often mistaken as hamstring muscle injuries.

In effect, fascia is like a tight body stocking. For instance, although there is no muscle extending the full distance, while the knee is held straight and the hip is flexed, the range of dorsiflexion at the *ankle* decreases. This is because the fascia restricts the motion. The so-called tight- or loose-jointed people are those with connective tissue differences and differences in fascia.

Superficial fascia is pretty well determined by inherited body type. Some people have soft protective fat layers, and some are lean and bony. Fat distribution varies with individuals. A person may be overweight and still have thin feet, and vice versa. This is why weight is not a factor in friction lesions on the feet. People with thin or very mobile fascia need additional protection. If you can feel the bones through the skin on the bottom of the foot, you need a cushioned insole.

Deep fascia functions along with muscles, tendons and joints. At points of major tendon movement, the fascia is thick. Where there is little movement, it is thin. There are specialized areas where the fascia is especially thick and specialized, and these have been given particular names, such as in front of the ankle where it is called the Y-shaped ligament. (It is not actually a ligament, which is a specialized tissue, but because it is thick and firm it has the appearance of a ligament.)

223

The Y-ligament or talo-crural (foot-leg) fascia holds the extensor tendons down, for maximum efficiency in an upward movement of the foot and toes. With the beginning of an exercise program, many people experience a tight or swollen feeling in front of the ankle, like a constricting band. This occasionally will produce a transient numbness on the top of the foot which often is mistaken for other, more serious problems. It can be prevented by proper warmup (flexibility) exercises before activity, by active massage during the symptoms and by warm, moist packs if the symptoms remain after activity. With the initial stages of training activity, there is some swelling of the tendons. In the presence of the firm, constricting fascia, there is pressure with nowhere for the swelling to go. The fluids must be mobilized in order to relieve this pressure. This phenomenon is usually present during the first 2-3 weeks of activity or a new event.

Loose fascia is another problem which often goes unrecognized. For those people with this condition, balance and stability are difficult. Many times, this shows as frequent tripping, falling and general clumsiness, with cracking or popping sensations and sounds like a "cracked knuckle." This is not serious, but it is disturbing. The sound is produced by movement of tendons snapping on each other or over joints. It can be eliminated by firm strapping support or stretch anklet supports.

With long-term conditioning, there is some decrease in this problem because of fibrosis, but in general these people will not do well in contact sports or those where fine movement and balance is essential, such as ballet or gymnastics. On the other hand, this is exactly the type of activity they need to resolve the problem. In order to excel at this type of sport, they will have to over-condition themselves in other areas, namely strength and endurance. This factor should be respected by the coaches and trainers who should tailor a special conditioning program for each member of the team. These patients should be more concerned with strength than flexibility.

224

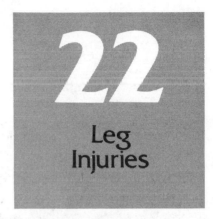

22
Leg Injuries

A quick review of few anatomical considerations of the leg will reacquaint you with the terminology to follow. The leg is that region lying below the knee joint and above the ankle joint. The leg is supported by two long bones. The tibia, which is the larger of the two, lies in the front of the leg and bears 90% of the weight transmitted through the extremity. The fibula lies lateral to the tibia and supports the remaining 10% of body weight.

The front border of the tibia can be felt all along its course from the knee to the ankle and is commonly called the shin bone. The lowest end of the tibia forms the medial side of the ankle joint and can be felt as a bony prominence called the medial malleolus. The top portion of the fibula can be felt as a bony protruberance just below the knee joint on the lateral side. The fibula also ends in a bony prominence called the lateral malleolus which forms the opposite side of the ankle joint.

The leg is divided into four muscular compartments. The front or anterior compartment houses the muscles responsible for raising the foot on the leg, the extensor muscles. The lateral compartment lies on the outside of the leg and contains those muscles largely responsible for pulling the foot away from the midline of the body (foot abduction), the peroneals. These muscles also function in supporting the ankle. The posterior compartment contains the calf muscles which are responsible for foot plantarflexion or that movement of the foot allowing us to stand on our toes. The deep posterior group contains the muscles responsible for flexing the toes and the posterior tibial muscle which helps maintain the arch of the foot.

So the leg unit consists of large muscles originating from either of two leg bones to exert their forces on the foot below. In a simplistic sense, most injuries in the leg stem from some irritating force to the muscles themselves.

THE OVERUSE COMPARTMENT SYNDROME

Each group of muscles is covered by fascia and is separated from the other groups. The overuse compartment syndrome of the leg occurs after unaccustomed sports participation and is most frequently experienced as a dull ache in either the anterior or lateral leg compartments. The ache is generalized within the entire leg compartment rather than being localized to a specific area. The cause of pain is excessive pressure in an unyielding compartment.

The leg compartments have little room for expansion, as each contains large muscle bellies. When muscle swelling occurs with exertion, it produces a sensation of fullness in the compartment, and if severe enough it can compress the small arteries supplying the muscles to cause a cramping sensation. Muscles that are in spasm to splint a painful ankle or foot can create a compartment syndrome as well. The pain associated with an overuse compartment syndrome usually begins within a few hours following vigorous sports activity. Pain can vary from a mild muscular soreness to an intolerable cramp made worse by bearing weight on the limb. This severe type, if not treated, can cause muscle and nerve damage.

Initial treatment should include ice massage and elevation. If symptoms warrant, remain non-weight-bearing with the extremity elevated until pain subsides. Continually monitor the pressure within the involved compartment by pressing on it manually. If pain is co-existent with marked firmness, seek medical attention at once. If a direct blow has occurred to the leg, causing the above symptoms of extreme pain and firmness, seek medical attention. A large, bleeding vessel can create substantial pressure to cause irreversible nerve damage if not treated at once. This condition is the classical anterior compartment syndrome, but is rarely seen without the history of a severe blow.

Self-treatment of ice and elevation should effectively reverse the swelling and pain within 24-48 hours. Most importantly, consider the causative factors and alter training to avoid recurrence. If ankle or instep pain is co-existent with lateral compartment pain, consider muscle spasm as a possibility. In this case, treat as directed and seek professional help.

Another frequent cause of the compartment syndrome is muscular overuse secondary to a mechanical fault or weakness of the foot. For that very reason we often see the overuse compartment syndrome as a forerunner of overuse injuries such as tendonitis and shin splints, which have similar causes. The compartment syndrome is an early warning of things to come.

Preventive treatment involves muscle flexibility and strengthening exercises to prevent acute reactions to overstress. If a mechanical weakness is predisposing a muscle group to early fatigue, orthotic devices can give these muscles a more favorable mechanical advantage through neutral foot control.

SHIN SPLINTS

The term shin splints is non-specific, but it is generally accepted to mean any pain in the lower leg brought on by activity. The Standard Nomenclature of Athletic Injuries written by the American Medical Association defines shin splints as "pain and discomfort in the leg from repetitive running on hard surfaces or forceable use of foot flexors; diagnosis should be limited to musculotendonitis inflammations, excluding fatigue (stress) fracture or ischemic (compartment syndrome) disorders."

The term is collectively used to designate any aching pain in the lower leg. It can occur in any sport and is usually associated with an untrained or unconditioned athlete, a change in footwear, an increase in jumping, a change in events or a change to a hard playing surface. Common sports associated with shin splints are running, football, basketball, hiking or forced marching. This type of injury usually occurs early in the season, so it is important that the athlete not push himself too much, too soon.

Shin splints usually refer to an overuse injury in which the leg muscles are microscopically pulled away from their bony attachment on the tibia, or there is pain within the muscle compartment itself. Shin splints can occur in two major areas, either in the front of the leg with pain down the outside (lateral) border of the shin bone, or in the medial side of the leg with associated pain under the tibia's inside border. These two areas respond differently to treatment so must be considered individually.

Anterior shin splints, in the front of the leg, occur secondary to a pulling action of the muscle responsible for raising the foot in relation to the leg (anterior tibial muscle). The cause here is most simply stated as one of overuse and can be attributed to predominantly one of the three following reasons: (1) muscular imbalance; (2) running on hard surfaces, and (3) pronated or flat feet. As in previous injuries, once we find the cause, the treatment is clear.

With anterior shin splints there is an imbalance occurring between the front or anterior muscles of the leg and the calf muscles in the back of the leg. The tendency toward tight calves in athletes is very common. The resulting imbalance tends to pull the foot downward (in plantarflexion). The equilibrium between muscles is lost, and the anterior foot lifting muscles must continually overwork to raise the foot during gait.

Running on hard surfaces such as concrete causes a jarring effect with every heel strike. To dampen this sudden insult, the anterior muscles tense up to splint the foot in preparation for the jolt and then gradually relax to lower the entire foot to the ground. The result again is muscular overuse.

Shin splints secondary to the flat foot is very frequently seen. The flat foot, when bearing weight, has a lesser amount of bony stability because the foot bones and joints are not aligned in their neutral or desired position. Therefore, instead of propelling from a stable bony formation, the muscles must work in an unconscious coordinated effort to stabilize the weak bony framework. Premature muscle fatigue and overuse are the results. This instability could be likened to one running across a mudslick. In this case, as with an unstable foot, one raises the foot rather than propelling forcefully from the toes because the underlying surface is unsteady.

The pain from anterior as well as posterior shin splints is initially felt as a tightness occurring after prolonged use. As the condition worsens, the pain may be present during normal activities or

228

in the absence of weight-bearing. Running a finger down the tibia usually elicits some tenderness. As the condition becomes more chronic in nature, numerous small lumps may be felt along the tibia border.

Treatment involves ice massage to the inflamed muscle to relieve inflammation and pressure as soon as pain is experienced. Workouts should be limited to pain tolerance and carried out on grass or soft surfaces to avoid an abrupt heel contact. Ice massage is particularly important after exercise when muscle swelling is the greatest. After the acute phase of injury, the anterior muscles should be exercised to overcome a possible muscular imbalance with the calf muscles.

Temporary, soft insoles should be constructed to lessen the shock of heel contact and to stabilize the foot. This usually involves a quarter inch heel lift and mild varus tilt. An orthotic device which provides neutral foot control should prevent the future development of shin splints so long as the training methods are not contributing to the problem. With foot control, the muscles that lift the foot need not work out of phase to help support the propelling foot. The stability and force is gained through properly stabilized joints and bones.

The second type of shin splints occurs in the posterior compartment or back of the leg and is called posterior shin splints. This can be caused by any of the deep muscles of the leg, especially the toe flexors and the muscle responsible for maintaining the arch of the foot (posterior tibial muscle). These muscles originate in the leg and then course around the inside of the ankle bones to enter the underside of the foot. As the muscle tendons swing around the ankle, they form a tunnel-like structure with bone making up the floor of the tunnel. This bend around the ankle works as a fulcrum so the muscle tendons have a greater mechanical advantage into the foot.

With the exception of very subtle foot deformities predisposing one toward posterior shin splints, we find simple foot pronation as being the most obvious cause. When the excessively pronated foot bears weight in activity, the inside arch flattens out. The flattening process overpowers the pull of the muscles coursing around the ankle, and the stretch is transmitted into the leg where the

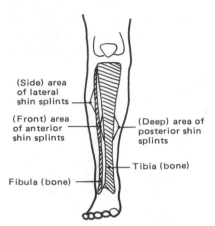

(Side) area
of lateral
shin splints

(Front) area
of anterior
shin splints

(Deep) area of
posterior shin
splints

Tibia (bone)

Fibula (bone)

Areas of the leg in which shin splints occur.

muscles attach to the leg bones. The posterior tendons involved have a limited ability to withstand this continued stretching above and beyond their normal function. The fatigue will either appear as tendonitis in the lower leg or ankle or shin splints near the muscle origin.

Treatment for "medial posterior" shin splints is much like anterior shin splints in its acute phase. Use ice before and after workouts, and before bedtime if necessary. Modify workouts to pain tolerance. Do not attempt to run through the pain. Orthotic devices reduce pronatory tendencies, including medial arch support and metatarsal pads. Muscle exercises increase strength and maintain flexibility in the injured muscle.

Another cause of posterior shin splints involving the toe flexors is overuse of the normal function of toe flexion. With certain foot deformities, the toes grasp more powerfully than is necessary with normal foot function. The reason is usually secondary to foot pronation but the problem can arise from other sources as well. If the toe flexor muscles seem to be involved, try to limit toe flexion, thereby decreasing the distance of tendon excursion. This is done by placing specially tailored felt to a similar device called a crest under the toes where they meet the ball of the foot. This lets the toes have something to grasp during gait.

In considering shin splints in general, we find the cause is usually muscular overuse (under-condition). Muscle overuse is generally secondary to a foot imbalance which necessitates greater muscle activity to compensate for the inherent weakness. The muscle, unaccustomed to the strain, fatigues—in this case, at its origin on one of the leg bones—ultimately to set up the classical inflammation which we know as shin splints.

STRESS FRACTURES

Stress fractures of the tibia and fibula are frequently seen in endurance sports. Their treatment is usually by means of plaster casting which is out of the realm of this book. We present the symptoms, however, to emphasize the fact that they are too frequently mistaken for soft-tissue injuries by the athlete.

Stress fractures can occur nearly anywhere on the two leg bones. There is no history of trauma and no audible crack or snap heard. Pain usually comes on after a period of activity and grows more severe with training. Pain is sensed as deep beneath the skin, with pressure on the bone and usually sharply with activity.

The most common interpretation of this type of pain is shin splints with a large component of bone involvement (periostitis). The pain of a stress fracture is commonly in the same general areas as shin splints. Diagnosis can only be made by means of x-ray, and x-rays are often negative for 3-4 weeks until the minute crack has condensed within the bone matrix and the bone bruise has begun to ossify. Therefore, pain in the leg giving similar symptoms as those presented above and not responding to shin splint treatment should be worked up medically to rule out the possibility of a stress fracture.

Certain activities, such as running tight figure eights or on a banked track, may bring on shin splints. As with stress fractures in the foot, the needs of the activity exceed the ability of the bone to handle stress. Following the healing process, the area of the fracture is stronger than it was prior to the injury. During healing, the athlete is advised to continue non-traumatic activities, such as cycling, flexibility and upper-body strengthening. Return from a stress fracture to full activity must be a gradual process.

23

Knee
Injuries

At the beginning of this chapter, we feel we should clarify why a podiatrist is writing on knee injuries. First, this section is limited to only overuse injuries of the knee; traumatic injuries of the knee are out of our field. In any condition where there is swelling, locking, giving way or limited motion of the knee, it is important that athlete be examined by an orthopedist.

What then comprises an overuse injury to the knee? This can be defined as any injury occurring around the knee joint, caused by repetitive microtrauma from normal sports participation. Any injury involving a direct blow would not fit within this category. We stress the word repetitive, meaning injuries resulting from over-extended use of the lower extremities. Adjectives often used describing this condition include: runner's knee, jumper's knee, tennis knee and hiker's knee. So this condition is quite common and, though seldom requiring surgery, can be chronically debilitating.

It is surprising to find that very little has been written on overuse injuries to the knee. It is obvious by reading the treatment objectives that very few observers have ever taken into consideration the body dynamics causing this overuse state. The American Academy of Podiatric Sports Medicine, since its inception, has been quite successful in disseminating information regarding the dynamic faults of the feet that predispose one toward knee injuries. It is through this rationale of treatment that many podiatrists have been having extraordinary results in the treatment of knee problems. Many cases of chronic knee pain are finding relief through appropriate biomechanical treatment.

The knee joint is the largest joint in the body and by itself functions solely in the production of forward acceleration. This is an extremely important concept to remember when considering knee injuries. Any motion other than straight ahead (sagittal plane) motion occurring within the knee joint is abnormal and can result in damage (this will be clearly explained later).

Think of the knee joint as the back wheel of a bicycle. The back wheel by itself has no capability of changing direction. The only way in which the bike can turn is through the combined effort of turning the front wheel and banking the turn with the entire bicycle. The human analogy to the front wheel is the hip joint. The hip joint changes body direction as the entire body tilts to adjust the center of gravity.

The anatomy of the knee joint in its entirety is complex. A basic understanding of the functional components involved in overuse injuries, however, is easily digested and necessary in the understanding of overuse syndromes. The knee joint is primarily made up of two bones, the thigh bone or femur and the larger of the leg bones, the tibia. Both bones are long and slender, but the ends that comprise the knee joint are enlarged, creating a greater surface to enhance stability.

The knee joint is not a ball-and-socket joint like the shoulder or hip, as this type of joint would allow unlimited motion. Instead, the knee can be thought of as two ball-and-socket joints in one. The femur ends in two ball ends (chondyles) side by side, and the tibial counterpart consists of two sockets side by side. They are cushioned by joint fluid and specialized cartilage, the medial and lateral meniscus (menisci). As long as all four parts of the joint are closely approximated, as they are in the living knee, motion can only occur in one direction. It is when forces are placed on the knee in other directions that injury to the supporting soft tissues occur.

The major soft tissues responsible for knee support are ligaments and muscles. It should be realized that the majority of force going through the normal knee is compression, which actually holds the joint in place. Therefore, soft tissues are more for secondary stabilization than for primary support. The major muscles responsible for knee stability are the quadriceps in the front of the thigh bone. This muscle group inserts into the kneecap, which in turn inserts into the tibia via a strong tendon called the patellar tendon.

The patella functions as a free-moving pulley to increase the efficiency of the quadriceps muscle as it crosses the knee joint. The patella is involved in a variety of overuse injuries. The quadriceps muscle functions to extend the knee joint and when flexed helps prevent any rotary or twisting motion. The hamstring muscles in the back of the thigh function in knee flexion and also help prevent twisting motions at the knee.

Four major muscles cross the medial and lateral sides of the knee joint. Three of these insert on the medial side and together are called the pes anserinus ("goose foot"). One called the biceps femoris inserts on the lateral side. These muscles help restrict side to side motion but can be prone to tendonitis with overuse states. They are collectively called the hamstrings (the muscles by which butchers hang meat on racks). All of these muscles, therefore, help keep the joint in its proper alignment by the pulling force they exert when crossing the knee joint.

The knee ligaments are even more important for maintaining knee alignment. The collateral ligaments are very strong and prevents sideways motion. There is one major ligament on either side of the joint, both medial and lateral. These ligaments are inelastic and tear if forces exceed their supporting limits. Unlike the medial side of the knee joint, the lateral side has additional ligamentous support.

A thick ligament called the iliotibial band extends down from the hip on the lateral side of the thigh and inserts across the knee joint. This added strength on the lateral side of the knee joint accounts for the fact that most ligament injuries occur on the medial side.

Within the interior of the joint, there are two more ligaments. One (the anterior cruciate) prevents forward dislocation of the joint while the other (posterior cruciate) prevents backward displacement. These two ligaments are vitally important in maintaining stability of the knee joint but are seldom involved in overuse injuries. Another structure often damaged in traumatic injuries is the meniscus (sometimes incorrectly called the knee cartilage). The menisci function like intervertebral discs to dissipate compressional forces coming through the knee joint. These structures are also seldom involved with primary overuse injuries to the knee.

The knee joint, although the focus of many athletic injuries, is seldom responsible for initiating the cause. Unlike the foot, most knees are indeed normal, but when continually subjected to abnormal stress they break down with fatigue. Therefore, when confronted with an overuse injury of the knee, look to the distal cause rather than the actual site of injury.

At a recent podiatric sports seminar George Sheehan, M.D., presented a lecture entitled, "How to Treat Runners Knee." In this lecture he began by saying, "I'm not going to keep you in suspense; you treat the foot."

This is the plan of attack we have found most beneficial. The most common foot problem predisposing an athlete to overuse injuries of the knee is abnormal pronation. Minor rotational changes in the leg and thigh occur with abnormal foot pronation. This twisting, when multiplied thousands of times with sports participation, can result in injuries to the knee. Therefore, before considering specific injury states, you may rightly guess that by preventing excessive pronation you will be reversing the distal injury process.

Clinically, we find that the overuse problems around the patella respond very well to balancing orthotic devices. Treatment of those problems around the joint line, or posterior to the knee joint meets with varied success, approximately 50%. We find that most medial anterior knee pains, especially under the patella, are associated with mobile, flexible foot types, and lateral knee pains are associated with the more rigid inflexible foot types with limited motion and increased shock up the extremity from the ground.

In those cases that do not respond to balancing devices, it is necessary to work along with the coach, trainer and orthopedist to design specific rehabilitation programs or corrective procedures. It is important to point out that, depending on severity and degree of damage, not all overuse problems can be reversed, and many must be rested. This is the last thing the athlete and coach want to hear.

In our podiatric practices, if the athlete does not respond to mechanical balancing devices very quickly, we consult with the orthopedist or personal physician. We clearly explain to the athlete that we are not authorities on knees, hips and low backs.

It is interesting to mention that we see a higher incidence of knee overuse injuries in women athletes than in men. This is because the relative width of the hips increases the angle of incidence from the femur into the knee joint. Also, in most cases these women do not have the years of conditioning upon entering the sport as their male counterparts.

RUNNER'S KNEE

The medical term for runner's knee is chondromalacia of the patella, with irritation and erosion of the undersurface of the knee-cap. Chondromalacia means "softening of the cartilage." Dr. George Sheehan states that out of a 1000-runner survey, some 17% stated they had suffered from runner's knee at some point in their running program. Although the strict definition of runner's knee only pertains to kneecap pain, it can also involve a host of ligament and tendon strains brought on by the act of running. Probably, a fair portion of the runners surveyed in this study suffered from the latter afflictions as well as chondromalacia.

The classical pain from runner's knee is felt under the kneecap. Pain usually is first noticed when running down hills or walking stairs. In these instances, the flexed knee puts additional pressure on the damaged kneecap. With more serious conditions, pain may be present when running on flat surfaces. A grating sensation is often felt with knee motion, and stiffness around the knee may occur after periods of rest.

Two simple tests may help in your knee evaluation: First, squat down with your knees flexed. If pain is present around your knee caps be suspicious. Next, sit down with your legs out straight and apply pressure on the kneecap with your hand. Contract the quadriceps muscle (straight leg raise) and allow the kneecap to slowly move under pressure.If you feel a grating sensation and pain, be particularly suspicious.

236

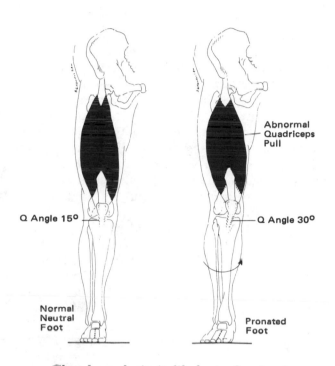

Abnormal
Quadriceps
Pull

Q Angle 15°

Q Angle 30°

Normal
Neutral
Foot

Pronated
Foot

Chondromalacia is likely to develop in the leg at right as a result of the pronated foot.

A functional look at the cause of chondromalacia allows a clearer understanding of the treatment objectives. The underside of the patella is V-shaped and fits into a similarly shaped groove in the femur. When the knee flexes ares extends, the firmly suspended patella moves down and up the femur in response to muscle activitiy. When the foot pronates, the leg rotates internally. This causes the suspended patella to ride on the shelf of the femoral chondyles, leading to erosion of the undersurface and pain.

Initial treatment involves reducing the existing training schedule to the level of pain tolerance and especially avoiding hills. If hills are unavoidable, either jog slowly or walk them. We often advise "quiet running" to eliminate the vertical forces as much as possible. Swelling is sometimes present and should be

237

treated with the ice method when necessary. In addition, aspirin can be used in conjunction to help reduce inflammation. Remember that aspirin is a systemic anti-inflammatory medication as much as a pain reliever.

Strengthening exercises for the quadriceps should begin at once. Good muscle strength is necessary to help prevent lateral drift of the patella. Do not do quadriceps exercises that involve flexing the knee beyond 90 degrees, as this may aggravate the problem. Start with straight leg raises, first without weight, for 10 repetitions (without pain) and then using sand bags or a similar device to weight the legs up to about 10 pounds. Progressive resistance exercises or isokinetic exercises can then follow, but knee movement should always be slow and not jerky.

Abnormal foot pronation should be corrected with orthotic devices. You can make a temporary soft orthotic yourself by using a medial arch pad and a varus heel pad. If this plan does not bring results in two weeks, consult a sports podiatrist about functional plastic orthoses. This modality is quite successful in conjunction with the other measures listed.

Future training should be carried out on relatively flat surfaces. Avoid running on roads that are noticeably crowned for water runoff, as this will cause even a normal foot to abnormally pronate on the higher side. If roads of this nature are unavoidable, keep the bad knee farthest away from the center line. Avoid running on beaches that are banked, as this will aggravate knees in the same manner.

INJURIES TO KNEE LIGAMENTS AND TENDONS

Let's consider ligament strains and tendonitis so often associated with the overused knee. The triad of chondromalacia, tendonitis and ligament strain can all be seen in the runners knee syndrome. Strains and tendonitis of the knee, however, tend to be more prevalent in sports requiring quick foot movement but less repetition than that of long-distance running. This higher incidence of strains is due to the frequent changing of directions which puts a greater twisting force on the knee. This type of overuse injury tends to emerge earlier in sports that require greater percentage of unnatural body motions.

Why do knee ligaments and tendons fatigue and become irritated in the face of increased activity? Three basic factors which are all responsible to some degree in overuse injuries to the knee are: (1) lack of proper conditioning in preparation for the activity; (2) unnatural activity leading to unnatural stresses; (3) inherent musculoskeletal weakness. These factors should be kept in mind as preventive treatment differs depending on the original cause.

When vigorous activity is attempted without preparation, the muscles are too weak to stabilize and coordinate knee motion effectively. This puts excessive stress on the muscle tendons and ligaments that are responsible for maintaining joint stability. This overstretching results in fatigue and damage to the soft-tissue structures. Pain can be experienced on either the medial or lateral sides of the knee as well, as above or below the kneecap. Except for a small difference in location, it is often difficult to differentiate between ligament strain and tendonitis of the knee. However, treatment for both conditions involves having adequate preparation for the activity.

Little needs to be said about point two other than that the further a sports activity deviates away from natural body movements, the greater the likelihood of sustaining injury. If we placed distance running and contact sports at either end of a graph, and plotted overuse injuries vs. traumatic injuries, we would see that as we approach contact sports overuse injuries would decline in frequency as traumatic injuries increased. So keep the sport in mind when considering treatment of knee injuries. For example, tendonitis of the knee in a rugby player is less likely to respond to postural correction than that of a long-distance runner. Little can be done to change the activities required in a sport to meet one's particular needs, but a more thorough conditioning program prior to serious participation will allow the supporting elements of the knee more time to adapt to the increased load.

Musculoskeletal weaknesses in the feet and legs are major contributors to overuse knee injuries. When faulty foot mechanics throw the leg and thigh bones out of alignment with every step, the supporting tissues cannot be expected to maintain stability in the face of vigorous activity without some signs of fatigue. A review of the self-evaluation of the feet and legs may help you in determining if you have any biomechanical weakness in the knee.

Treatment for tendonitis and strained ligaments of the knee involves these basic measures: (1) treat acute stages of injury; (2) cut back on activity to allow healing; (3) substitute non-traumatic aerobic activities to maintain condition; (4) rehabilitate as needed to prevent recurrences.

The acute stages of this type of knee injury usually appear with localized pain on weight bearing. Most frequently, the pain is only present after some period of vigorous activity. If swelling is present, the pain is often longer lasting. Cut back on your activity, particularly the first week, using the emergence of any pain as a signal to stop.

We usually recommend a temporary layoff, then progressive resistance (strengthening) exercises of the major thigh muscles and then a be done without pain, jogging in a figure-eight pattern can be attempted. A progressive program of jogging will allow the previously damaged tissues time to adapt to the increased load asked of them.

Quadriceps strengthening exercises are particularly important, so that resumption of activity finds the stabilizing muscles ready to accept the stress. Appropriate flexibility exercises are important during periods of rehabilitation. Massage the painful area with ice for 10-15 minutes after activity to suppress inflammation. Ice again before bedtime if pain is present. Aspirin may be of help in reducing inflammation. Elastic knee braces may be purchased at a drugstore and used during periods of activity. They do little to stabilize the knee but offer localized compression. If foot abnormalities are suspected, construct a soft orthotic device using a Spenco insole or a Dr. Scholl's arch support as a base, and apply a varus heel pad and an additional medial arch pad to help maintain the foot around the neutral position.

JUMPER'S KNEE

Jumper's knee is a tendonitis of the quadriceps tendon as it attaches to the kneecap or as the patellar tendon inserts into the leg bone. This condition is the same as that previously discussed

240

regarding tendonitis, but is brought on by the specific act of jumping. The fast knee flexion and then propulsive extension necessary to gain vertical height in a basketball or volleyball player puts a great deal of stress on the quadriceps muscle and inserting tendon. The impact of landing also requires great strength in the quadiceps and patellar tendons to avoid knee collapse. With continuous jumping, the tendon begins to fatigue and tear near its insertion. It's this tearing process that leads to the pain and swelling of jumper's knee.

In moderate cases, pain is usually greatest after activity and may appear either below or above the kneecap. When pain arises, vigorous activity should be discontinued, and athletic participation should be reduced to pain tolerance. Ice massages should be used as with other knee injuries, and exercises, beginning with isometrics, are carried out to strengthen the quadriceps. (Remember to avoid fast knee flexion and extension with these exercises.)

The athlete should be examined to determine if a mechanical malalignment is predisposing him toward this injury. He should be instructed to jump with less vigor while the knee is still growing stronger. Landing should occur on the ball of the feet and with the knees slightly flexed to dissipate the sudden shock.

In the treatment of all overuse knee injuries, it is very important to consider the causative factor or factors and base your treatment regimen along these lines. Be patient with your treatment plan; results are sometimes slow. But consider any reduction of pain as a step in the right direction. Seek professional care when your condition does not respond to self-treatment. The longer you neglect treatment, the harder it is to reverse the injury process.

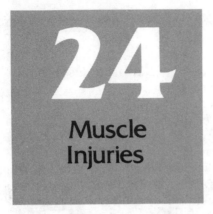

24

Muscle
Injuries

Most muscle injuries in the leg and thigh are primary; that is, not secondary to foot problems or imbalance. Therefore, we do not feel they are within the scope of this book. We mention these major problems only so they can be recognized and treated by the appropriate professional.

The muscle pull, a very common injury, is the result of an actual tear in the muscle. There are degrees of injury, but the tear is usually incomplete, preserving the integrity of a majority of the muscle fibers. It occurs most commonly in those muscles that cross two joints. In the lower extremity, they are the hamstrings and the gastrocnemius.

In general, a weak muscle will tear in its belly and a strong muscle will tear at its insertion. The mechanism of injury is the contraction of the muscle under a heavy load. The muscle becomes overstretched and finally gives way. It is common in those sports where quick, sudden movement is necessary—sprinting, football, hockey, basketball, etc.

When this happens, the muscle gives way and the athlete feels as though he's been hit with a baseball bat. A bulge in the muscle may be evident. If the muscle is strong, warm and well conditioned, the chances of injury are small, so the best prevention is conditioning and flexibility.

Pulls of the hamstring muscles are most common in those events where explosive speed is necessary. The mechanism is that the anterior (quadriceps) muscles are the strong extensors of the

242

Length-Tension Ratio

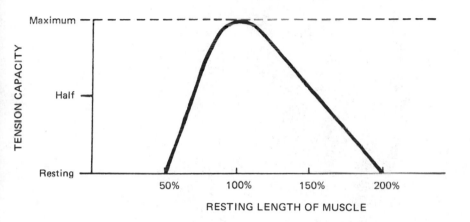

knee in running activities. They become more developed than the posterior compartment (hamstrings). In this situation, aggravated by firm, inelastic muscles and tendons from improper warmup, the hamstrings are overpowered and the pull occurs.

Initial treatment is ICE, the massage, mobility progressive resistance exercises and the gradual return to activity. If there is any scar tissue in the healing process, the muscle pulls can become chronic because of the inelasticity of the muscles.

A charleyhorse is a contusion of the thigh, with bleeding into the muscle. It is beyond the scope of this book, but it must be recognized and treated as soon as possible to prevent disability.

25

Hip
and
Sciatic Nerve

Any sharp, shooting pains around the hip joint, either from the back or down the side of the leg, should be considered as possible nerve compression problem. Seek medical attention as soon as possible. Some sciatic nerve pains and specific low-back pains may be related to posture. With postural improvement, these problems will diminish. Most low-back rehabilitation exercise programs consider the effect on posture.

As described in Chapter Three, as the foot pronates, the leg internally rotates. As this happens, there is a forward (anterior) tilt of the pelvis, and with this anterior tilt, a lumbar lordosis. This cramps the low-back discs of the spine, and stretches and strains muscles around the hip, which can press on the sciatic nerve as it passes under the hip joint. This is now far away from the foot, but with control of excessive pronation it is possible to reverse this process and relieve some low-back and sciatic nerve problems which may be causing pain.

If there is any limb-length discrepancy causing a tilt of the pelvis, or a rotational problem from above or below, causing a twist on the pelvis, these low-back and hip problems can become complicated. In examining the athlete we compare the non-weight-bearing measurements to the stance and gait function to see how much compensation has taken place. We then consider the additional specific braces brought on by the individual event, and attempt reversal of the overuse syndrome. This often brings dramatic reduction of symptoms.

244

HIP INJURIES

Injuries to the hip joint are less common than knee injuries because the hip joint allows motion in all three directions, rather than the single, forward and backward motion of the knee. We limit our comments to overuse injuries of the hip which might be helped by foot treatment.

All injuries of the hip should be examined by a physician. Again, if there is evidence of primary injury such as swelling, locking or giving way, this must be considered a primary joint injury and not related to foot imbalance. If there are recurrent pains brought on systematically with activity, consider the overuse syndrome.

Dr. Donald Johnson of the Sports Medicine Clinic of Carleton University in Ottawa, Canada, has stated, "It must be emphasized that the patient as a whole must be looked at. When one is examining the hip, it is important to look at his feet, to look at his footwear and to ask what type of training he is doing to more accurately diagnose the type of chronic overuse syndrome to his hip."

Balancing of the foot can change the rotation of the femur within the hip joint. We do not mean to imply that foot balancing will help all overuse problems, but in those cases where a specific lower extremity imbalance is measured non-weight-bearing, and observed in stance and during gait, then orthotic therapy should be considered along with specific rehabilitation of the hip itself. We have been gratified, and often surprised, by our results.

Dr. Johnson has said, "The worry has always been present with runners that long years of training are going to lead to degenerative osteoarthritis of the joints. From a recent study of Finnish long-distance runners, there is felt to be no increase of osteoarthritis with running. It is theorized that the pumping action of the synovial fluid with running nourishes the articular cartilage of the femoral head and acetabulam, and actually prolongs the life of the cartilage. A recent study of the Finnish long-distance runners years after their high performance years, demonstrated that runners had 4% incidence of osteoarthritis of the hips whereas controls or non-runners had 8.7% osteoarthritis of their hips. (The reference for this is the *British Medical Journal*, May 24, 1975.)

245

"However, it is also of interest to note that most of the Finnish and Scandinavian running is done on soft surfaces or fitness trails. This is compared with most of the running done in North America which is done on pavement. I think that it would be well to advise that whenever possible one should run on soft surfaces to avoid the chronic pounding on the roads. To the best of my knowledge, there has been no long-term study done on runners here in North America."

Several other hip problems related to chronic overuse have been observed:

1. *The Snapping Hip.* This is caused by a chronic trochanteric bursitis with thickening of the iliotibial tract. The iliotibial tract then snaps back and forth over the posterior aspect of the trochanter and causes the snapping when the leg is brought from flexion into extension.

Treatment consists of ice, rest, local injection of cortisone, anti-inflammatory medications and stretching exercises. Surgery for the resistant case consists of excision of the bursa and lengthening of the iliotibial tract. (This condition can sometimes be helped by foot balancing.)

2. *Trochanteric Bursitis.* Local pain and tenderness over the greater trochanter is aggravated by running and may be severe enough to limit running. It is important to examine for the short-leg syndrome. It is also important to test with active abduction exercises. There should be no pain on active abduction. If there is, then one is dealing with a chronic muscle strain as opposed to a trochanteric bursitis.

Treatment should be ice massage, oral anti-inflammatory drugs, a heel lift to balance the short leg if necessary, stretching exercises for the iliotibial band, local injections of cortisone and surgery for the resistant case only. This consists of excision of the trochanteric bursa and possibly lengthening the iliotibial tract.

3. *Muscular Strains.* Chronic muscular strain usually occurs in the runner with a chronic overuse syndrome. Examples are gluteus maximus and gluteus medius strains about the hip. These are differentiated from trochanteric bursitis by the pain on active ab-

duction of the hip. The local tenderness is usually somewhat higher than the greater trochanter.

Treatment involves Ultrasound and stretching exercises. Occasionally, injections of cortisone are used into the area.

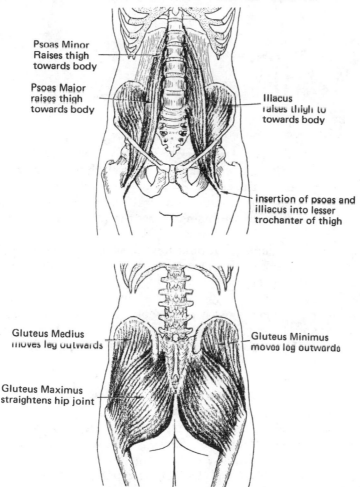

Two views of the hip area, in which a number of injuries can develop.

26

Leg-Length Differences

Consistent low-back strain on one side or recurrent problems on one leg may indicate a difference in leg length. This may come from above or below the pelvis. Problems above the pelvis causing imbalance include congenital structural scoliosis, muscle spasm and many others. The problems below the pelvis may be structural or functional. They may take place at any level—the hip, femur, knee, tibia, ankle, subtalar joint, heel bone or any combination of these. Major discrepancies are noticed at a young age, but the minor ones go unnoticed.

Approximately 80% of symptoms of limb-length discrepancies show up on the short side. Most people have some inherent difference in limb length, and this causes them no problems through normal life. However, in certain endurance activities and those situations where the particular sport requires fine balance or equal leg strength and control, symptoms will begin to show up.

Most of the time limb-length differences go unnoticed. When they are noticed, they are often over-treated. We recommend treatment for only those limb-length differences that are causing symptoms. If we attempt to balance a non-painful situation, we are liable to *produce* problems, especially low-back strain.

In examination for a limb-length discrepancy, review the principles described in Chapter Two. In stance, if one hip is lower than the other, support that side, but if there is any doubt as to where the limb-length difference is, try support on the symptomatic side; 80% of the time you will be correct. As a general rule, begin by supporting half of the measurable difference. In other words, if you suspect a two-centimeter difference, first give a one centimeter of support. Ideally, this should be a full shoe lift, but as a practical matter, it is easier to provide a heel lift. This can be done with a felt pad inside the shoe, building up gradually to one centimeter. If additional support is found necessary, it can be attached to the sole of the shoe itself. The disadvantage of a full shoe lift is the increased weight; the disadvantage of a heel lift alone is that the foot is put into an equinus position, causing a sagittal plane imbalance (you have then changed from a frontal plane tilt to a

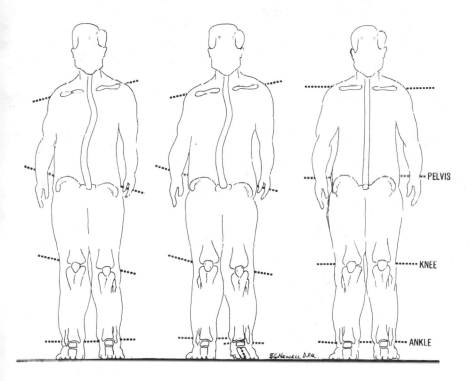

Left: Anatomical short leg. Center: Functional short leg. Right: Legs of equal length.

forward imbalance). You might consider reducing the height of the longer limb by removing layers from the heel of the shoe. A lift can be built into an orthotic device for more comprehensive control.

After the lift is in place, watch the person stand and walk with and without it. Keep him walking for at least five minutes to see if there is significant strain or relief. If there is any increased strain at this time, or during the first two days after its application, remove the lift and seek medical evaluation.

It is very rare to have a pure single-plane osseous abnormality. There are bone and soft-tissue compensations in all three body planes.

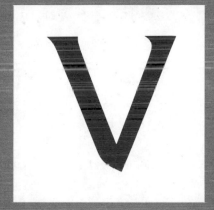

V

CORRECTIVE
METHODS

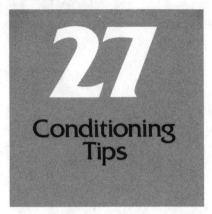

Conditioning
Tips

Athletic performance is based in motivation (desire and attitude), training and conditioning, and inherent structural ability (genetics). This section deals with training, (the use of repetition and practice in the development of skills) and conditioning (the development of the body for strength, endurance and flexibility).

Performance in sports requiring specialized movements can be improved by conditioning specific muscles and joints for strength and flexibility. Movements become more fluid, and therefore more efficient, with training. The athlete gains a level of confidence in his body so that he involuntarily relaxes those muscles which are not necessary for the particular sport (the antogonist muscles). Also through training and conditioning the athlete gains a sense of "where his body is" at all times so that balance and control are improved. For this reason, we emphasize the development of style before the development of speed.

Inherent genetic structure will help or will limit athletes. Some athletes are "natural" to sports, and others must train to reach the same level of skills. Since most tissues of the body can be conditioned, performance improves with time. The rate of conditioning varies with each individual, so that coaches and trainers should respect this fact.

Health can be promoted by educating athletes, coaches and trainers and preventing the "common injuries" which sometimes debilitate the athlete. We also know that the athlete will develop an attitude of self-realization by questioning, seeking answers and learning from his or her very personal experiences. To understand and know yourself is the key. Your body is a sensitive, responsive system. As your training program continues, you will begin to listen to your body which will tell you the things that are good and those that are not.

When studying conditioning, stretching and sports technique, we invariably are studying human motion or kinesiology (since all these activities are based on moving the body or some part of it). When we think of the forces which act on the body to create motion or alter human motion, we are studying biomechanics. We realize that when we study biomechanics or kinesiology, we are observing human motion from an outside or external point of view.

In order to evaluate your own level of conditioning, decide how you will achieve these goals, and keep a record (diary) of your improvement. The intent of the information is to give the reader some idea of what to expect when observing if the athlete is conditioning properly and progressively. It gives exercises which can be used for the purpose of recording the daily progress of the athlete according to the exercises. This performed chart informs the athlete, coach and trainer if there is gradual improvement in the condition of the athlete by the number of reps the athlete performs. Correlated with other data, this can be helpful in determining the status of the conditioning athlete.

For medical reasons, also consider several physical signs. If there is an improvement in the blood pressure—for example, if athlete A began his conditioning program with blood pressure of 155/85, and after weeks of conditioning his blood pressure dropped to 138/80 and levelled off—this would indicate the athlete is gradually conditioning himself. The plateau of blood pressure reading may correlate with the athlete's closeness to peak condition. We know that the normal blood pressure values vary as one gets older, but generally anything above 140 systolic (upper number) and above 90 diastolic (lower number) is considered abnormal. As one gets older, these values get larger, too, so what may be normal values for a younger athlete may not be normal for the older athlete.

Make an individual assessment, meant for the athlete's subjective views on how he "feels." This is a tool for the athlete, coach and trainer to assess how effective the training program has been in conditioning the athlete. It is normal to feel fatigue, pain and stiffness when you begin to workout. But repeated, localized pain or soreness may require examination and treatment.

A fourth area entails the subjective and objective observations of the coaches, trainers or athlete to see if improvement has been made by the athlete.

Hence, this record is a "check and balance" system to inform us of any minor or major change occurring to the athlete. If, for example, we find an athlete who is decreasing in repetitions of exercises, has lost 15 pounds in two weeks, and feels fatigued and has a hard time completing school or job assignments and can't sleep at night, and, lastly, his perfromance has noticeably declined, there is something adverse going on and we want to know what it is in order to correct it. If the individual has been following a certain conditioning program faithfully, but did not have a physical exam that year, the athlete should be examined by his physician. Even if we find that the athlete is physically and mentally normal, with persistent questioning about "extra-curricular" activities we may reveal the athlete doesn't get enough sleep. In any case, we are concerned with the proper health and maintenance of good health. This information is a feedback mechanism that tells what's going on at all times.

Our nervous system (brain, spinal cord, nerves), cardiovascular system (heart, arteries and veins), respiratory system (nasal passage, trachea, lungs), muscles, tendons, ligaments, bones and joints all are coordinated simultaneously by our brain to create motion. Therefore, any loss of function in any of these organs may result in the overall decrease in the performance of the athlete, depending, of course, on the nature and degree of injury and the organs involved.

However, despite injuries or abnormalities resulting in the loss of normal function, our bodies have a built-in mechanism to compensate for many bodily abnormalities (or losses of normal function). This compensatory ability is different in each individual.

An annual physical examination is essential for the athlete in detecting early signs of impending disease, disease states already existing, structural abnormalities and previous injuries. The ideal structural examination should include a comprehensive review of the hips, knees, ankles and feet in terms of function, abnormalities and pathology observed, and compensations. (See Chapter Two). Past injuries should be evaluated to determine if the injuries have completely healed and returned to normal function.

TERMINOLOGY

The science of biomechanics has developed a specific terminology. Certain definitions will help our explanations of lower extremity function.

• *Center of mass gravity.* This is the point at which the weight of the body may be concentrated and at a point of balance.

• *Displacement of the center of gravity.* This is the end result of all forces and motions acting upon (and concerned with) the motion of the body from one point to another.

• *Agonist muscle.* A prime mover, this muscle is opposed in action by another muscle, the antagonist. (Biceps flexes the forearm to the arm while the triceps opposes that motion).

• *Antagonist muscle.* This muscle acts in opposition to the action of another muscle.

• *Types of Body Movements*

1. *Sustained force movement.* This force is generated by the muscle against resistance by contracting agonists while relaxing antagonists.

2. *Passive movement.* (Sub-divided into manipulation, coasting and gravitational movements [falling]).

a) *Manipulation* is the application of an outside force other than gravity against a part and that part moves without resistance (such as a trainer flexing and extending the knee of an athlete who is relaxed and not resisting).

b) *Coasting* is the continuation of movement of a part caused by initial muscular contraction or outside force (such as throwing a baseball).

c) *Gravitational or falling movement* is the continuation of movement of a part without muscular contraction caused by the force of gravity of the part (such as holding an arm overhead and letting the arm fall down to the side).

3. *Ballistic movement*. Defined as rapid movement this is initiated by muscular contraction and then that muscle relaxes and permits coasting movement to complete it (such as a karate punch or hitting a baseball with bat).

4. *Guided or tracking movements*. These are described when great accuracy and steadiness, but not force or speed, are required during a movement. Both agonistic and antagonistic muscles are active to maintain skillful movements.

5. *Dynamic balance movement*. Described as the process of maintaining body balance by noticing imbalances producing the appropriate muscles to contract or relax, the effect is the production of oscillating movements to regain balance, (such as a gymnast doing a front single leg lever). The movement just performed is then rapidly reversed at the end of each movement by contracting antagonistic muscles alternating in dominance with agonistic muscles.

- *Classification of Body Levers*

1. *First-class lever*. The fulcrum is situated between the force arm and resistance.

2. *Second-class lever*. The resistance is situated between the force arm and the fulcrum. This type of lever requires more force to do the work and decreases the speed at which it is accomplished, similar to opening one's mouth against pressure.

3. *Third-class lever*. The force arm is situated between the fulcrum and the resistance. This is the most common type of lever described in the body, like biceps flexing the arm to lift a weight.

- *Body tissue function and purpose.* Each body tissue and skeleton has a specific function. This section identifies these parts and explain their general and specific function in the body.

1. *Skin or epidermis* protects the underlying body tissues and bones from harmful chemicals, radiation, foreign bodies, bacterial, viral and fungal organisms and trauma. It allows for regulation of body temperature for heat loss or preservation; skin responds to friction and pressure by thickening.

256

2. *Fat* protects the underlying body tissues and provides insulation to preserve heat. Excess carbohydrates are converted to fat by the body for storage until the body needs energy. Fat serves as a reserve supply of energy.

3. *Fascia* is a sheet or band of fibrous tissue which lies deep to the skin (superficial fascia) or forms a covering around the muscles and organs (deep fascia).

4. *Muscles* provide stability and support for our bone architecture. Contraction and/or relaxation of muscles crossing joints produces body motion and the ability to do work and provides protection against trauma to underlying organs and tissues.

5. *Ligaments* arise from bone and attach to bone to provide elasticity, strength and stability to the bony architecture.

6. *Tendons* arise from muscle and attach to bone to provide motion by crossing joints of the hands and feet when the tendon contracts or relaxes. The difference between a tendon and a ligament is that a tendon is the elastic extension of muscle, attaching muscle to bone, while a ligament is an inelastic band of tissue (made of collagen) attaching bone to bone.

7. *Bones* protect and house our body organs. Our bony architecture allows us to stand erect, walk and run bipedally (two feet). Movement occurs between bones at joints where two bones come together, separated by cartilagenous surfaces and covered by soft tissue. Bone marrow produces red blood cells and white blood cells which are essential in providing oxygen and nutrients to our body tissues and protecting our cells from foreign bodies, bacteria, viral and fungal invasions.

8. *Nerves* stimulate the muscles to contract or relax, detect pressure and temperature and relay nerve impulses to and from the brain. Nerves connect the brain to other internal organs.

9. *Arteries and veins* provide a passage way for oxygenated blood and nutrients to be transported to all body tissues (arteries) and return deoxygenated blood to the heart and lungs for re-oxygenation and distribution (veins).

CONDITIONING PRINCIPLES

Since there are many types of conditioning programs for

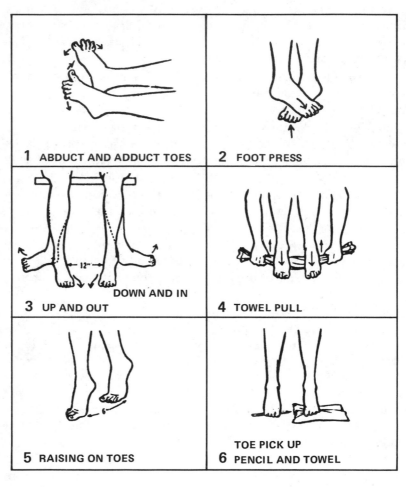

1 ABDUCT AND ADDUCT TOES	**2** FOOT PRESS
3 UP AND OUT DOWN AND IN	**4** TOWEL PULL
5 RAISING ON TOES	TOE PICK UP **6** PENCIL AND TOWEL

Exercises 1 to 6

Move ankles, feet and toes slowly through these exercises.

Exercises 7 and 8

Raise one leg at a time, lowering slowly. Then raise both legs together and lower slowly.

Exercise 9

Raise legs up 2'' from floor or bed and slowly cross and uncross them.

258

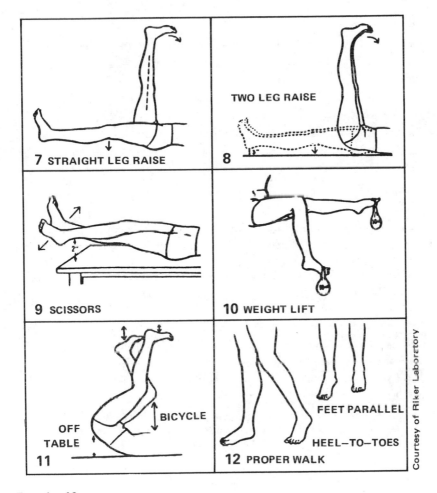

7 STRAIGHT LEG RAISE	**8** TWO LEG RAISE
9 SCISSORS	**10** WEIGHT LIFT
11 OFF TABLE — BICYCLE	**12** PROPER WALK — FEET PARALLEL — HEEL–TO–TOES

Courtesy of Riker Laboratory

Exercise 10

With 10 pound weight across foot, elevate alternately the right leg, then the left leg, to 90°.

Exercise 12

When walking, keep feet parallel and finish step on the toes (not on ball of foot.

Do's, Don't's and Why's of Track

Common Injuries

• Sprains (ligaments at joint), such as sprained ankles.

• Strains (tendons between muscle and bone), such as achilles tendonitis, hamstring pulls, or shin splints.

• Overuse problems such as cramps, stress fractures, Jogger's heels, Runner's knee (chonchonalacin patella).

• Muscle imbalances from improper total conditioning.

• Blisters, bruises, and friction problems.

Do:

• Work out on varied surfaces, mixing pace and direction for best overall conditioning.

• Do specific flexibility and warm-up exercises which copy the motions in your particular event, especially before competition. Warm-up with yoga stretching exercises. Emphasize endurance running at the beginning of the season to avoid the type of injuries which you may get from doing speed work. Build up your strength with isometric exercises, isokinetic exercises and weight training.

• Use ice rather than heat on inflamed areas.

• Use good equipment to prevent injuries; examine equipment closely for flaws; replace worn-out equipment. Use a pair of shoes for training which give you more support than the track or competitive shoe. Apply hot glue to heel to avoid unnecessary wear.

• If you have a blister or friction problem, use vaseline, or skin toughness, or wear double socks with natural fabrics like cotton or wool-thin inside, thick outside.

• To prevent recurring injuries, strengthen the surrounding muscles as well as the opposite limb; if a joint or muscle feels unstable, use elastic support or tape.

• When repeated muscle or joint overuse symptoms occur with activity, consider functional foot orthotics to prevent inefficient motion.

• Consider professional advice if injuries are not healing quickly.

Don't:

• Don't try to "run off" pain: Stop and evaluate the problem.

• Don't attempt a 100% work-out under extreme conditions of heat or cold, after meals, if you have a fever, or if you are just back from a lay-off or injury.

- Don't compete without a complete warm-up.
- Don't attempt to "cover-up" pain or injuries with pills.
- Don't "over-race."

Why:

- Muscle pulls, knee and ankle injuries can result from insufficient flexibility exercises or warm-up before competition, overuse or over-extension of muscles and joints, muscle and bone imbalances.
- Jogger's heels, fatigue or stress fractures, and plantar fascial (arch) strains occur with repeated overuse associated with running on the ball of the foot, running on hard surfaces and with prolonged strenuous effort by unconditioned athletes, or with improper shoes.
- A slight difference in limb-length, may be enough to unbalance the stride, so slightly as to be imperceptible to the runner, but nevertheless enough to throw that extra and unusual sideways thrust into the joints.
- Running off pain in the foot or leg can lead to further damage and injury from increased inflammation and to further pull or strain of the muscle or ligament.
- Overuse syndrome and pronatory gait patterns tires the feet quickly and subjects them to increased injury from fatigue and instability.
- Inadequate shock absorption in back of shoes of joggers involved in hard heeled contact may result in heel, knee, hip, or low back pain.
- Muscle overload and fatigue may lead to ischemia of the muscles subsequent cramps or muscle spasms.

The coach and his athletes must know that peak ability means exhaustion and staleness are close at hand. (**George Sheehan,** The Athlete's Dilemma)

Do's, Don't's and Why's of Swimming

Common Injuries

- Usually soft tissue injuries and imbalances, rather than bone problems.
- Pulled or strained muscles, "horse-rider's" strain.
- Abrasions.
- Skin burns or bruises from water impact.

Do:

● Proper warm-ups, flexibility exercises, and conditioning before competitive events.

● Develop endurance and good muscle tone through aerobic conditioning; consider jogging during the off-season.

● Proper breathing.

● Institute proper hygiene of foot against "athletes foot" infection, keep skin injuries clean: use antiseptics when out of water.

● Become familiar with the pool in which you are to race. Inspect the sides of the pool before entering.

● Learn to do a technique right first, then improvise or stylize, if necessary.

● In the front and back crawl, develop gradually and sufficiently the Flexors/Extensors of the Hip-Knee-Ankle joing for rhythmic movement.

● Work on calf muscle strength and flexibility.

● In the breast stroke, develop the adductors of the legs in order to avoid medial knee strain or "horse-rider's" strain.

● Develop a style of swimming that suits you and not necessarily someone else.

Don't:

● Indulge in excess periods of leg work when training.

● Swim immediately after eating.

● Hyperventilate.

● Run on the pavement or dive head first into unexplored waters.

● Don't take pills to "cover-up" pains.

Why:

● Leg cramps are due to insufficient oxygen and the build up of lactic acid.

● While racing or during timed training, hurried or careless contact between the hands/feet and the tiled, metal or cement walls of the pool may cause injuries.

● Occasionally minor strains of the quadriceps are seen in swimmers who indulge in excess periods of leg work when training.

● The thrust obtained by vigorous adduction of both legs in the breast stroke with full extension of hips, knees, and ankles, from a position of

262

wide abduction, may result in "horse rider's" strain or occasionally tear of the medial collateral ligaments of the knee.

● Over-development of the calf muscles from training with the feet and toes pointed downward must be offset with stretching to prevent strain in feet and legs when standing and walking.

General Hints for Care of Feet and Legs

1. Relax twice a day in a tub of *warm* (not hot) water. Keep spray running under water, as you massage and manipulate feet and toes. Wash feet gently with soft cloth and mild soap. After 5 minutes lift feet under warmer spray for a minute; then re-immerse in bath. Repeat 6 times.

2. Gently apply rubbing alcohol and dry thoroughly, but gently. Then gently massage with special ointment, diluted liniment, lanolin, cocoa butter or oil. Dust on talcum powder.

3. Avoid extremes of temperature. Keep feet warm and dry. Change socks twice a day. At night wear loose-fitting bed socks.

4. Always wear properly fitted shoes with low heels and wide toes, or soft leather or lined with moleskin. (Do not wear rubber shoes or bedroom slippers or walk with bare feet.)

5. Once a week have feet examined and nails trimmed after washing. Cut straight across. For brittle nails apply lanolin and bandage loosely.

6. Do not cut corns, callouses or ingrown nails. Have this done by your podiatrist.

7. Adhere to prescribed diet—high protein, moderately low fat, low carbohydrate.

8. Do not use tobacco in any form.

9. If skin is broken or inflamed, do not bear weight; wash carefully and apply sterile, dry gauze. Never use antiseptics, iodine, lysol, creosol, formaldehyde or phenol preparations. If in doubt, consult your podiatrist.

10. With foot swelling or previous phlebitis, elevate foot of bed four inches. When sitting, elevate legs on a stool.

11. Do not wear constricting garters or bandages. Do not cross legs when sitting or standing for long periods. Keep off feet for five minutes every hour; remove shoes, massage and exercise toes.

various sports, this chapter is a discussion on the principles of conditioning rather than multiple and elaborate descriptions of conditioning programs being utilized today. This section provides various suggestions and aids to the athletes, coaches and trainers who may be in the midst of modifying or selecting a conditioning program, on what to look for in a conditioning program.

In maintaining the integrity and optimal function of body tissues, athletes, coaches and trainers should be very concerned about the prevention of illness and/or injury caused by overuse syndrome and poor conditioning of the muscles, tendons, ligaments, heart and lungs of the athlete.

The term "overuse" implies "undercondition." Attention to proper conditioning programs becomes mandatory for athletes, and awareness of all the subtle and intricate details on how to condition and maintain this state is questioned by athletes, coaches and trainers. There is a fine line between enough and too much training. Athletes functioning at this optimum are close to the brink of disaster (overtraining) and should respect it.

Most conditioning programs (as with the actual sporting event) should provide the athlete with time to engage in warmup exercises. The purpose of these exercises is to increase the body temperature and to stimulate muscles, heart, lungs and nervous system for action.

Although past research has been inconclusive as to the efficiency of warmup exercises on the optimal performance of athletes during competition, we should not forget the importance of these exercises in the prevention of injuries. It is recommended that specific exercises for each sport be utilized as opposed to a generalized warmup regimen. The specific exercises will allow the athlete to rehearse precise, intricate movements, and to increase efficiency and coordination as well as prepare the body tissues for the stress and strains of the athletic activity.

The athlete, coach and trainer also should be aware of the duration, intensity and elapsed time between the warmup exercises and the actual performance. Exercise for a long period (and with great intensity) fatigues the athlete unnecessarily before the actual competition. The intent of warmup exercises is for flexibility, not strength.

264

Warmup exercises should be done as closely as possible to the actual performance, which prevents the "cooling down" phase of readiness. In terms of performance, the so-called cooling-down effect has not shown to be highly reliable (since many athlete's coming off the bench a considerable time after their warmup have performed optimally within seconds). This suggests a mental emotional factor which allows the athlete to perform optimally, even if he or she has cooled down. However, individuals are more prone to injury when they have cooled down and should warmup again before entering into the competition.

The athlete, coach and trainer also should be aware of environmental conditions and make the necessary adjustments according to the temperature and weather conditions. For example, if the temperature is 100 degrees or more, warmup exercises should not be as rigorous, and duration should be adjusted to a shorter time period. There should be frequent rest periods, the athletes should be observed for signs of heat exhaustion or heat stroke, and they should wear lighter clothing.

When we speak of warmup exercises, we can subdivide them into two categories: (1) passive exercises, which are any external agent stimulating the athlete while he remains motionless. (This is exemplified by heat treatments, massage treatments, or "buddy-assisted" stretching); and (2) active exercises which are those movements which require exertion or motion on the part of the athlete without external forces and passivity.

Most exercise programs are in the active category and increase body temperatures much faster than the passive exercises. The passive exercises produce a more soothing feeling, and are effective in alleviating tension and promoting physical and mental relaxation. This is good for both loosening up and cooling down the body gradually after a vigorous workout.

Every conditioning program, regardless of the sport, should include a stretching regimen. Stretching is essential in warmup exercises as well as during the cooling-down phase of exercising. A regular, well-understood stretching routine will maintain or increase muscle, tendon and ligament flexibility, help prevent injury and create a feeling of well-being. Stretching is important from both the psychological and physiological point of view.

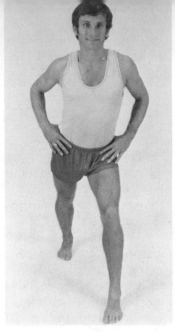

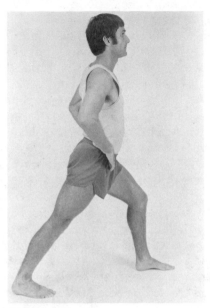

General warmup exercises to stretch the calf, hamstring and low back. Increase the degree of stretch only after muscles loosen.

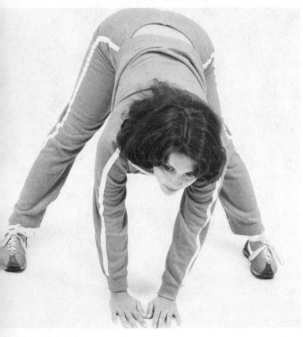

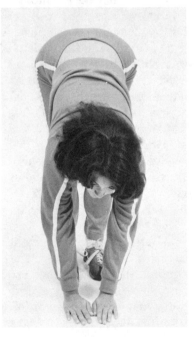

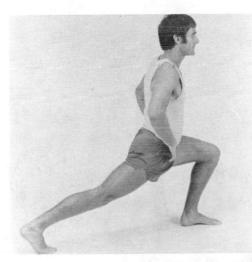

*More advanced varia-
tions of the exercises on
page 266. These in-
crease the flexibility of
muscles which athletic
training may have
tightened. Additional
exercises are shown on
pages 268 and 269.*

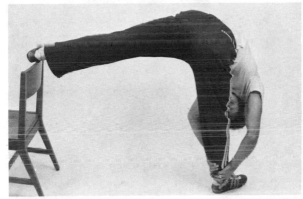

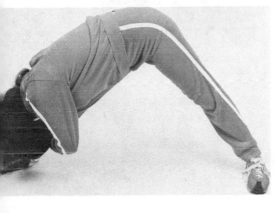

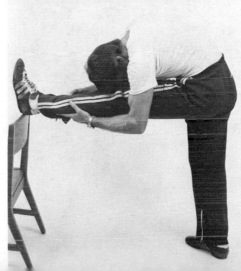

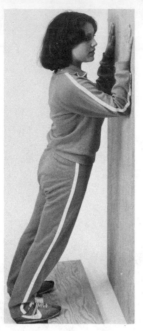
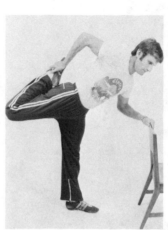
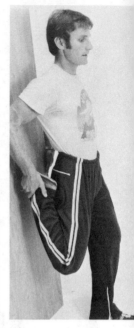
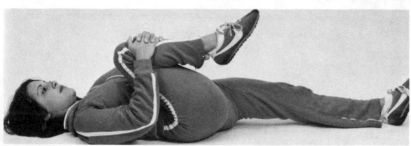
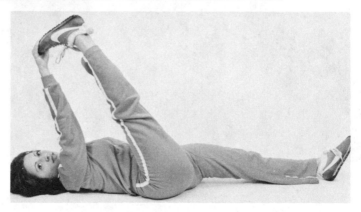

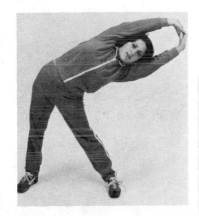

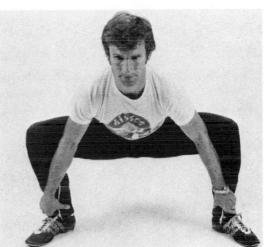

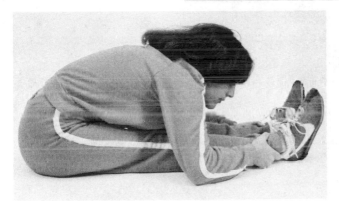

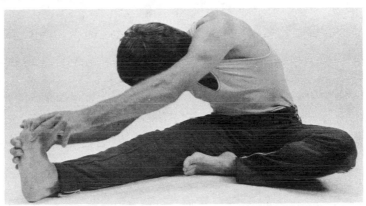

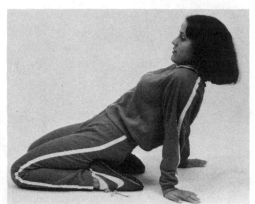

Stretch to the edge of discomfort—even if it isn't as far as this woman can go. She is more flexible than most athletes.

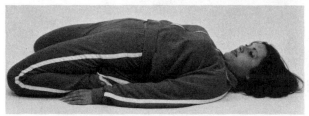

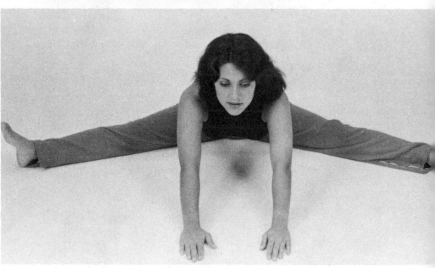

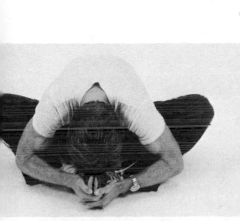

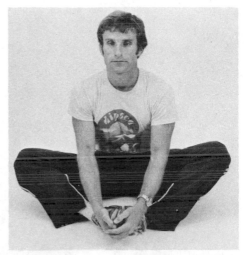

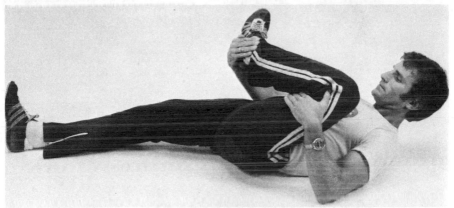

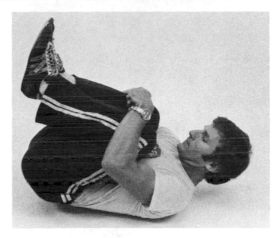

This series of sitting and lying stretches (beginning here and continuing on pages 272-273) provides a highly recommended stretching routine for runners.

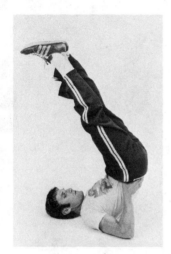

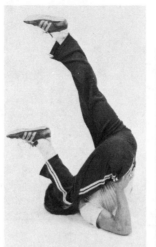

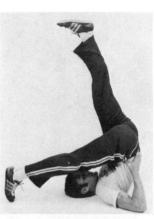

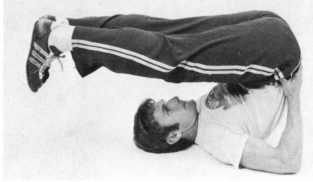

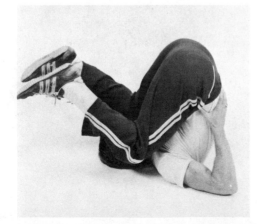

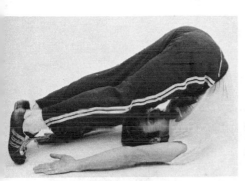

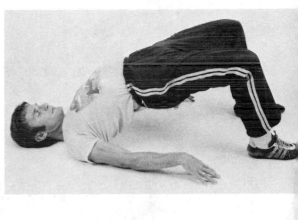

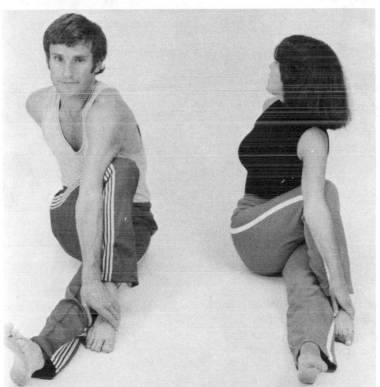

273

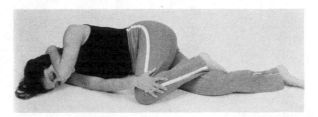

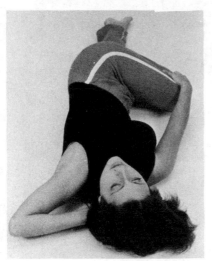

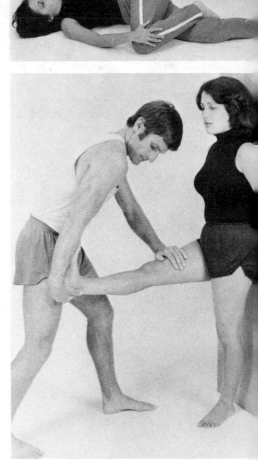

The top three photos illustrate
the spinal twister exercise. The
remaining set shows assisted
stretches to be done with a
partner.

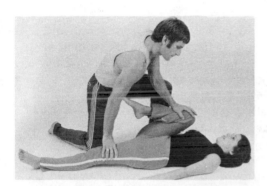

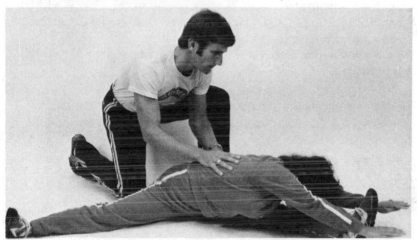

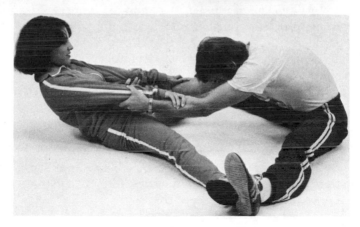

Stretching should be done with a proper attitude. It should be done in a relaxed, non-competitive manner and individualized to the athlete's own rhythm and pace. It should be done gradually and *never* forced to the point where pain or discomfort is the paramount experience (as in over-stretching).

Thus, the object of stretching is to feel relaxed and good, as well as receive the benefits of exercising. So when you begin to stretch, stretch to the point where you are still relaxed and comfortable. Then, gradually stretch farther until you can feel the stretch or pulling but without a lot of pain or discomfort. Try to hold the stretch for 10-20 seconds, and relax and breathe slowly without tension. Do not bounce. Once this practice is done routinely, stretching will become an everyday, healthy habit which you will enjoy and learn from even beyond the years of athletic competition.

A few points to keep in mind while stretching:

- It is essential that you know how flexible you are.

- Do the stretching exercises in a non-competitive and non-comparision attitude.

- Develop or find your own natural pace and rhythm which is comfortable for you.

- When you stretch, do so in a relaxed manner, concentrating on your breathing and feeling. Holding your breath only creates tension, so breathe gradually, slowly and in a relaxed manner.

- Stretch in a gradual manner and don't hurry. First, stretch to the point of least tension with maximum comfort and relaxation. Gradually increase the stretch until you feel the stretch or pull but not experiencing any associated pain or discomfort. "Overdoing it" stretches the soft tissue too soon, when it has not been conditioned to do so, and can leave the muscles, tendons and ligaments susceptible to injury.

- A patient attitude is necessary for gradual progress in developing a good feeling about stretching regularly.

- Remember, there is a difference between pain and the feel of stretching or pulling of the muscles, tendons and ligaments, so be able to distinguish between the two.

276

- Remember, some of you will experience mild to moderate pain when you stretch or exercise. This is natural for you. But don't overdo it, overstretching or hyper-extending your muscles, leg and tendons.

- If you don't know how to do a particular stretching exercise, get help, preferably from a competent athlete, coach or trainer, or seek professional help.

We often recommend a specific "flex" program for a specific period of time. On the first day, the athlete states what his goals are, such as doing a "hurdlers stretch" on the floor and "reaching the head to the knee." At that point, we set a specific time period, such as six weeks, during which time the athlete stretches his hamstrings, low back and calf muscles twice daily for at least 10 minutes.

Within six weeks, he achieves his objective or changes his goal. At that point, he can stop the repeated twice-daily stretching and stretch only often enough to maintain that level of achievement. This way, the exercises do not become boring and do not continue "forever." Also, the athlete receives the reward of achievement.

To be more specific in our discussion of conditioning, some basic principles should be kept in mind when we assess our conditioning programs.

- Since the range of motion may be limited by tight muscle, fascia or ligaments, it may be increased by stretching these tissues. For example, do toe touching or do push-ups against a wall with the feet slightly apart and in-toed. The athlete must keep his heels on the floor while he performs this exercise. This stretches calf muscles.

- The stretching of tight muscles, fascia or ligaments should be done gradually and should be preceded by warmup exercises. For example, stimulate and prepare the body by doing jumping jacks, running in place, etc., for 10-15 minutes, then perform specific stretching exercises.

- The gain in range of motion or flexibility of the soft tissue will be lost unless deliberately retained by means of repeated exercise and stretching. For example: athletes on weight training programs in combination with long-distance running; work on leg lifts and running will contract hamstrings (muscles of the back of the leg), unless stretches such as the hurdle exercise are done.

• Flexibility at weight-bearing joints should not exceed the ability of the muscles to maintain the body segments in good alignment. For example: flexibility and stretching exercises which work on the muscles, tendons and ligaments of the knee should not be continued when the athlete, coach or trainer notices hyper-flexibility which leads to instability during performance. All flexibility training should be done with the normal function of joints in mind. For example, the knee joint is a hinge which bends forward and backward, and it should not be stretched from side to side (such as the "lotus" yoga position).

Most of these principles are obviously common knowledge and taken for granted by athletes, coaches and trainers. An important point to remember is that muscles which flex or extend must be exercised equally in order to maintain equilibrium (unless the athlete is exercising the injured part to regain strength and flexibility previously lost). Contracting one set of muscles and not stretching them produces a state of muscular contracture and muscular imbalance. The antagonistic muscles may become over-powered unless they are exercised and stretched equally.

It is important to maintain flexibility and muscular equilibrium because as the athlete de-conditions and ages, any imbalance may create problems in the future. For example, an individual doing deep knee-bends with weights will abduct his knees (move outward), which puts increased stretch on the medial meniscus and ligaments of the knee, and maximally pronates the feet (the arch collapses). The quadriceps femoris muscles may strengthen, but if the hamstrings are not attended to, there will be a muscular imbalance and weakness in knee joint function, as well as increased susceptibility to injury.

Certain principles which should be kept in mind concerning muscular and neuromuscular functions include:

• Muscles contract more forcefully if they are first put on a stretch (not overstretched). For example: throwing the hip and shoulder forward before throwing a javelin.

• Increase in the muscle strength is brought about by gradual increase in the demands made on the muscle (the overload principle). Example: swimming two laps of an Olympic-sized pool and gradually increasing the distance.

• Unnecessary movements and tension in the performance of a motor skill mean both awkwardness and unnecessary fatigue (inefficient motion). This should be eliminated by developing awareness of body position, muscle tension and learning how to relax muscles not in use. Example: hitting a golf ball.

• Skillful, efficient performance in a particular technique can be developed only by practice of that technique. Example: hitting a tennis ball over the net and keeping it in bounds.

• Fatigue from overpractice diminishes skillful performance. Example: karate men practicing katas or forms after a certain period of time begins to tire which shows in his movements which lack the precision and skill compared to his earlier performance.

• The most efficient type of movement in throwing and striking skills is ballistic movement. Example: football, tennis, baseball and karate.

• Develop body awareness in terms of positioning, balance and forces required in the skill.

• Reflex responses of the neuromuscular system should be recognized and utilized when clearly indicated.

• When there is a choice of anatomic leverage, the lever appropriate for the task should be used.

In the conditioning and development of the athlete's skills, these principles reinforce the importance of practice and developing kinesthetic awareness of what the athlete's body is doing at a given moment. The continued practicing produces an awareness of such perceptions as rhythm, balance, center of gravity and dynamic changes of center of gravity, judging distances and utilizing one's anatomy efficiently and effectively as in leverage.

By developing skilled movements, one decreases the wasting of energy by increasing efficiency and control. This specifically means relaxing muscles during a precise movement and simultaneously using just enough muscular action to move the part or parts skillfully. Furthermore, physiologically, skilled movements

279

reduce the consumption of oxygen and decrease the production of lactic acid in muscles, subsequently delaying fatigue.

A conditioned and skilled athlete who has developed kinesthetic awareness of joint position decreases the possibility of injury. Skills which are primarily ballistic movements, for example, should be practiced ballistically even in the earliest learning stages. This means that emphasis is on form or style rather than accuracy is practiced, with accuracy being developed through continued practice. If, however, the emphasis is on the latter, the beginner tends to perform the skill as a moving form or slow, tense and deliberate form. Once this pattern develops, it is extremely difficult to change to a ballistic movement, thus resulting in a decrease in the skill and efficiency of the movement.

CONDITIONING CHECK

The information here will give the athlete, coach or trainer some criteria with which to contrast other programs in terms of strong and weak points. The conditioning program of your choice should emphasize areas where specific muscular and kinesthetic awareness should be developed. Generally speaking, a good conditioning program develops strength, speed, endurance, flexibility, agility and faster reaction time.

This reinforces certain facts about properly conditioned athletes: (1) They rarely require medical treatment during their years of conditioning and activity; (2) if injured, the conditioned athlete recovers from injuries quicker than an unconditioned athlete; (3) most injuries to athletes occur when fatigue becomes a major factor; hence, a properly conditioned athlete can resist fatigue longer and can recover from fatigue quicker than a poorly conditioned athlete; and (4) the athlete's heart and lungs also respond to proper conditioning by working efficiently and maximally, and during the rest they slow down markedly without losing their efficiency.

The intent of this chapter is to give the reader some idea of what to expect and observe in determining if the athlete is conditioning properly and progressively. Any additions or modifications by the athlete are encouraged.

In short, it is very important for the recreational athlete entering into competition to be properly conditioned in order to maintain his health and well-being. This includes the prevention of injury which may affect the athlete in his maturing years. As the athlete de-conditions with age and inactivity, old injuries may play a vital role in the physical and psychological well-being of the individual.

Certainly, it is important, especially in our society, to stress winning, but not at the cost of jeopardizing the health of an athlete during questionable circumstances. The athlete must demonstrate full functional ability of the injured area before he is allowed to return to competition. This is also true for those individuals maintaining some degree of conditioning for reasons of health.

Thus, the role of sports medicine is, in fact, a vital one in the overall management of the athlete's health and well-being. In order to succeed in maintaining health, physical examinations are necessary, as well as continued emphais in the proper care of the athlete in terms of diet, general conditioning, proper maintenance of athletic equipment, proper management of the athletes during practice and games, and professional consultation for any problem which could potentially jeopardize the health of the athlete.

28
Additional Support

When a person has conditioned himself properly, and he still has inherent structural weakness, what can he do? One thing is to undergo a surgical correction of the problem, but this has drawbacks. For many reasons, the chance of success is not 100%. So what are the alternatives?

First, the athlete can stop what he's doing. Second, he can try another sport or event. This type of advice is often given by the non-athletic doctor. Both of these alternatives are not acceptable to the athlete. Third, he can attempt to support weakened areas and balance unbalanced structures with the use of protective and supportive devices—specifically, selection and use of the proper training equipment, shoes and socks, padding and strapping materials and devices, arch supports and orthotic devices.

An increasing number of articles on orthotic devices (foot appliances) are appearing in sports medicine literature. Each article by such authors as Drs. Sheehan, Subotnick and Hlavac have their own individuality, but each is trying to relay a similar message. The fact is that sports-minded physicians and podiatrists are finally getting to the source of many long-misunderstood problems. Problems such as shin splints and tendonitis, once regarded as injuries an athlete paid for participation, are now being treated with a remarkable percentage of success.

Treating an athlete routinely with drugs, injections and a layoff period while ignoring the underlying cause of his ailment is little better than not treating him at all. We must treat the cause of injury. It has been said that a tincture of time will heal most wounds. But in the athlete's case, he not only lacks the time for a "temporary" recovery, but he often is anxious to increase the quantity of their injury-producing "addiction." This can prove to be quite frustrating for the doctor who is getting poor results with his treatment, but even more for the athlete who is temporarily laid up and going through a mental "withdrawal" syndrome. The athlete may feel physically recovered, only to find that resumption of full load activity brings on his problems again. Thus, the athlete is plagued continually with his injury whenever he pushes himself towards quality or quantity performances.

An athlete's injuries must be looked at in a different light than the average individual. Using a distance runner as an example, since this sport requires physical endurance, you will see that injuries are usually secondary to mechanical stresses. Architectural variations in the foot, leg or hip which might function quite well in everyday life are now proving inadequate for the spiralling distances a runner puts on his feet. Dr. Sheehan states that "the athlete has provided medicine with the new normal...man at his maximum."

Each individual's extremities have an inherent efficiency quota for locomotion. The further one deviates from this ideal state, the sooner overuse injuries arise. One runner may be plagued with shin splints when he approaches 25 miles per week, while another quite similar athlete may enjoy trouble free running at 150 miles per week. The sum of all mechanical and structural abnormalities of the foot and leg creates an injury spectrum.

The lower end of the spectrum for the runner is usually trouble free in everyday life. The upper limit, without undergoing long adaptive soft tissue changes or correcting abnormal mechanical stresses, is that point at which the body gives out with an overuse injury at its most vulnerable location. To reduce or eliminate these abnormal motions and stresses is the goal of the functional orthoses. An orthotic device can best be defined as a foot appliance, transferrable from shoe to shoe, that effectively changes the manner in which the bones and muscles of the extremity function during gait.

Normally, when the foot first strikes the ground while walking or running, the heel contacts just to the outside or mildly inverted position. Heel wear on the shoe is influenced by ankle of gait as well as tilt of the heel bone.

Immediately thereafter, while the ball of the foot begins to descend toward the ground, the heel bone rotates outward or everts as the foot pronates. This pronation or flattening out of the foot is necessary when the entire foot meets the ground to allow for greater mobility in the rear part of the foot for adapting to varying and uneven terrain.

After this time and continuing until toe off, the heel bone rotates in the opposite direction (inverts) as the foot supinates which allows the foot to become a rigid lever from which to propel.

The phase of gait when the foot is actively resupinating is vitally important so that the foot may propel as a rigid lever and the greatest efficiency during propulsion is realized. There is an interlocking and simultaneous motion of the foot and the leg. Mechanical or structural pathology as described in Chapter Three invariably will disturb this delicate balance during gait.

The most common foot abnormalities such as forefoot varus, subtalar varus and tibial varum may not allow the foot to become rigid or resupinate when it should. The foot under these abnormal states will remain pronated or highly unstable and mobile during the later stages of gait, and cause muscles to fatigue in their attempt to stabilize an unstable foot. The participating muscles of the foot, leg and thigh work longer and harder than normal, and often result in the more common overuse complaints of the endurance athlete. Even without acute overuse symptoms, a runner propelling from an unstable foot is losing both energy and valuable seconds if participating in a race.

Many podiatrists explain the mechanism of orthotic control as a "balancing of the abnormal foot." This phrase is simple but actually quite precise in meaning. The joint allowing for inversion and eversion (side-to-side motion) to occur, the subtalar joint, can be thought of as a universal joint in the way that it functions. The combined motions of inversion and eversion create a continuous arc of potential positions. Where the leg bones transfer the body weight on this arc is dependent on the soft tissue and bony support of the foot beneath.

284

If the foot pronates excessively, weight falls to the inner side of the arc. Conversely, an in-turned ankle or ankle sprain is the result of body forces suddenly falling to the outer limits of the subtalar arc. This mechanism can be simulated by standing on the foot. Closely note the bone and muscle movements. There is a continuous battle in a weak foot for support and balance to maintain body weight over the central portion of this arc.

The orthotic device centers body weight correctly over the foot and allows it to regain the normal stages of gait with the desired pronatory and supinatory components. It sets up a balance between the foot and the ground. It reduces abnormal side-to-side motions that occur in the leg and thigh with excessive pronation and allows the entire extremity to function more efficiently during forward progression. The muscles of the foot, leg and thigh will function to their maximum capabilities around more stable joints and the foot will become a stable propulsive mechanism.

Foot orthoses function very much like eyeglasses or contact lenses. They do not correct but only balance. Eyeglasses correct vision, not the eyes; orthoses correct gait, not the feet.

One unfortunate drawback of orthoses is their cost. The entire session of visits including examination, casting, dispensing of the orthoses and follow-up usually range anywhere from $100-300. The casting procedure and construction of the orthotic device itself (usually sent to a special orthotic lab) accounts for a good portion of the total cost.

Initial measurements of the joints of the foot and leg are taken, and a plaster cast impression is taken of the foot. This cast is the most critical, as the doctor must hold the foot in the position most conducive to efficient alignment and function while the cast is drying. If the cast is too high in the arch area or supinated, the orthoses will not allow for enough motion in the foot and the athlete usually complains of running on the outside of the foot, sliding off the orthotic, or blistering in the medial arch area. If the orthotic is excessively low in the arch area or pronated, it will allow too much abnormal motion and little if any therapeutic control is achieved. It is generally agreed, however, that a slightly pronated cast allowing for greater motion in athletic endeavors is superior to overly restricting foot mobility. Running as compared to walking requires this greater amount of freedom of the foot as the surfaces encountered are more variable, the force of body impact on the foot is greater, demanding more shock absorption.

The negative cast impression is then poured with plaster to form the positive cast which is used as the mold for the orthoses. The thermoplastic is heated and pressed over the mold. The plastic generally used in orthotic construction is thermal labile (soft at 250-300 degrees) in nature and measures three millimeters (approximately one-eighth inch) in thickness. The plastic orthoses has a slight amount of "give" to it which enhances comfort, but also allows it to change shape in time. Orthoses should be checked for proper fit and re-pressed over the cast if necessary every 2-3

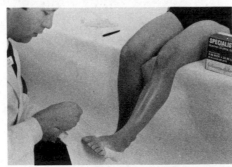

Fitting an athlete for orthotic devices starts with making a negative cast of the foot.

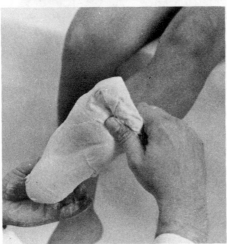
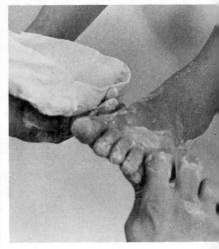

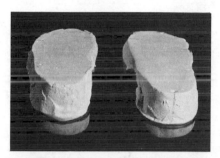

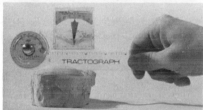

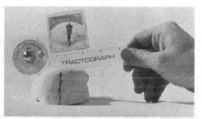

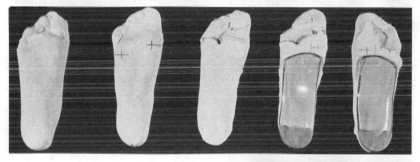

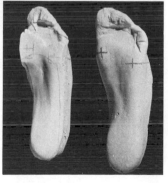

Plaster molds are taken from the negative casts, the molds are adjusted to the individual's needs, then orthoses are formed to fit these duplicates of one's feet.

287

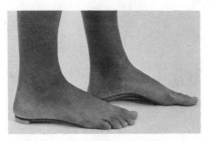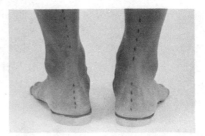

The finished orthoses support the athlete in his neutral position.

years, depending on the degree and severity of use. The conforming orthotic device is then often balanced or "canted" at specific angles to provide balance through all phases of weight-bearing movement.

The rigid orthotic, although offering optimum control is not the answer for controlling the foot in all athletic endeavors. Rigid plastic orthoses appear to be best suited for those activities which allow for heel contact during gait and where most activity occurs in a straight line of forward progression. As the sport's gait requirements deviate from this state of forward progression with a heel-contact phase, the chances of achieving control and stabilization are decreased.

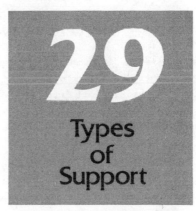

29
Types of Support

Orthoses are custom-made devices or supports made for the foot which are readily transferred from shoe to shoe. The functions:

1. Provide stability and maximum efficiency of the foot during stance and gait.

2. Prevent excessive or unwanted motion in the lower limb that results in foot-knee-back disabilities; prevents the overuse syndrome.

3. Increase shock absorption.

4. Accommodate painful bottom-foot lesions and limb-length differences.

5. Support fallen and strained arches as well as inherited muscle and bone imbalances of the foot.

6. Provide relief for knee and back pain resulting from muscle-bone imbalance of the foot.

7. Possible relief for achilles tendonitis, heel spurs, shin splints and muscle inflammation.

There are three basic types: (a) soft orthoses which temporarily relieve and support the weak and painful foot; appropriate for sprinters and jumpers; (b) semi-rigid orthoses which provide longer support and greater flexibility; appropriate for competitive athletic events and athletes with limited motion in the foot and exceptionally tight back leg/thigh muscles; (c) functional rigid orthoses are longest lasting; appropriate for everyday walking, distance training, skiing and other forward sports.

The semi-rigid and rigid orthoses are pressed over a positive cast made from a negative cast of the foot out of plaster of paris. Proper specifications are based on a full biomechanical examination of the foot in a neutral or almost neutral and stable position of the foot. Podiatrists are specially trained to perform this examination and cast the foot in the proper position.

The objective of all functional orthoses is to support the foot around its ideal neutral position and to prevent compensation. They are effective in controlling the following problems:

1. Structural foot and leg imbalances (compensated and uncompensated).

• Forefoot varus—with a functional orthotic, support the medial side of the foot, so that it is perpendicular to the rearfoot. This may be done by balancing the cast or adding a wedge to the completed orthotic.

• Forefoot valgus—support the lateral side of the foot to perpedicular.

• Rearfoot varus (subtalar varus and tibial varum)—after balancing to the forefoot position, balance the heel bone by using a rear foot post to support the foot in its inverted neutral position.

• Rearfoot valgus subtalar valgus and genu valgum)—theoretically post this is in its measured valgus position with an everted heel post. In practice, we usually post these flat in order to help the appearance of the foot.

• Talipes equinus—with osseous equinus, add heel elevation to neutral orthotic. It may be necessary to allow some pronation in the cost and the orthotic. With soft tissue egrinus, use flexibility exercises plus neutral orthotic.

2. Abnormal foot types:

• Pes cavus—a symptomatic high-arched foot which does well with support. If the range of joint motion is limited, it may be necessary to use a softer material for the orthoses.

• Pes planus—if the flat foot is the neutral position of that foot type, it does not need functional rigid orthoses. But if it is a compensated foot type, it should be controlled in its uncompensated position.

• Pes valgo planus—this is a deformity indicating compensation for another deformity and must be supported in its uncompensated position.

• Morton's foot—if associated with imbalance, treat the same as forefoot varus. If necessary, use flexible extension (morton's extension) under the first metatarsal head to the sulcus of the toes.

• Plantarflexed first ray, flexible or rigid—if rigid, protect with soft accommodative extension. If associated with forefoot valgus, treat it as a forefoot valgus. If flexible, cast and support the foot in the neutral first ray position.

3. Secondary compression syndromes:

• Tarsal tunnel syndrome—a varus support may release tension on the medial ankle retinadulum.

• Mortons neuroma—a metatarsal elevation under and behind the third and fourth metatarsal heads may relieve the compression syndrome.

• Some stress fractures—when caused by a long or depressed metatarsal, or stress fracture of the leg caused by imbalance, a functional orthotic will relieve the stress.

4. Muscle imbalances causing overuse:

• Anterior shin splints—functional orthotics provide heel lift and frontal plane balancing. They will relieve shin splints caused by muscle imbalance.

• Posterior shin splints—varus support relieves posterior tibial and long flexor muscle overuse.

• Achilles tendonitis—if caused by equinus foot type, a functional orthotic with heel elevation will help. If caused by frontal plane rearfoot imbalance, tendonitis will be relieved with heel cupping and posting.

• Peroneal muscle spasm—helped with rearfoot posting.

5. Heel problems—the plastic heel cup maintains the body's protective fat pad around the heel bone. Posting prevents strain of muscle and ligament attachments to the heel bone.

6. Ankle problems chronic sprains and weak ankles caused by imbalance are helped a great deal with a heel post.

7. Knee problems—especially those around the patella, they respond well to functional orthoses. Medial patellar problems are

associated with excessive motion; lateral knee problems are associated with limited joint motions. Both are helped with heel cupping and rearfoot posting. Most overuse and imbalance problems of the knee are helped, but internal derangements of the knee are not helped.

8. Hip problems—overuse and imbalance problems causing excessive or limited motion of the hip joint are helped with functional control. Prevention of excessive foot pronation stops excessive internal hip joint motion associated with "snapping hip" and bursitis. Arthritis and internal hip joint problems are helped.

9. Low-back postural problems—those problems associated with lumbar lordosis, anterior pelvic tilt, some disc syndromes, some sciatica and postural fatigue symptoms are helped by prevention of excessive pronation. Warning: functional orthoses, because they are rigid, will tend to aggravate most other types of low-back problems. Low-back problems on one side of the back, caused by limb-length imbalance, will be helped with a straight lift or incorporated into a functional orthotic device.

10. Combined problems—there may be multiple imbalances from the feet and legs, throughout the lower extremity, with and without compensation in various joints and muscles, making the diagnosis unclear. It is often necessary to establish a neutral control with a functional orthotic. This eliminates variables and helps the correct diagnosis, treatment plan and resolution of the problem. Fortunately for the patient and unfortunately for the doctor, many problems are resolved in this manner before an accurate diagnosis is made!

The knowledge and control of biomechanics of the lower extremity through functional orthotic therapy is unique to podiatric medicine. We hope to relate and share this knowledge with other professions for the benefit of our patients.

PADDING

The purpose of padding on the feet is to provide direct protection from areas of repititive pressure and friction, such as corns, calluses, abnormal toes and bone bruises. Pads are used to protect irritated areas and to provide support of specific joints of the feet.

292

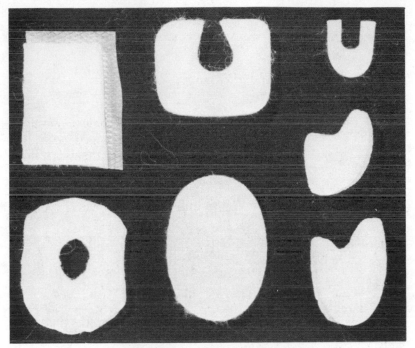

Various types of felt and foam padding

They are used on a short-term basis and should be replaced daily. If a more permanent protection is necessary, it can be made into an orthotic device for simple transfer from one suitable shoe to another.

Professional specialty materials are available through surgical supply retailers. Many other materials are available in sporting goods shops and pharmacies. It is not the material itself that works in relieving the problem, but the manner in which it is applied.

The material most commonly used in padding and strapping are: alcohol to cleanse the skin; pre-tape spray adherent or balm to help the tape stick; one, 1-1/2 or two-inch wide adhesive tape; eighth- or quarter-inch thick adhesive felt; quarter- or half-inch thick plain felt; scissors; razor.

Materials that are helpful if available: moleskin (two-inch wide rolls with thin adhesive backed material to decrease friction); lamb's wool may be used instead of tape—to separate and protect toes; "skin-guards" tape; quarter-inch foam.

In private podiatric practices, we often wish to keep pads on the feet for several days at a time, through normal bathing. We do not recommend this for athletes. We recommend daily replacement of new protective materials.

We recommend that the athlete talk with his trainer, if available, about the proper application of padding and strapping, and the selection of materials. It is important to use good equipment and avoid the rubber-based tapes that might be irritating. In sports, with perspiration there is a high chance of irritation and infection, and the pad or strap does more harm than good. If there is irritation, pain or blisters, remove the tape immediately. Never apply tape over cuts or in areas of previous infection.

In preparing skin: (1) be sure the skin is clean and dry; (2) use alcohol to remove surface skin oils; (3) use pre-tape balm or solution.

In general, select a material about as thick as the area (corn, callus, swelling) you are trying to protect. Since there is movement of the foot within the shoe during activity, place the pad behind or around the sides, but not in front of the area; do not place it where it will be rubbed off; never place it on top of a sore area, unless you are trying to reduce friction only rather than protect the area from pressure; if there is a cut or blister, do not put tape over it, but cover it with a dry sterile material and then pad around it.

When cutting and applying the pad and tape, follow this procedure:

1. Cut the pad to the appropriate size, avoiding other bone prominences (fill the non-weight bearing area).

2. Taper (skive, bevel) the edges before applying.

3. Apply pad and press; this should be comfortable for the athlete.

4. Cut tape to cover the pad; this prevents rolling of the edges.

5. Avoid any folds in the tape or pad.

After finishing, apply powder or household wax to prevent rolling and sticking on extraneous surfaces, and apply sock or shoe slowly to prevent rolling of padding.

Pads may be purchased pre-cut or may be custom-made at the time of application. The simplest pads for regular use are:

• Aperture pads (complete circle to protect specific area).

Crescent pads (half-circle to protect around and behind an area; most common type).

• Crest pads (to lift or separate toes).

294

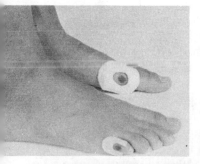
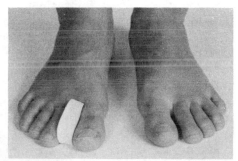
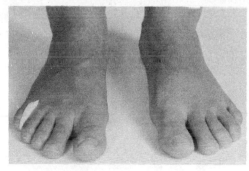

Top left: Bunion pad (left foot), corn pad. Top right: Separator to help align big toe. Left: Separator for corns between toes.

- Balance pads (to support one side of foot or other).
- Short metatarsal pads (to provide lift behind metatarsal heads).
- Long rotational pads (to provide lift behind metatarsal heads and provide arch support).
- Arch pads (to put bulk under a specific area).
- Heel pads (to elevate or cup the heel area).

STRAPPING

Pads may be used alone or in conjunction with a supportive strapping, or the strapping may be applied by itself. There are many manuals and pamphlets available through tape companies to describe the standard tapings—the Figure-Eight wrap, the Louisiana wrap, the Gibney boat, the basket-weave, the "J" strap, etc. Each trainer has a favorite tape method, which works well in his hands. Most trainers have developed these over years of experience.

If you know how a joint should normally function, you can support it with tape. Tape is most efficient when it is perpendicular (90 degree angle) to the axis of motion of a joint. This is the basis of the "Dye" straps that is described in the next chapter. We show one strap for midtarsal joint problems, one for subtalar joint problems and one for ankle problems.

The main objective of taping is to align the bones, support the joints and therefore relax the muscles in specific areas of the foot.

The main objective of taping is to align the bones, support the joints and therefore relax the muscles in specific areas of the foot and ankle. The Low-Dye support is useful in support of the arch, support of the plantar fascia, heel problems, fatigue problems and in combination with padding. The High-Dye support combines the Low-Dye foot control with balancing of the Subtalar joint for the control prevention of sprains of the ankle and subtalar joints. The

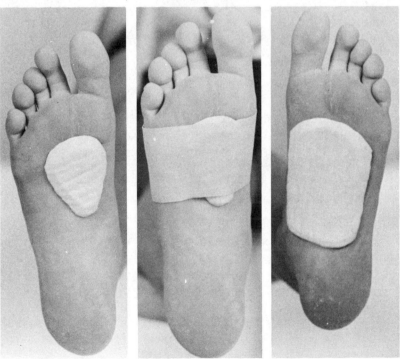

J-strap elevates the heel, and therefore relaxes the achilles tendon in the relief of tendonitis.

Note that each strap acts as an "outside muscle" to support the foot specifically where it needs that support. Tape loses its effectiveness very quickly, in terms of tension, but the pressure of the tape on the skin "reminds" the athlete when there is imbalance. Before the propriocentive sense has been registered, the athlete can feel that he is just beginning to lose balance, because the tape pulls on his leg. Therefore, he never gets to the point of loss of control.

Studies have shown that, although tape stretches and loses control over joint position, those athletes who are taped or even wear high-top shoes have a much lower incidence of ankle joint injuries. We feel this is because the athlete now has earlier cues as to where his joints are.

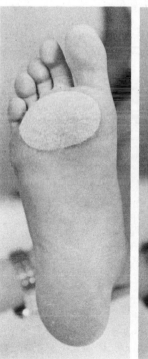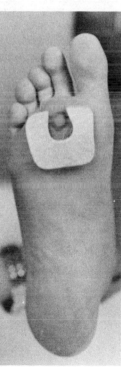

Accommodative padding (left right): For second metatarsal; long metatarsal pad for arch support; moleskin to decrease friction; pad to take pressure off metatarsal heads; short metatarsal pad.

30

Wraps, Straps and Pads

In general, "wraps" are used in a standard manner to protect joints from exceeding their normal ranges of motion. They prevent injuries. "Straps," or the use of tape to support a previously injured part, are used in a specific manner to maintain bone and joint alignment, and to assist imbalanced muscles. They are used for external support where the internal support system of the body has been altered. Most trainers have developed specific methods of their own. We do not mean to question any taping method which has proved to be successful, but only provide examples which we have found successful throughout podiatric medicine and in our clinical practices.

LOW DYE STRAP

Dr. Ralph Dye is a podiatrist who has developed classical taping methods incorporating functional mechanical support of the foot and ankle. This technique in taping is used predominantly for injuries or pain attributed to excess pronation in stance or during gait. Any injury that is aggravated by or secondary to abnormal stresses from pronation should benefit to some degree with this strap, if properly applied. It reduces subtalar joint motion. An overuse injury responding favorably to this temporary method most frequently responds very well to permanent orthotic therapy. (Note: This method does not require shaving the skin.)

The patient is sitting with the leg extended and the foot at right angles to the leg. The foot is grasped gently and the first of three

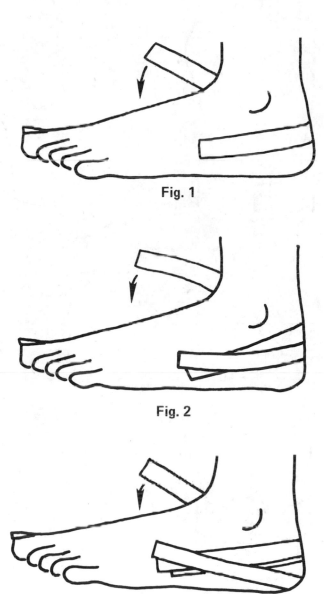

Fig. 1

Fig. 2

Fig. 3

Low-Dye Strap

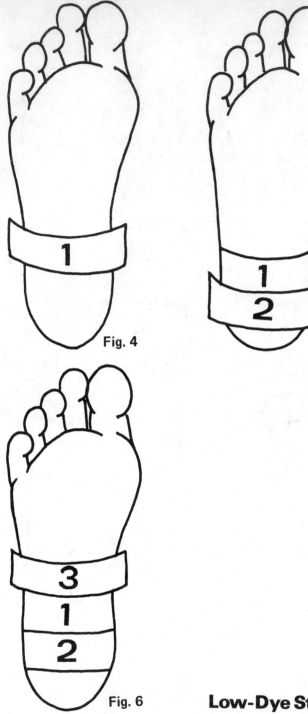

Fig. 4

Fig. 5

Fig. 6

Low-Dye Strap

strips of one- or 1-1/2-inch tape is applied, starting proximal to the fifth metatarsal joint. After the tape is secured on the outside of the foot, grasp the end in one hand and wrap it around the heel while simultaneously inverting or turning the heel in slightly. Attach the other end of the tape just behind the big toe joint on the inside of the foot. Repeat this two times (Figures 2 and 3), overlapping the first piece of tape by about two-thirds both above and below.

For taping the bottom of the foot (as in Figures 4, 5, 6 and 7), two-inch adhesive tape is cut in pieces approximately five inches long. Grasp either end of the two-inch rest straps firmly. Forcefully press against the bottom of the foot, making contact with the bottom-outside first. Continue to press even more firmly so the bottom inside is applied with more force. The application of these strips is not done in a pulling fashion; pulling the tape from the bottom outside to inside would cause wrinkling of the skin and subsequent discomfort. Cover the bottom of the foot extending out to within two inches of the ball of the foot.

Figures 8 and 9 illustrate a side view of the foot and the application of one last side strip in the same manner as Figure 1 to cover the ends of the rest straps. Now, apply a strip of two-inch tape over the top of the foot so the adhesive side is away from the skin. Finally, apply another two-inch strip directly over the first (Figure 10) to anchor the previously applied tape, and prevent initiation to the hair and skin.

THE HIGH-DYE STRAP

This is used for specific support of the sides of an unstable ankle or subtalar joint. First, apply a standard Low-Dye Strap.

Following inversion injuries, where there is or was pain under the outside of the ankle joint, and the heel bone, ankle or subtalar joint are unstable in an inward direction, prevent inversion. With the foot held at right angles to the body:

1. Apply three strips of one- or 1-1/2-inch tape from just under and inside the medial ankle bone, overlapping each strap by two-thirds, extending under the foot and around the front of the ankle and lateral ankle bone, up across to the lower one-third of the leg.

Apply each piece one at a time, with tension and no folds, so that the person can now evert but not invert the foot.

2. As a balancing support, apply two pieces of one- or 1-1/2-inch tape, in the opposite direction but with much less tension.

3. Apply a light, circular retaining wrap around the leg covering the ends of the tape. This prevents rolling of the edges with loss of support.

Following eversion injuries, where there is or was pain under the inside of the ankle joint, and the heel bone, ankle or subtalar joint are unstable in an outward direction, prevent eversion. The tape is first applied from the outside to the inside. With the Low-Dye Strap in place and the foot held at right angles to the leg:

1. Apply three strips of one- or 1-1/2-inch tape from just under the outside ankle bone, overlapping each strap by two-thirds, ex-

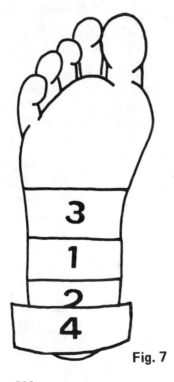

Fig. 7   **High-Dye Strap**

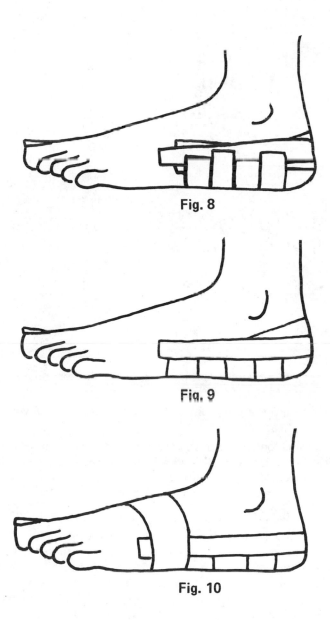

Fig. 8

Fig. 9

Fig. 10

Louisiana Wrap

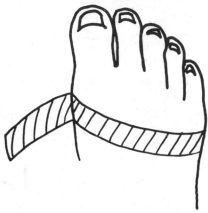

Fig. 11

2. Apply two strips in the opposite direction for balancing support.

3. Apply a retainer around the top strips (at sock-top level) to prevent rolling of the edges.

tending under the foot and around the front of the ankle and the medial ankle bone, up across to the lower one-third of the leg. Apply this firmly and with no folds, so that the person can now invert but not evert the foot.

LOUISIANA WRAP OR SUBTALAR WRAP

(Note: both the Louisiana and the High-Dye straps require shaving the ankle area.) This wrap is relatively easy to apply with practice and very good as a pre-game tape for sports such as basketball, football, soccer and rugby. The functional basis for this wrap is to act as an external ligament to help prevent ankle sprains. The heel is repeatedly taped, therefore stabilizing it in a fixed position to help maintain foot stability and support. Pre-game taping with the subtalar wrap can be done directly over the

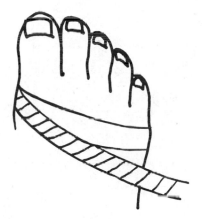

Fig. 12

athletic sock, gauze or pro-wrap with minimal loss of strength.

Figure 11 illustrates the one-inch tape being wrapped once around the foot to function as an anchor. The tape is then brought up around the dorsum (top) of the foot and around to the side (Figure 12). The tape is firmly applied around the heel and across the bottom of the heel to come up the opposite side (Figure 13).

Care must be maintained in applying the heel locks beneath the achilles tendon which inserts into the back of the heel. The tape is again brought up across the dorsum of the foot and secured around the heel bone, making an "X" (Figure 14). Tape is then taken across the bottom of the foot and started in the original position (Figure 15).

The process as explained is repeated a number of times to enhance the strength of the subtalar wrap.

VARUS HEEL PAD

We use this pad for both athletic and non-athletic patients. The use of a varus heel pad along with a Low-Dye Strap gives greater

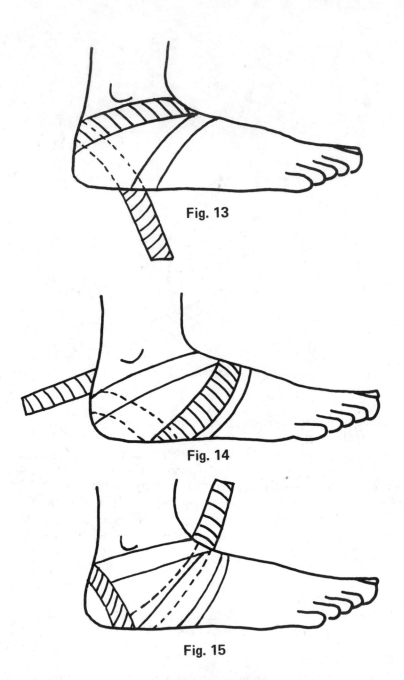

Fig. 13

Fig. 14

Fig. 15

Louisiana Wrap

control against abnormal foot pronation and allows us to better evaluate the cause of a mechanical problem. The varus heel pad is easy to fabricate and can be placed directly on the skin as incorporated in a Low-Dye Strap or placed inside of the shoe (placement in the shoe will allow longer use).

Figures 16 and 17 give two views of its shape and application. The biomechanical basis of the varus heel pad is to wedge the heel bone in an inverted position. This helps prevent heel pronation and the subsequent foot pronation. As with the Low-Dye Strap the tapered varus heel pad can be used to help determine if foot pain is related to biomechanical dysfunction. If positive response is noted, appliance (orthotics) therapy is indicated.

The varus heel pad is placed in the shoe so the thickest portion is on the inside of the foot or the same side as the big toe (Figure 16). If the pad is placed opposite to that shown, foot symptoms may increase. The other pad shown in Figure 11 is a medial arch or lower metatarsal pad. The best materials to use for the varus heel pad are firm quarter-inch felt or compressed cork if available. If the material used is compressible (such as felt) the wedge should maintain about three-sixteenths of an inch to be of value. Foam is not recommended because of its ease of compressibility.

MEDIAL ARCH PAD

The medial arch pad is essentially the same as the pads found in most athletic shoes. However, we often make them larger. There is little biomechanical value, but this small pad often relieves muscle or joint aches on a temporary basis. It is often used along with a varus heel pad in a shoe or in combination with a Low-Dye Strap.

If the medial arch pad is used in conjunction with the varus heel pad (Figure 11), cut one end of the pad off so it is essentially a continuation of the heel pad. This enhances the heel pad's ability to maintain a more neutral position of the foot. If the arch pad is used alone in the shoe, place it a half-inch closer to the heel than is normally seen. This better supports the heel bone and has a greater functional value. The medial arch pad is shaped like a half moon and tapered on all rounded sides. Felt is satistory for this type of pad. Compressed width on the inside should be approximately one-quarter inch.

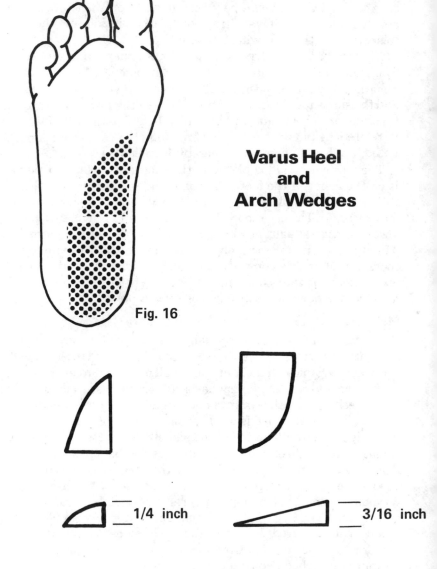

**Varus Heel
and
Arch Wedges**

Fig. 16

1/4 inch

3/16 inch

Fig. 17

In any of these uses of temporary support, if the tape is uncomfortable, causing increased problems, it should be removed immediately. If there is doubt, seek professional attention.

31

Orthotic Materials

SOFT (FLEXIBLE) ORTHOSES

In general, the soft appliances are best suited for people who need the protection of a soft-tissue supplement. Soft appliances cushion the foot and protect prominent areas, the same way an adhesive pad does when it is applied directly to the skin.

The advantage of any soft appliance is that it may be transferred from one shoe to another. The disadvantage is that, because it is soft, it compresses and loses its shape with use, so it must be replaced. An entire book could be written on the subject of flexible orthoses, as the list of materials currently used in their fabrication is endless.

Each particular device (and there are many) has its own inherent ability to control the foot which is a direction reflection of the rigidity of the material used in its construction. Soft orthoses offer some support and will minimally change the gait so that the foot functions in a more neutral position. On slow-motion film analysis, no demonstrable difference is seen in a runner's foot function with or without soft orthoses in training shoes. The only remarkable changes in gait control occurred when rigid plastic devices were used. The successful use of soft devices, however, proves that more foot control is being achieved than what meets the eye through film. As stated previously, just stopping the last few degrees of abnormal motion often gets the athlete over the acute phase of his ailment and on the road to recovery from his injury.

310

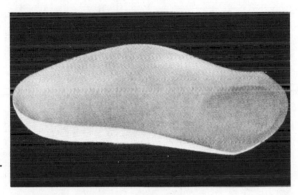

A type of semi-rigid orthosis.

SEMI-RIGID (SEMI-FLEXIBLE) ORTHOSES

Semi-rigid orthotics are used for accommodation of lesions and for bulk support. Functional rigid orthotic principles of forefoot and rearfoot wedging may be used with semi-rigid devices, but in order to achieve the same functional control, we must use more bulk, so it fills up the shoe.

Semi-rigid orthoses are made from a casted model of the foot in much the same way as a rigid plastic device. The classical and still popular semi-rigid device is constructed by using laminations of leather and cork around a thin layer of fibrous material called celastic that retains its shape. This laminating process often produces excess bulk in the shoe. We must try to keep bulk to a minimum while still retaining a fair degree of rigidity.

Current trends in semi-rigid orthotic construction for athletes are showing that fiberglass and flexible plastics are retaining their shape longer and offer more control than their leather and cork counterpart.

Regardless of material, the semi-rigid device has earned a place in sports medicine by achieving favorable results for athletic injuries and allowing greater comfort during participation.

RIGID (FUNCTIONAL) ORTHOSES

The third category of orthotic control includes the rigid or functional devices, which by definition maintain their structural form with weight-bearing and allow for neutral control of the foot throughout the gait cycle.

311

Foot Appliances: General Considerations

TYPE	INDICATIONS	AGE RANGE	EXAMPLES	REQUIRES	MATERIALS	VALUE
1. SOFT A. Static	Soft Tissue "Supplement" (Diffuse Lesions)	OLDER	Mo-Lo	Nothing	Mo-Lo + Leather, celastic	?
			Plantarform	Nothing	Open cell foam	No!
			"Spenco"	Nothing	Closed cell foam	Yes
			Liederman	Print	Grinding rubber	?
			Celastic, felt	Nothing	Celastic base, layers of felt	Yes?
B. Dynamic	Soft Tissue "Control" (Esp. Forefoot)		Urethane	Nothing	Poly-urethane, Vultex	Yes
			Contura-Mold	Nothing	Contour Mold	?
			Adhesive felt, Latex	Nothing	Cover; activated felt	?
			Acrylics (Soft)	Nothing	Plastics; Malleable	Yes
			Rosemount	Nothing	Malleable	?
2. SEMI-RIGID	"Accommodation"	Varies	Levy (Rubber Butter)	Slipper Cast	Oak Chips, Latex	Yes
			Podiasin (3M)	Slipper Cast	Mix, Monomer and Polymer	Yes
			(Leather) –	?		
			Shaffer, S-Mayer, Mayer	Cast	Leather, Celastic, Korex	Yes
3. RIGID	"Balance" Struc. & Funct. "Control"	YOUNG Usually under 30	Prenyl	Cast	Prenyl (Hot water soft)	No?
			Whitman	Cast	Steel (lab)	Yes?
			Roberts	Cast	Steel (lab)	Yes?
	"Correction" (Esp. Rearfoot)		Silverman	Full Foot Cast	Fiberglass, heel posting	Yes?
			Functional	Slipper Cast		Yes?
			(Rohadur)	(Non W-B)	Plastic (Small oven)	Yes!

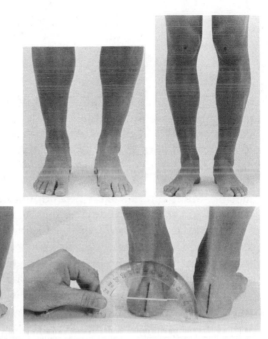

Correction of abnormal gait patterns through functional orthoses has been available for about 15 years. Prior to this time, normal foot function and methods of measurement to determine abnormal from normal were not well understood. Today, excursion patterns of most bones and joints of the extremities are defined so a doctor can measure the severity of a deformity and know the correction desired to achieve optimum function. Most mechanical problems seen today by podiatrists can be corrected via orthotic control.

Rigid orthoses are designed to control motion in the joint directly below the ankle joint (the subtalar joint) and secondarily control the joint responsible for maintaining the metatarsals in a stable and correct alignment (midtarsal joint). This joint lies slightly forward on the foot from the area of the subtalar joint. Achieving joint control in these areas by maintaining them around their neutral position will allow the entire foot, both rear-foot and forefoot, to function in a stable manner.

Stabilizing posts to correct abnormal positions of the ball of the foot to the rearfoot and posts to correct abnormal joint positions in the rearfoot can be applied to the orthotic device. If either the rear or forefoot is twisted (inverted or everted) on the other, the post will not correct the relationship in the foot, but will maintain it in this position during gait. That is, neutral orthotics prevent

313

compensation and maintain the foot in its individual neutral position. Posts are used for such deformities as forefoot varus, valgus, rearfoot varus, valgus as described in Chapter Three. Rearfoot posts are frequently used even if no structural problem exists in the foot. Posts in these instances are used when a deforming force is overpowering the heel, causing unwanted motion. Many injuries such as tendonitis and shin splints respond favorably to this type of device.

Rigid orthotic devices are permanent. They do not change shape, and they are unbreakable. They achieve the best control of motion, but because of this they sometimes limit activity to the point of irritation. The rigid functional orthotic must be very accurate in its construction, or the athlete will not be able to tolerate it. There are many stages of evaluation and construction that must coincide to produce the ideal neutral orthotic. Each measurement must be accurate, the cast must duplicate the measurements, and the correction built into the cast and the resulting orthotic device must control motion without producing irritation.

Successful results may be achieved with any of these materials. The doctor must be the one to decide which material, which cast, how much correction and which orthotic laboratory to use. In skilled hands, any material will work to achieve the desired results of pain-free, controlled, efficient function.

There are many guidelines in the selection of materials. In general, for flexible foot types, use rigid materials; for rigid foot types, use flexible materials. As a person grows older and the range of motion in his joints decreases, use less rigid materials.

There is an on-going discussion within podiatry as to which materials are the best for athletes. The problem is that in different sports and in different phases of gait we need different types of control. At heel contact, we need rigid control for support and balancing. During mid-stance, in standing and for side-to-side mobility, we need semi-rigid arch support. And for the propulsive phase where the athlete is up on the ball of his foot, we need cushioning and flexibility. The ideal material has not yet been found. When so-called ideal material is found, it will only be ideal for some athletes and for some doctors.

314

32

Support
by
Sport

SPRINTING AND DANCING

Certain actions have limited potential for gait control in that the footgear worn is not conducive to a functional device. Sports such as sprinting, some field events utilizing lightweight spikes, ballet and modern dance are included in this category.

These sports have similar problems, one being that the shoes worn have no intrinsic support to accommodate a rigid appliance. Plastic appliances require a flat-soled shoe and a reasonably firm shank. A second problem is that the majority of their event is spent either on the ball of the foot or on the toes. Therefore, these events would not benefit with a plastic orthosis which aims its initial control at the rear part of the foot.

Gait control to alleviate symptoms of overuse and stress in these selected cases would be aimed at providing control in training and helping to develop proper muscle and joint function. Temporary substitution from street or training shoes into a competitive-type shoe without support shows foot function to be improved from previous states, prior to treatment. Modifications of the competitive shoe may be helpful in special cases where the ball of the foot is twisted on the rearfoot (forefoot varus, forefoot valgus). In these cases, felt or cork wedges or cants can be applied under the ball of the foot either to the inside or outside of the shoe if possible.

Sports such as football, soccer, tennis, basketball and baseball have a greater potential for achieving gait control and relieving problems. Each sport utilizes a fairly rigid shoe, so orthotic accommodation in each particular type of shoe would be no problem. The activities involved in each sport more closely resemble the desired gait. However, each of the above sports requires an important component of either extremely quick side-to-side movement or quick acceleration.

FOOTBALL

Football is a game involving many variations in motion. Linemen would surely benefit from orthoses if indicated since they are not required to accelerate, run and cut as the ends and backs do. A lineman with flat feet not only has foot instability but also instability of the entire lower limb. This instability limits power and propulsion which is greatly needed in meeting a defender at the line of scrimmage.

Football backs and ends may find plastic orthoses (especially with stabilizing posts) too restricting for the quick side-to-side movements necessary. Orthoses shift a greater proportion of weight-bearing to the outside of the foot which increases stability intrinsically but brings the foot-to-leg relationship slightly closer to a potential ankle sprain. Balancing the rounded heel with rigid plastic ("posting") to control heel pronation problems affords a more stable platform but can be overpowered if the force is sufficient.

A soft appliance which allows more foot mobility would be indicated if the rigid device is undesirable. It is frequently observed, however, that the restriction of movement is not a problem. Plastic orthoses are often preferred by football backs with moderate to severe pronatory problems for the additional stability they provide.

TENNIS

Activities involved in tennis are much the same as those described for a back in football. Quick movements in all directions are essential, and as with the preceding example, rigid orthoses may prove to be somewhat restricting. Preference in this sport usually points to a more pliable device. An avid tennis player, if in need of gait control, should seriously attempt to wear the prescribed or-

316

thoses during hours of participation. This is essential since tennis has been known to cause a disproportionately high number of foot and leg injuries related to faulty foot mechanics.

BASKETBALL

Basketball is a game of continuous forward accelerations at nearly top speed, quick side-movements and many jumps when nearing the basket. Each of these factors is a moderate contra-indication for rigid orthoses, but when coupled together again point to the use of a softer device. The quick forward motions eliminate the heel contact phase of gait and, most importantly, a player who jumps on inherently weak ankles may have a greater tendency to sustain ankle injuries with plastic orthoses. Studies have shown that high-top tennis shoes and the use of ankle strapping prior to participation do minimize ankle injuries in basketball players.

SOCCER

Soccer involves many of the same maneuvers as football. Semi-rigid orthoses would be first choice on our list for this sport. Rigid orthoses must be considered for the more troublesome feet. The top of the foot may also be protected inside the shoe with custom-molded protective devices. Most soccer players want to feel the position of the ball, so this is a temporary measure to protect the foot as it heals from injury.

BASEBALL

The activities involved in baseball participation would fall into two categories from a biomechanical standpoint. The first would be the running requirements of the outfielder and base runner, the second being the act of batting itself. The running aspect of the game would benefit from rigid control, whereas the batter would achieve greatest efficiency with semi-rigid appliances. Batting is a complex sequence of weight transference to achieve maximum momentum and force with the swinging arms. Maintaining the foot in its neutral position allows for greater leg stability and force when swinging and meeting the ball. We recommend semi-rigid orthotics for most players.

GOLF

Golf involves the most natural gait to basic activities: natural walking and swinging the club. Walking allows for maximum gait control with no contraindications to rigid orthotic use. Mechanical faults of the extremities causing early fatigue of the feet and legs can be resolved by the realignment of the foot in a properly fitted orthotic device. The golf swing also benefits from foot stability in a similar manner as the baseball swing, but a rigid device will limit the side-to-side motion necessary for the backswing and follow-through. Therefore, we recommend the semi-rigid device.

SNOW SKIING

Balancing the foot over the snow ski can be achieved two ways. A familiar way to compensate for bow legs (tibial varum) is to cant the skis, or put a wedge between the skis and the boot. This process is effective for structural problems outside of the foot and allows for even weight distribution on the skis and snow. Ski boots are very rigid, but without a proper cant the foot will still flatten out to meet the supporting surface of the boot. The other means of balancing would be through orthotic use, which in skiing is most effective only for structural problems within the foot. To cant for a foot problem will not prevent the foot from excessively pronating, but an inside-the-boot support will transfer rotation of the leg to edge motion of the ski.

Why cant or use orthoses for skiers? Two words: edge control. A skier who skis with maximally pronated feet has a limited ability to set the inside edges of his skis. When turning, edges must be set with precision to allow for smooth, symmetrical turns. A skier with poor edge control will have difficulty maintaining a parallel turn and will find the tail of his downhill ski stemming out, or he will begin tucking the downhill leg behind his uphill knee.

A good test for ability to set edges is to simply traverse a moderate slope with correct form. If you find it necessary to continually jam your downhill knee into the uphill knee to prevent your downhill ski from drifting, chances are you have a problem with edge control. Serious skiers should have a screening examination to rule out some of the more common mechanical imbalances of the feet and legs. Results after balancing are dramatic, and a skier often finds it takes a full day to readjust to the change.

The most frequent initial comment after insertion of orthoses will be that of catching the outside edges, which is quickly modified. Problems that have arisen in the past with canting are usually due to improperly selected and placed cants. Most ski shops do this and know little about what they are trying to achieve. If orthoses are needed for the ski boot, it is best to take them in to the podiatrist's office for a correct fit or better yet take the orthoses along when buying a new pair of boots.

ICE SKATING

Ice skating utilizes a suitable shoe for appliances, although since total body weight is transmitted onto a single blade, this adds a different angle for consideration. Controlling various phases of gait as in most other sports is not important here, but more so the angle at which the blade meets the ice.

When standing on the ice, the feet should be in their neutral position within the ice skates. Deviation from the normal state may not be visible as a change in blade angle to the ice, but compensation by the extremities to maintain the body over the skate may alter normal expression of limb rotation during movement. More subtalar joint motion is necessary in this sport than most others. The foot does not move excessively in the skate itself, but the leather of the skate gives slightly to allow for "banking" of the blades throughout the turns.

WATER SKIING

Dr. Subotnick has constructed cant-like devices for water skis so the foot maintains a more neutral position while skiing. Again, for the serious competitive skier edge control for cutting through a slalom course must be precise. Balancing the foot of the water skier is not as crucial as the snow skier, because the water skier's feet remain stable and cutting is achieved by leaning with the entire body. Control for the water skier is centered more on stability. Favorable results have been achieved in this newly explored area of practice.

BICYCLING

A cyclist has limitations very similar to the sprinter. Propulsion is achieved by force through the forefoot or ball of the foot without using the heel. As with the sprinter, forefoot abnormalities are balanced by canting the forefoot. This can be done by canting the pedal itself. Such problems as forefoot varus and valgus can be controlled in this manner. It is our feeling that a slight cant of approximately two degrees may increase the structural stability in even a normal foot and increase the propulsive capabilities as force is applied to the pedal.

Many podiatrists, while agreeing that rigid orthoses are well suited for everyday wear, feel a softer appliance is the more realistic approach for many of the fast-moving activities mentioned. This type of supporting device only partially corrects abnormal pronation of the foot, but it has the benefit of being generally more comfortable in the shoe.

This option in treatment is well taken if one holds to the thought that abnormalities magnified by excessive trauma of distance running or related sports should respond favorably to subtle modifications in foot support and control. This statement is well supported by the great number of runners who find relief from arch pads found in most running shoes today or by using felt correctly positioned into the running shoe.

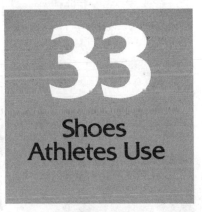

Shoes
Athletes Use

As with all your equipment, the selection of the right shoes will help your performance. Actually, the shoe will not make you better, but a shoe should not keep you from improving or make you worse. In those sports that require shoes, the selection of the proper shoe will aid your traction, support protection, leverage and balance. It might make that small difference between excellence and despair. As podiatrists we prefer to serve as *foot* doctors rather than *shoe* doctors, but it is often necessary to pay attention to this question. In today's society, there are many shoe styles that are the cause of problems, rather than the cure.

Always use the right shoe for the sport. Shoes are designed with function in mind. There is no ideal shoe for all sports under all conditions. As described, there are certain significant foot actions specific for each sport. The shoe should be efficient through all necessary movements and help eliminate inefficient action.

Shoes have a variety of purposes depending on the activity. Some of the most common are: (1) protection; (2) support; (3) increase traction; (4) cushion the ground; (5) balance foot deformities; (6) accommodate foot injuries.

WEAR PATTERNS

The ideal normal sole wear pattern occurs from the rear outside of the heel, moving toward the middle of the shoe as it approaches the ball of the foot, and then out under the big toe.

Wear along the inside or outside of the shoe can indicate imbal-

321

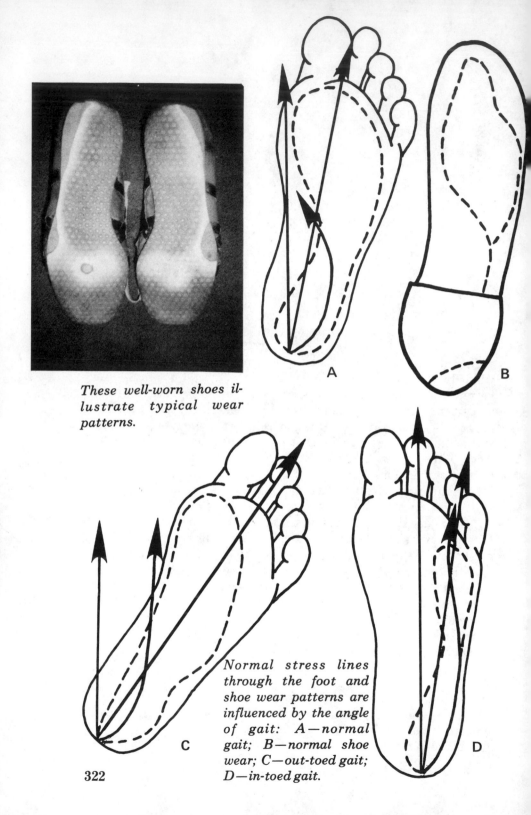

These well-worn shoes il-
lustrate typical wear
patterns.

A

B

C

D

Normal stress lines
through the foot and
shoe wear patterns are
influenced by the angle
of gait: A—normal
gait; B—normal shoe
wear; C—out-toed gait;
D—in-toed gait.

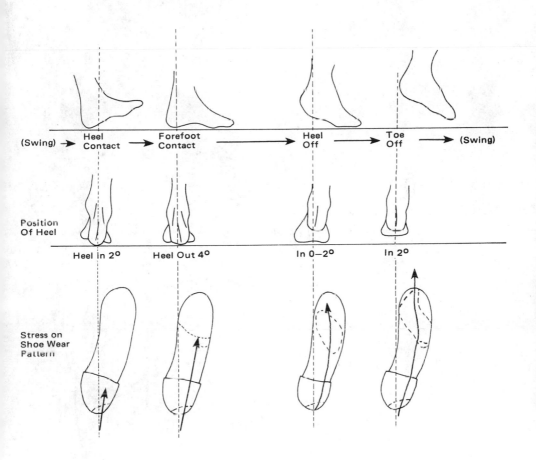

(Swing) → Heel Contact → Forefoot Contact → Heel Off → Toe Off → (Swing)

Position Of Heel

Heel in 2°   Heel Out 4°   In 0–2°   In 2°

Stress on Shoe Wear Pattern

Motions of the foot through the weight-bearing cycle during running, and related shoe wear patterns.

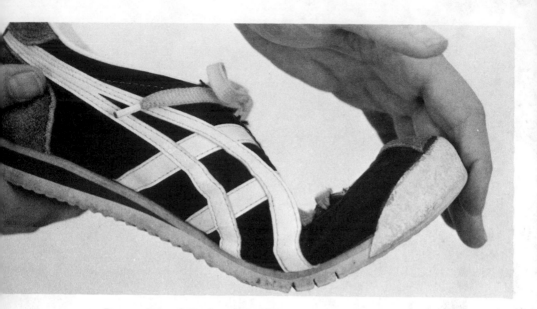

In a solid-soled shoe, flexibility may be increased by cutting the sole.

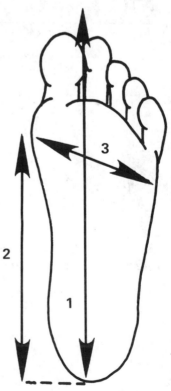

Measurements for proper shoe fit include (1) heel to toe length; (2) heel to ball of the foot at the widest point of forefoot; (3) width at widest point of forefoot.

324

ances in the foot or lower limb. These imbalances can cause undue stress to a part or parts and decrease efficiency of performance.

SHOE CARE

Never wear a brand-new shoe for competition. Wear it a few times to allow it to form to your foot, and to find out if there are any pressure points.

If a leather shoe gets wet, use a shoe tree during the drying time. Don't start a training session with wet shoes. Don't attempt to dry shoes with heat; they will shrink and become stiff.

Use powder in shoes to prevent friction, absorb moisture, and prevent transfer of fungus infections.

Shoes, no matter what the purpose they are intended for, can do the job best if they are properly fitted and properly cared for and maintained. Further, your shoes can be a barometer, telling you when something is out of balance by abnormal wear.

SHOE VARIATIONS

There are many factors that can be built into shoes. These will help some athletes and hinder others because each individual is different. Shoe manufacturers construct shoes over a standard last (wooden foot model) which is an average of various foot types. If a shoe is constructed over a faulty last, it will injure the average foot.

As podiatrists, we are often asked to recommend sizes, but most of us will not do that because each manufacturer builds his shoes over a different last, and the sizes and shapes vary somewhat. We often request that the athlete return to me with his shoes to check for proper fit. A proper shoe should provide support and cupping of the heel, firm arch support, cushioning of the ball of the foot and flexibility of the front sole for easy push-off.

There is no ideal shoe for all feet and for all foot problems. People with normal feet and no injuries are able to wear almost all types of shoes with no pain or disability. If a person has recurrent overuse or imbalance injuries, then certain types of shoes may help, and certain types of shoes may aggravate his problem and increase his disability.

In order for a shoe to fulfill its function, it must fit properly.

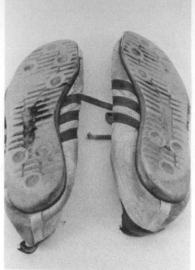

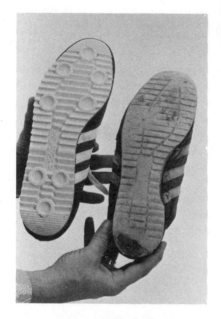

This is what happens to all shoes after hundreds of miles of wear. They wear down, of course, but they also compress from pounding and even shrink with washing.

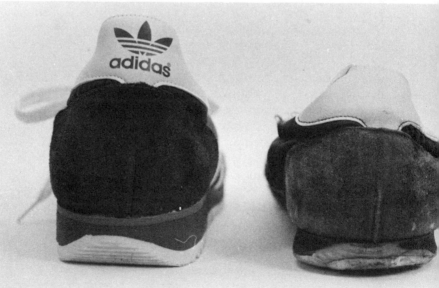

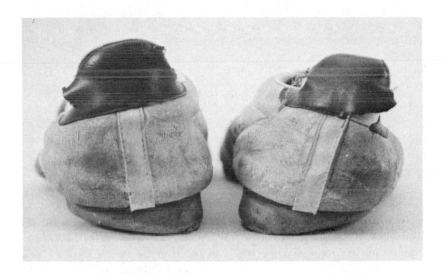

Most shoe salesmen are concerned more with sales than with proper fitting. Many are not trained in measurement techniques so it is up to the athlete himself to decide how a shoe fits. Given the choice between a slightly larger or slightly smaller shoe, select the larger shoe; if one foot is larger than the other, choose the larger size. When being measured for shoes, compare the sitting and standing size of the foot.

Most measuring devices measure three things: length from heel to longest toe, heel to the ball of the foot and width. It is best to fit the foot from the heel to the ball of the foot, rather than the toe, especially if you have a Morton's foot (short first metatarsal). Very few athletic shoes provide widths, so if you have an exceptionally wide or narrow shoe, be very careful.

The heel counter (cup around the heel) should fit snugly yet not be so stiff as to cause irritation. A loose fitting counter can cause blisters or possible tendon irritation from excessive motion. The vamp of the shoe (part that covers the forefoot) should be wide enough to accommodate the forefoot without being too loose (causing blisters) or too tight (causing corns, toe deformities and cramping of the muscles. The toe box should allow free movement of the toes without pressure. Pointed toes or toe boxes that slope can cause irritation to nails and the digits themselves. Also, toes should not hit the end of the shoe. Remember that feet swell and get larger during activity.

GOOD SHOES FOR BAD FEET

Certain factors in shoes will aid in the relief of chronic overuse, imbalance or traumatic problems of the feet. Many sports, such as running, have a very large selection of shoes so that the runner has a choice. Other more specialized sports offer only one or two types of shoes so the athlete himself must modify the shoe or protect his foot if it does not conform to the standard last.

Some of the more common foot problems will be helped by certain shoe structure or modifications:

Relief from achilles tendonitis needs a flexible shoe with a cushioning of the bottom of the heel and good elevation. Ankle sprains and instability need a shoe that will provide support and balance at heel contact especially a shoe with a wide heel. Arch problems and flexible flat feet require shoes that have a good shank and conforming arch. Calluses on the bottom of the foot require good cushioning. Corns on the top of the foot require a deep toe box, proper fit and no pressure from "stretch" socks. Problems in the back of the heel usually require cupping and elevation, while problems at the bottom of the heel (heel spurs, bruises, plantar fasciitis, "jogger's heel") require all of those plus flexible cushioning. Forefoot pain or metatarsalgia, whether caused by forefoot imbalance, stone bruises, neuritis or lack of normal protective fat padding will be helped by thick but flexible cushioning. Negative-heel shoes do not have much part in sports medicine. In general, they will help low-back postural problems in standing and tend to help stretch the heel cord, but they are not functional during most vigorous activities.

These comments are generalities and are meant as guidelines for those athletes who are searching for a better shoe. Each person should select the shoe that is the best for him. If he is happy with one, he should not experiment with others. Proper shoes will not make him a better athlete, but the selection of the proper shoe may allow him to graduate through his conditioning program so that better performance is the result.

328

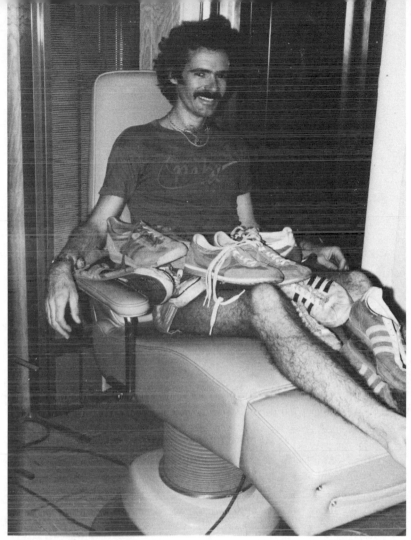

Runners typically own a large assortment of shoes.

SOCKS

In general, stay with natural fabrics, like cotton and wool. Try to find sock which fit properly. Avoid the tube-type stretch socks or "one-size-fits-all" type because they will tend to cause pressure on the toes and toenails.

Use clean dry socks daily. Use mild soaps and detergents to prevent skin irritations. If there are any cuts, blisters, abrasions or infections, use white socks so there is no chance of increased problem from irritation of the dyes.

If there is a problem of friction or cold feet, as in skiers, consider double socks, with the thin, form-fitted type on top. This retains warmth, decreases friction and draws off any moisture.

Choosing the Right Shoes

Choosing a good running shoe is similar to ordering a fine steak. The quality of what you choose may depend on your personal taste, preference and needs. The final choice involves deciding which features are important to you. In choosing your shoes, we recommend the following:

● Acquaint yourself with what generally is required of a running shoe and which shoes meet these requirements.

● Decide what you require from a shoe, and which shoes meet your requirements.

● Buy a pair of shoes that fits your feet.

Again, a proper shoe should provide support and cupping of the heel, firm arch support, protection of the ball of the foot and flexibility of the front sole for easy push-off. Shoes are for protection, support, traction, cushioning from the ground balance of foot deformities and the accommodation of foot injuries. Once you have realized the general requirements of running shoes, ask yourself these three questions to further reduce your choices:

1. What kind of runner are you? The shoes should accommodate your individual needs whether you jog around the block on the sidewalk after work, run cross-country or during lunch hour.

2. What kind of running do you do? If you race competitively, weight of the shoes will be of some significance, but if you jog around the block occasionally, a cheaper, sturdier model might do just as well.

3. What kind of problems do you have? Certain types of shoes may help recurring foot problems while others may aggravate these problems.

In selecting a running shoe, as reported in *Runner's World*, it is important that you consider the following factors:

● *Sole makeup.* The most durable and well-cushioned soles have a tough outer layer of rubber with a softer layer under it and adequate thickness under the forefoot.

● *Sole bend.* At toe-off, the foot flexes about 30-35 degrees along with the shoe. If the shoe does not bend easily, the shins, achilles tendons and calves become over-stressed. A balance should be present between adequate cushioning and flexibility.

● *Heel width.* Runners in training land on their heels. Consequently, they need a wide, stable platform. A wide heel makes the shoe more stable. Flared heels have the added advantage of extra cushioning at footplant. Shoes that measure around three inches at the heel are considered good.

● *Shank support.* The shank (area under the arch) of a shoe needs to be rigid and lie flush with the ground. The shank must not buckle at foot contact or possibilities of heel and arch injury increase.

● *Heel lift.* The elevated heel relieves strain in the backs of the legs and some "lift" seems essential to runners. Measurements are taken by subtracting the thickness of the sole beneath the forefoot from the maximum thickness of the heel.

● *Inside support.* Runners still assume they need arch supports and manufacturers continue to supply them on the assumption they work. Shoes with good inside support have built-in arch supports, heel cups or both.

● *Upper softness.* Leather and suede have disturbing tendencies of growing brittle from weather and age. Brittle shoes can cause blistering. Nylon shoes, however, remain soft.

● *Heel counter.* The counter (the hard piece wrapping around the back of the heel) is designed to stabilize the heel, and minimize foot and lower leg injuries. Look for a full, rigid counter.

● *Weights.* The effect of weight is obvious, but you can't get support and cushioning without it.

Analysis of Popular Training Shoes

	Achilles Tendonitis	Ankle Sprains, Instability	Arch Problems, Flat Feet	Calluses (Bottom of Foot)	Corns (Top of Foot)	Fatigue (Heaviness)	Heel Problems, Back	Heel Problems, Bottom	Metatarsalgia (Forefoot Pain)	Shin Splints	Width
ADIDAS COUNTRY	B	A	B	B	B	B	B	B	B	B	C
ADIDAS SL 72/76	B	B	B	B	C	B	B	B	B	B	C
BROOKS VILLANOVA II	?	B	B	B	B	C	B	B	B	B	A
E.B. (LYDIARD) ROADRUNNER	C	A	B	A	A	A	B	A	B	B	A
ETONIC	B	A	B	B	B	B	B	B	B	B	B
KARHU 2323	A	B	C	B	B	B	C	A	B	B	B
NEW BALANCE 320	B	B	B	C	C	?	B	B	B	B	A
NEW BALANCE TRACKSTER III	B	C	A	C	C	B	A	A	C	C	A
NIKE CORTEZ, ROAD RUNNER	D	B	B	B	B	C	A	C	D	B	B
NIKE LD-1000	?	A	B	B	D	?	B	B	B	B	B
NIKE WAFFLE TRAINER	C	A	B	B	B	B	A	B	B	B	B
PUMA 9190S	D	A	B	B	B	B	C	C	B	B	B
TIGER MONTREAL	C	B	C	C	B	B	B	C	C	C	B

A = excellent; B = good; C = fair; D = poor; ? = effect unknown

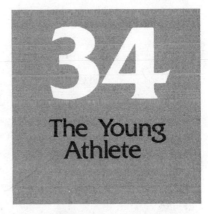

34
The Young Athlete

The primary measurable bone abnormalities (described in Chapter Three) are the frontal plane abnormalities of rearfoot varus and valgus, forefoot varus and valgus; the sagittal plane abnormality of talipes equinus, and the transverse plane abnormality of metatarsus adductus. There are many other specific abnormalities such as the Morton's foot, and it is possible to have a combination of several abnormalities present in the same foot.

In the very early stages of development, during the first years of life, it is possible to correct congenital foot and leg problems. When a structural problem is recognized by the pediatrician, orthopedist or podiatrist, or the parents themselves, such as in the case of a clubfoot (talipes equinus varus) this can usually be corrected with firm taping or casting to maintain proper alignment. It is best to do this before the child has begun walking. Corrective positioning takes 4-8 weeks.

Once the child is 3-4 years old, the bones are quite well formed and difficult to correct with conservative methods. At this point, it is possible to examine structural problems very clearly and to begin treatment. Treatment at this age will allow proper development. It will prevent the common problems seen in adults, like bunions, hammertoes and some types of flatfoot. Through this measurement procedure, we determine the single plane imbalances of the lower extremity. The objective of treatment is to support the foot in its neutral position. This prevents inefficient compensations.

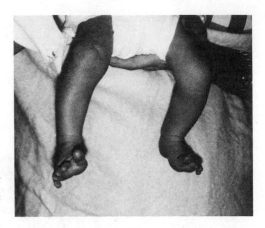

This one-week-old baby shows the normal infant pattern of bowed legs and inverted feet.

Most children pronate to some degree. How do we know which ones need treatment and which ones will outgrow the problem? The children themselves usually can't explain exactly what's wrong. As described in Chapter Three, there are many reasons for pronation, as normal motion and to compensate for other imbalances. As a general rule, we recommend treatment to all children who evert past five degrees (which is cosmetically disturbing) and to all those who pronate maximally, to the end of the range of motion at the subtalar joint (which causes stress on joints, strains on muscles and long-term bone changes).

Through proper measurement and casting procedure, we construct an orthotic that supports the foot in its individual neutral position. Orthotics then allow the foot to function around their individual neutral position, prevent compensation, and promote normal stance and gait without stress.

In treatment of adult foot imbalances, the same thing is true. Once the correct diagnosis is made, we support the deformity. With a rearfoot varus or valgus, forefoot varus or valgus, or talipes equinus, we support the deformity. The result is that we do not correct the foot. We accept the abnormality and prevent compensation. This allows normal motion and function of the foot, and controls the function of the limb above.

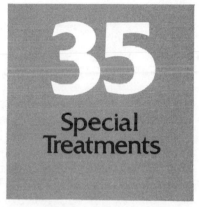

35

Special Treatments

In addition to the first aid measures and treatment plans we have described for the care of athletic injuries of the lower extremity, there are many other ways to aid the healing process. We often get questions on the validity of these procedures. When used with common sense, all are helpful. Some of these methods help attitude as much as produce physical benefits.

We find a great deal of help through the physical therapy procedures. Not all teams and individuals have these available to them, so we did not include these procedures previously. But they are an excellent adjunct to the prevention, conditioning, healing and rehabilitation processes.

The mention of some other, more exotic treatment approaches will raise some eyebrows, but many athletes have benefitted and owe their success to these methods. The author and contributors to this book have not been formally trained in all of these methods, but we have seen clinical results, attended demonstrations, lectures and classes, and heard reports from the athletes themselves. We are open to the use of any method that will help the athlete, treat him with integrity and do him no harm.

PHYSICAL THERAPY

The common used physical therapy methods we find most helpful in consultation and referral are ultrasound, hydrotherapy, ice therapy, weight training through progressive resistance exercises and flexibility training. A few words about each:

Ultrasound is produced by a high-frequency electrical machine that makes sound waves beyond the range of human hearing. The unit is usually portable and has a handpiece that can be used directly on the surface of the skin or under water along with or following hydrotherapy. The purpose of ultrasound is to establish high-frequency vibrations which mobilize fluids to decrease swelling and speed the healing process. It is especially useful in the treatment of strains, sprains, and contusions. Because of the high-frequency vibrations (like a microwave oven), the more solid structures like bone are stimulated.

Ultrasound is the best way to mobilize deep tissue problems. However, ultrasound should be used only by a trained person and never on a person with nerve or bone damage, or any person with poor circulation. Otherwise, an actual burn can result. When ultrasound is used on the skin, it should be used with a massaging motion with a transfer medium of ointment or gel, which itself may be therapeutic, and never on bone prominences. The normal dosage should not exceed one watt per square centimeter unless under special controlled conditions. Improper use of ultrasound does more harm than good. When applied properly and used several times a week (not more than once each day) during the healing process, it helps minimize pain, swelling and scar tissue, and aids in the rehabilitation process.

Hydrotherapy is the use of moving water, with or without additives, for its soothing and massaging effect. It is helpful following strains, sprains and stiff joints. It permits mobility without full weight-bearing. The hydrotherapy tank may be small and portable for use on the extremities, large and fixed for use with larger body parts or even the total body. For chronic injuries and for its soothing effect, it is usually used at 100-103 degrees F. The power and the direction of the water jetstream are adjustable. The hydrotheraphy tank should be kept scrupulously clean, because it is a source of transfer of infection.

Hydrotherapy is also used to heal recent injuries. The main disadvantage is that the body part must be held down (dependent) which produces swelling. For this reason and for some others, hydrotheraphy is often used today with an ice bath, which stimulates the reflex massaging action.

336

Both ultrasound and hydrotheraphy machines are effective electrical units. But the use of electrical equipment around water is dangerous. Each unit must be inspected and approved for use, as well as the area. Injuries have resulted from improper use and maintenance of these devices.

Ice therapy can be used by anyone, but its proper use increases the effectiveness and the results. The use of ice (cryotherapy) is effective in decreasing swelling and pain by constricting surface blood vessels, numbing the nerve endings and by producing reflex deep circulation.

Ice should be available near the field of play for immediate application to the injured area. Cold packs that become cold when crushed are good but quite expensive; it is better to have a filled ice chest there on or near the field. At home, in the office, or in the training room where a refrigerator is handy, fill styrofoam cups with water, freeze them, and then they can be used by peeling off the top layer of foam and using the base of the cup as a handle.

For those athletes who find it necessary to ICE regularly, this method works out well. Remember that it helps to keep the part elevated. When we say elevation throughout this book, we mean to try to keep the part at or above the level of the hips, and ideally above the level of the heart.

The mechanism of ice therapy is simple but fascinating. Ice does much more than make things cold and numb. As mentioned, it constructs the superficial vessels, thereby limiting swelling and pain; it dulls the nerves and numbs the area, which breaks the cycle of pain to give mental relief; and, when the superficial circulation is inhibited and the cold sensation is felt deeper, it causes a reflex dilation of the deep vessels to bring in healing cells and move out the damaged cells.

When used with a massaging action in line with the direction of blood flow, the massage itself is soothing. It helps pump the fluid, and there is no danger of freezing or frostbite to the skin or deeper structures.

Conditioning of the body involves three things, the development of strength, endurance and flexibility. The best way to achieve each of these is by doing them. More strength is developed by stressing an individual muscle group than by stress through a gross movement. When we are able to move heavy weights with effort, we are able to move light weights with speed, agility and confidence. Weight training can be done through isotonic exercise, stress with movement or isometric exercise (stress without movement).

Weight training can be used to develop strength to prevent injury and to restore strength during rehabilitation after injury. There are many theories as to the best methods and the best weight machines. It is accepted that for development of muscle bulk use heavy weights with few repetitions, and for development of muscle definition use light weights with many repetitions. All weight training should be done aerobically, with good ventilation. In rehabilitation from injury, first work on a full, pain-free range of motion, then begin with very light weights, with very gradual progression of the resistance.

Flexibility training has been one of the main emphases of this book. There is a difference between maintenance flexibility, which athletes attempt to achieve throughout their training programs and we have described well, and therapeutic flexibility, for those situations such as deep adhesions of scar tissue, chronic contractures or spasms of joints, or joint conditions limiting normal motion. If you find a specific point of tension, problems with an area of previous injury or a difference in flexibility between your two limbs, consider having physical therapy to help re-establish normal function and range of motion.

MANIPULATION AND MASSAGE

Manipulation is a form of corrective action to maintain, re-establish or produce motion in one part on another to change joint alignment. Done properly, manipulation is corrective; it aligns joints and often relieves pain immediately. In order to manipulate bones and joints properly, one must fully understood the anatomy, or damage can result.

The simplest and safest form of manipulation for the non-trained person to do is to put direct tension on a joint, to separate the opposing surfaces—that is, pull on it in a straight line; many times, this will cause a "pop" and relieve tension on a joint or nerve. If unskilled in manipulation, do not attempt any more, but

338

consider professional help. Never attempt manipulation on a suspected bone injury.

Massage is a well accepted form of therapy that stimulates local tissues and mobilizes fluids. There are many different forms of manual stimulation, ranging from rubbing of the skin surface to deep percussion. Massage is helpful in the relief of muscle pain, and there are psychological relaxing effects.

"ROLFING" AND STRUCTURAL INTEGRATION

These systems of treatment attempt to achieve harmonious body balance of the individual body parts to each other. They are helpful in achieving relaxation and an awareness of what the function of each part of the body does.

"Rolfing" is a deep form of massage evolved through the work of Ida Rolf. The technique of Rolfing is to deeply knead the muscles at their attachments to bones and in large muscle masses over bone prominences. This is usually done with the application of the knuckles vertically down to the bone. The objective is to break adhesions and to stimulate blood flow. Even when done properly, this is a painful procedure because the bone covering (periosteum) is sensitive.

Before the Rolfing procedure is done, the person is evaluated structurally. Any areas of tension, resistance or previous injury get special care. Because it is traumatic, the person should be advised of what to expect, and there should be no Rolfing done on areas of acutely traumatized tissue. Rolfing is an adjunct to rehabilitation, especially where chronic adhesions exist. It can be done on any part of the body and is usually achieved through a series of treatments.

Structural integration applies the studies of anatomy, physiology, logic biomechanics, etc., in making an individual aware of the structure and functional ability he has within his own body. The objective is to achieve body balance which results in a feeling of well-being. Many of these methods, including diet, posture control and attitude modification do achieve this feeling of well-being and body balance.

The critics to this approach say that it is impractical (impossible) in today's society. One major problem with the achievement of structural integration is that we must walk on hard, flat unnatural surfaces; our bodies must adapt to our environment to some degree. One of the results of structural integration and the other new approaches to life-style is that they will begin to change our environment, first through attitude, then through design. It is interesting to note that a person may be structurally integrated yet still out of balance with the earth (the supporting surface) and with society.

REFLEXOLOGY, ACUPUNCTURE, ACUPRESSURE

The Western approach to medical treatment procedures has been through science. Each step along the way is logical and the result is the proof or rejection of the truth; there are no half-truths. Some of the methods of Eastern medicine easily can be absorbed into this scientific approach, and some cannot. Some Eastern methods achieve good results (the patients get better) but not for known scientific explanations.

Reflexology is the manipulation and massage of the foot to achieve relief of organic problems in other parts of the body. The advocates state that nerves and meridians end in the feet. Therefore, stimulation of these lines of communication will stimulate normal function of the body tissues and parts. Reflexology is also called zone therapy. Foot reflex zones are not acupressure points but serve as reflex points.

Acupuncture is the application of needles to trigger points and meridians of the body. Many times, the needles themselves are stimulated with heat or mild electrical current. Acupuncture is especially helpful in the relief of pain and in anesthesia. Over the past few years, as scientific evidence gives support, acupuncture has gained acceptance from traditional Western medicine.

Acupuncture is often helpful in treatment of foot and leg problems. The areas of communication and flow are well understood. A specialized form of acupuncture is called osteopuncture. In those cases where deep joint or bone problems are encountered, the area may be stimulated directly with irritation to the local bone and joint tissue. Advocates report a relief of pain and increase in range of motion of joints.

Acupressure is acupuncture without needles. The meridians are stimulated with manual pressure rather than with needles.

340

As you have probably derived by now, all these forms of manipulation and massage achieve similar results. They defy standard scientific explanation, and this is where the traditional Western medical researchers find it difficult to accept.

36

Medications

Many medications are available without a prescription. State, national and international laws vary, but it is generally accepted that those drugs which are available "over the counter" are safe to take. All medications are forms of drugs; all drugs are toxins, (poisons, to some degree). If a drug is strong enough to be effective, it is strong enough to do harm.

America is a drug-oriented culture and our attitudes are molded by advertising and peer-group pressure. Most people feel that if they have an annoying, unwanted, unnatural or painful sensation, they should "take something" to make it go away. We have tried to emphasize throughout this book to first understand the problem and reverse the cause of that unwanted sensation, and to *do* something rather than *take* something. We have stressed that pain is a natural and good response to tissue injury and that it should be respected. We have said listen to the responses of the body, and don't attempt to cover them up. We feel that drugs, medications, and injections must be used selectively and carefully.

Many conditions are helped by over-the-counter medications, but these medications must be used with caution. Not all people react the same to drugs. It is not the purpose of this book to extend beyond our scope of practice, but there are certain common sense statements that must be made.

When purchasing medications over the counter, be careful. If there is any doubt about the proper use of a medication, talk it over with the pharmacist. Read the label carefully. Make sure you are not allergic to any of the ingredients. If you have any known medical problems, or you are taking regularly prescribed medications, talk this over with the pharmacist or your doctor before taking new medication so the two drugs do not interact.

ATHLETE'S FOOT REMEDIES

This disorder is caused by a fungus that lives in the superficial (surface) layers of the skin. It will not penetrate deeper into the body but can spread to other body skin areas. Many preparations are available for its treatment. Some ingredients kill the fungus directly, some inhibit growth, some merely cause sloughing of the superficial skin layers in which the organism lives.

Carfusin, Tinactin, Iodine, Gentian Violet 1% solution and 20% formaldehyde solution will kill the fungus. Gentian Violet and Carfusin are dye solutions which color the skin temporarily. Sodium and Calcium propionates, Desenex and benzoic acid inhibit growth but do not kill. Salicylic acid is used to remove surface skin layers where the fungus grows. Salicylic acid and benzoic acid are combined in a preparation called Whitfields ointment which is also very effective. Potassium permangentate solutions in a 1-10,000 concentration or Domeboro soaks are useful in acute, weeping stages of fungal infection which frequently occurs.

Some of these preparations are also available in powders which are useful to keep feet and socks dry. Some commonly used products are Daliderm, Maseda foot powder, Deso-Talc foot powder and Soloex. These preparations are available at most drug stores, but a podiatrist should be consulted if symptoms worsen or persist.

CORNS AND CALLUSES

Products available for treatment of these disorders fit into three categories: pads and dressings to protect the area from irritation; chemicals to remove the thickened skin overlying the lesion, and mildly abrasive stones and sandpaper to remove the thick skin mechanically.

Corns and calluses are caused by increased intermittent friction and pressure over a localized area of the foot. This results because of a structural abnormality in the bones of the foot which causes increased pressure on the skin overlying the prominent bone.

343

Placing protective pads over the irritated area will reduce the friction and is one mode of treatment. Numerous varieties are available for this purpose, Dr. Scholl's products being one of the more common. Various materials are used in their construction including felt, sponge rubber, moleskin, latex foam, lamb's wool and leather. These materials are used in insoles, aperture pads, called cushions, bunion pads, metatarsal cushions and arch supports. Lamb's wool is useful for corns between the toes.

Metatarsal cushions supposedly raise the metatarsal bones to reduce their pressure on the ball of the foot, but their effect is questionable. The arch supports are leather and felt or foam, and come in one shape with different sizes. Since each person's foot is a different shape, the effectiveness of this performed uniformity of shape is also questionable. Some people even construct their own pads using bandaids, tape, gauze, moleskin, felt and whatever else is handy. These pads and dressings help temporarily, but they do not treat the cause and the problem eventually returns.

Salicylic acid is included in most solutions sold to remove corns and calluses chemically. It is also imbedded in some pads which are then called medicated. Lactic acid, acetic acid and silver nitrate will also accomplish the same result. These chemicals simply remove the hard, thick skin which builds up and aggravates an already tender area. They can cause burns and should be used with caution.

Pumice stone, sandstone and sandpaper are available to remove thick skin mechanically. They are more efficient if the skin is softened first by soaking or applying emollient creams.

Removing the thickened overlying skin also does not treat the cause, and the problem eventually returns. A podiatrist should be consulted for professional definitive care of these disorders.

WARTS

Warts are common benign lesions of the skin caused by a virus. When found on the sole of the foot, they are called plantar warts. Other names apply to warts in other areas of the body. The warts can become painful, especially on the feet, and should be removed if this happens. Many procedures are available, with some more effective than others, and in many cases the warts may disappear on their own without treatment. It is not known why some people are more susceptible than others, but it is known that the virus can spread.

There is no "best" treatment for warts, and many products have been tried. A podiatrist or physician can offer the best forms of treatment, but some over-the-counter products are available. It is important to prevent scars forming as these can be a problem in themselves. Some products available are Wart-away, Vergo and Compound-W.

The ingredients most effective are glacial acetic acid, salicylic acid, ether and acetone. Again, these agents simply remove the superficial skin layers and can cause burns to normal skin, so they should be used with caution. They should not be used by people who have diabetes, circulatory problems or healing problems.

DEODORANTS AND ANTIPERSPIRANTS

Perspiring is a natural process that may occur to a greater or lesser degree depending on various factors. Emotional stress, physical activity, humidity and temperature are some. Sweat is broken down by skin bacteria into odiferous products. Therefore, frequent washing and sock changes will remove bacteria and breakdown products from the skin preventing odor.

Deodorants merely mask the odor but don't decrease sweating. Antiperspirants contain ingredients that act on skin to decrease sweating. The most common active ingredients are aluminum hydroxychloride, aluminum sulfate, aluminum chloride and zinc phenolsulfonate. These are found in most commercially available preparations. Twenty-five percent aluminum chloride solutions and 20% formaldehyde in alcohol solutions are also effective.

Some products are produced specifically for feet and come in sprays, powders and spray powders. Along with the active ingredient, the drying effect also is helpful.

DRY SKIN AND CHAPPING

Dry skin has many causes, but in all cases it is a loss of water from the superficial skin layers. The water originates from the deeper layers of skin and slowly diffuses to the surface where it is released as normal skin is shed. Several environmental factors remove moisture faster than it can be replaced from below. Air currents, high temperatures and low humidity are the main ones. Water itself is a drying agent and is why "dishwater hands" are dry and cracked. Another good example of the drying effect of water is the prune-like appearance of fingertips after soaking in the bath for a long time. There are also occupational reasons for dry skin such as exposure to chemicals, solvents, paints, etc.

The main way to soften dry skin is to put the lost water back or prevent water loss. The use of petroleum jelly (Vaseline), mineral oil, vegetable oil, lanolin and shortening, coats the skin with a greasy film to prevent water loss and soften but is not very pleasing to use. A less effective way is the use of cold creams which are more pleasing products that contain some water in an oil base.

Vanishing creams, body lotions and most hand lotions are the most pleasing and creamy, but they are effective due to a high concentration of water in an oil base. Bath oils usually contain mineral oil or vegetable oil, but their effectiveness when put in a tub of water is questionable. It is probably better to soak as little as possible and apply the oil directly to the skin upon drying.

Vitamin A has been included in some skin preparations but there is very little evidence for its effectiveness on dry skin, and overdoses of Vitamin A can be dangerous. There is almost universal agreement that hormones in skin creams have little effect on dryness or wrinkling. The use of glycerin as a moisturizing agent is doubtful since at low humidity it will extract moisture from the skin. It is effective at high humidity but most dry skin occurs in the opposite situation.

ECZEMA AND PSORIASIS

Eczema is a term that encompasses a wide variety of skin diseases that may have similar appearances but very different causes. Some skin changes universal to these overlapping disorders include itching, redness, blisters, hives, scaling, weeping and oozing. The well-known skin disorder psoriasis, with no known cause or cure, may loosely be called a type of eczema. A podiatrist or dermatologist should be consulted for a definite diagnosis of what is causing the problem, but some products are available to alleviate discomfort until that time.

Areas of eczema should be kept very clean since the skin is sus-

346

ceptible to infection, especially if cracked or raw. Mild soaps for sensitive skin, such as Lowila, should be used. Emollients can be used to keep affected skin soft and supple. Alpha-keri, Lubriderm, Keri lotion and Nutraderm are some examples. Other products may also contain more active substances such as camphor and menthol to decrease itching; tars and related compounds to sooth and calm down psoriasis; antiseptic agents to reduce infections, and benzoic acid, salicylic and resorcinol to remove thick skin.

In cases of weeping or oozing, cool wet soaks or compresses are very soothing. A few such products are Polytar, Zetar, Alphosly, CZo lotion, Daxalan, Mazon and Diasol. Using such products can by no means guarantee results but may help if the problem is transient or mild.

ALLERGIES

Allergic reactions may take a systemic total body rejection or a simple irritation. If you have any past history of reaction to an ingredient in a medication, do not take it. It may be possible to build up a resistance to this ingredient through medical evaluation and treatment. If untreated, systemic reactions usually increase each time you take this ingredient. It is not the scope of this book to discuss foot allergies or types of shock, but these are possible reactions to medications. There are no OTC medications to help this.

The most common skin allergy is skin irritation at the point of contact of the allergen, called "contact dermatitis." There are many rubber products, dyes, metals and leather tanning processes that can produce skin irritation. If you have a rash, recurring or increasing in specific areas, consider the possibility of an allergy to something touching your skin, or making "contact" through perspiration. Change socks, shoes, use mild soaps and detergents, and use drying powders. If things don't get better within one week, see a doctor.

ITCHING

Itching is a precursor of pain; it is an inflammation of the surface layer indicating that a tissue has been irritated. To relieve the itching, you must relieve the cause of the irritation. Some specific disease processes must "run their course," but some can be reversed and relieved. Itching brings on scratching, a counterirritant which substitutes pain for the itch.

Itching may be relieved with cool compresses or ice on accessible body areas. There are many effective products available as local, topical or internal medications. Discuss this with the pharmacist.

POISON IVY AND POISON OAK

Poison ivy and poison oak are the principal causes of allergic reactions to plants in the United States, although there are others. Contact of the plants to the skin allows compounds present on the plant to enter the skin and cause an allergic reaction. First exposure takes more than 12 hours to show a reaction, while subsequent exposures are quicker and more severe. The symptoms include blisters and hives arranged in linear fashion as well as intense itching and redness. The treatments mentioned here may be used for any case where itching is a problem.

Prevention is the best form of treatment. Once skin contact has occurred, the resulting reaction cannot be stopped. Keep all skin areas covered when running or hiking in unfamiliar terrain. In case of exposure, the affected areas can be treated with cool compresses of Burow's solution or mild saline (salt) solution. Calamine lotion, hydrogen peroxide and isopropyl alcohol are also good. Washing with soap and water or solvents does not remove the effect of the plant.

There is no effective preparation that, when applied to the skin prior to contact, will prevent the skin reaction. Many preparations are available to treat the skin reaction and each has some effectiveness. However, the reaction subsides on its own in 10-14 days, so it is difficult to evaluate the effectiveness of these products.

EXTERNAL ANALGESICS

External analgesics are pain relievers which are applied to the skin surface. Pain is a natural, protective sensation mediated by nerves. It usually signifies damage to cells or tissues and as such should not be disregarded. The source and cause of pain should be sought, located and understood before measures are taken to eliminate the pain or discomfort. There are a multitude of pain-relieving drugs, and in this section we discuss products applied to the skin surface to reduce pain below the skin surface.

Most of the over-the-counter products employed to relieve deep-seated pain by topical application contain irritants and relieve pain by a counter-irritant action rather than by a direct pain-relieving effect. The term rubefacient is used when these products are applied locally in proper concentration to induce heat and redness. In either case, when rubbed into the skin a local irritation is caused which overrides or alters the pain sensations produced by deeper structures. The actual mechanism of effect is uncertain, but application is often followed by pain relief. The rubbing, massage-like action also has an effect to stimulate circulation and relax muscle tension.

Counter-irritants have been used most successfully in neuralgia, arthritis, bursitis, sore and aching muscles, bruises, sprains and sciatica. The active ingredients are provided in lotions, liniments, ointments and creams. In addition, some products also contain alcohol, kerosene, acetone and pine oil which also have some irritating effect. Most products contain similar active ingredients, and their effectiveness is basically similar.

Methyl salicylate is most frequently used and is the main constituent in oil of wintergreen. It may have some effect by the salicylate being absorbed into the blood stream through the skin. It is poisonous if swallowed and should be kept from children. Menthol actually gives a feeling of coolness when it is applied. Camphor and thymol are also common ingredients. Turpentine oil, clove oil, cinnamon oil and chloroform are well known active ingredients. Allyl isothiocyanate is better known as volatile oil of mustard. Capsicum deoresin is one more common ingredient. Benzocaine has a direct local anesthetic effect on skin nerves to numb the area temporarily.

Some of these products can cause allergic skin reactions and should be discontinued if this happens. If the pain persists or worsens, it should be regarded as a warning of a more serious problem.

INTERNAL ANALGESICS

Internal analgesics are pain relievers taken into the body, usually as tablets. The effect of analgesics is to relieve pain and to decrease inflammation. They should not be taken to "cover up" pain, but as anti-inflammatories which help speed the healing processes. Many athletes take pain-killers to cover up deeper problems which only get worse.

This group of products includes aspirin and a large group of similarly related compounds. In spite of the claims made for the disorders they are effective against, there are actually only a few problems for which they have a proven value. Strictly speaking for the athlete (and this eliminates many common disorders not athletically related), the use of these drugs should be limited to sprains, strains, some joint conditions such as arthritis and some muscle problems such as pulled muscles.

The choice of which to use should be made on the basis of the action of its ingredients and not subjective claims made during advertising activity. In this light, we list common ingredients in most of these preparations and their pharmacologic actions and uses.

Acetaminophen (for people who are sensitive to aspirin) and acetylsalicylic acid (aspirin, ASA) are anti-inflammatory agents effective in reducing body temperature in cases of fever which are usually disease-related and not where excess heat energy is generated from exercise. ASA tablets can cause irritation and even bleeding from stomach lining when swallowed. The solution is to chew or crush the tablets before swallowing, take with food or use a suppository. Acetaminophen is less irritating to the stomach. Gastric upset can be decreased when these compounds are in a buffered form. The buffering agents include sodium bicarbonate, aluminum glycinate, magnesium carbonate, aluminum hydroxide, magnesium hydroxide and calcium carbonate. Incidentally, these also make up the bulk of antacid preparation ingredients. You can also take a tablet with a glass of milk, which also has a buffering and antacid action.

ASA and acetaminophen, along with salicylic acid, salicylamide and other salicylates, have the ability to alleviate mild to moderate pain. Pain in this category would include the moderate pain of

350

headache, neuralgia, muscle pain arising from stretching or overuse, slight trauma, shin splints, sprains, strains, joint pain and pain following minor surgery. Aspirin and the salicylates are probably most effective for rheumatic conditions, arthritis and inflammatory conditions.

These drugs have toxic side-effects which can be exacerbated if the drugs are taken too long or in too high a dose. So use these drugs for the above-listed conditions, but if symptoms continue consult a physician.

We caution against using products with Phenacetin, as it has been found to have a deleterious effect on the kidney and has been removed from the market in some countries. Read the label on the bottle very carefully.

Caffeine is included in many of these analgesic preparations. Its exact usefulness is unclear, as it has many actions in the body. It is thought to potentiate the action of the main stimulant ingredient.

Athletes would probably have a more frequent need for these products due to the stresses and strains they place on their bodies. An objective choice and proper use of the products will help attain their maximum effect.

"UNDER-THE-COUNTER" DRUGS

Many athletes are tempted to increase their motivation or physical ability through the use of illegal drugs. There are long-term bad effects from these types of poisons, and there are no drugs that improve performance on a long-term basis. The following information is issued as a warning. We pray that you consider the effects of taking drugs on yourself, your team, and your family.

Drugs have been used in the past by athletes to increase athletic performance by: (1) decreasing fatigue; (2) decreasing pain due to injury or stress on muscles, tendons, ligaments, joints and bones; (3) increasing alertness; (4) dissipating tension and anxiety from the stress of athletic competition; (5) allowing sleep; (6) elevating the psychological mood to make the athlete feel stronger; (7) increasing muscle bulk.

Grade school, high school, colleges, universities, amateur and professional athlete associations and unions bar the use of drugs to enhance athletic performance. Furthermore, current research factually states that drugs used specifically to enhance athletic performance do not improve performance of the athlete. Continued use of drugs for this purpose may be damaging to the athlete physically and mentally because of the effects of the drugs with long-term use.

The use of some drugs to improve athletic performance is illegal unless done so under the strict supervision of a physician for the sole purpose of treatment of an injury, illness or disease.

DIET SUPPLEMENTS

In general, the natural forms of medications have been more effective than the synthetic form. The normal diet contains all the necessary vitamins and minerals. It has been jokingly said that if food intake would increase athletic performance, then the winner of a marathon race would be the one who eats the most. It is our opinion that diet and diet supplements have been "overplayed," and that the use of these should be a well studied and well understood decision.

Vitamins. Vitamins are essential for maintenance of normal growth and development. With the emphasis being placed on vitamins in the media, we wonder how early man ever survived without his daily vitamin supplements. He did it by eating a balanced diet. It is true that many of the processed foods produced today have had much of the vitamins and minerals leached out during preparation, but in many cases these losses are replaced artificially or the vitamins can be obtained from other diet sources.

In the case of a normal diet and a healthy individual, vitamin deficiences are rare unless some other disease process is present. A healthy body can occasionally experience an increased tissue demand for vitamins and minerals during processes of growth, pregnancy, menstruation and vigorous physical work or stress. Hence, the question of vitamins for athletes. The increased activity of athletes will demand a greater food intake which, if balanced, will supply most vitamins. If the diet is in question, then a multivitamin supplement in the recommended dose is probably a useful addition.

352

Vitamins A, D, E and K are fat-soluble vitamins, which means they are absorbed along with fat in the diet. The minimum daily requirement (MDR) of Vitamin A is 4000 units for an adult. (All the following figures will be adult dosages.) The MDR is a federal standard based on proven conservative research, so is often questioned. Vitamin A is required for normal functioning of the skin and the retina of the eye. It is obtained from most vegetables, especially the green leafy type, as well as fruits, liver, milk, butter and eggs. Vitamin D, E and K also come from these sources.

Vitamin D is necessary for absorption of calcium and phosphorus from the intestine to allow proper bone development. A rich source of D is fish liver and fish vicera. Cod liver oil is an example of such a preparation. The MDR is 400 units, and an absence of Vitamin D will cause rickets in children and osteomalacia (soft bones) in adults.

The controversial Vitamin E is found in vegetable oils, vegetable shortenings and margarines in addition to the sources stated above. The MDR is 12-25 units. In spite of the many and varied claims for the usefulness of Vitamin E, it has not been proven to enhance athletic performance. In fact, the only definite use of Vitamin E at present is in premature babies and in patients with diseases that impair fat absorption.

Vitamin K is necessary for the body to form factors that allow normal blood clotting. It is not included in available over the counter preparations.

The water-soluble vitamins include Vitamin C and the B vitamins. For this reason, overdoses of C and B are very rare; the excess is excreted unchanged. The MDR for Vitamin C is 70 milligrams. The best sources of Vitamin C or ascorbic acid are raw vegetables and citrus fruits. Vitamin C has many functions in the body involving growth, tissue repair and maintaining integrity of cartilage, teeth and bone. Inadequate intake of C causes scurvy. It is purported that British sailors were nicknamed "Limeys" because they used the juice from limes to prevent scurvy on board ship. The present practice of using high doses of Vitamin C to prevent colds or increase athletes' performance is gaining acceptance through clinical and pure research studies, but is still very controversial.

The B-complex vitamins include Vitamin B1 (thiamine), Vitamine B2 (riboflavin), niacin, Vitamin B6 (pyridoxine), folic acid, Vitamin B12 and pantothenate. The MDR are 1.2 milligrams, 1.7 miligrams, 1.4 milligrams, 0.5 milligrams, 0.3 milligrams, and 0.2 micrograms, respectively. There is no known recommended dose for pantothenate. The foods supplying most of this group of vitamins include green vegetables, liver, heart, kidney, grains and lean meat. B-complex vitamins are required for proper functioning of the cardiovascular, nervous, and gastro-intestinal systems.

Minerals are also required by the body in specific amounts supplied by the average diet. Some vitamin preparations are supplemented with minerals. Sodium chloride tablets can be taken to replace salt lost through excessive perspiration. The use of mineral supplements is beyond the scope of this discussion.

The ingredients of almost all vitamin and mineral preparations exceed the MDR. Thus, preference of one product over another is arbitrary. You should be cognizant of the expiration date on the package, as some vitamins will lose their potency over a period of time. Therapeutic vitamins and minerals should be prescribed by a physician.

Electrolytes and Fluid Balance. Over the past few years, there have been important changes in the theories of treatment and prevention of electrolyte imbalances, dehydration and heat disorders resulting from strenous exercise. This has resulted mainly from research work done by exercise physiologists and physicians who study body chemistry changes resulting from athletic activity. This work has produced treatment and prevention regimens based on scientific evidence rather than theory.

As a basic review of body compensating mechanisms, a discussion of perspiring is in order. During exercise, the body's workload increases and more energy is required. This energy comes from recently eaten food as well as food stored in the body in the form of fat and sugar. As the body processes use this form of energy, heat is given off as a by-product.

The amount of heat produced rises in direct proportion to the severity of exercise occurring and in turn raises the body temperature above the normal. Body temperature can also rise due to high

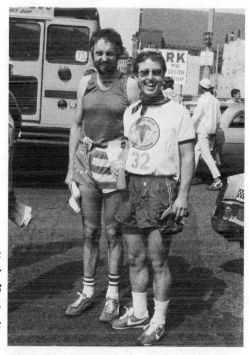

Electrolyte replacement drinks are helpful during long, hot runs like the 1976 Boston Marathon. Pictured is Dr. Harry Hlavac (right) with Mel Kotter.

surrounding air temperature in the absence of exercise. So there are two factors that will raise body temperature. The body compensates for this rise in temperature by increasing the flow of blood to the skin to dissipate heat from the blood to the surrounding air. If this is inadequate, then sweating occurs to cool the skin by evaporation of water.

However, if the air temperature is higher than body temperature and the relative humidity is 100%, these processes will be ineffective and body temperature will not decrease. In such cases, the body temperature may rise up to 104-105 degrees and cause severe heat problems. The temperature must then be returned artificially. If the problem is not checked, heat stroke and death can result. Less dramatic effects of heat disorders are cramps, fatigue, exhaustion, dizziness, headache, incoherence and collapse.

Exercising in heat should be worked into gradually since the body can become acclimatized and able to withstand higher tem-

355

peratures for longer time periods. It is also helpful to wear light clothing and expose skin to the air so that breezes can aid the cooling process of sweating.

Sweat contains salt (sodium chloride), as well as water, which is lost from the body once it is shed onto the skin. If lost in a sufficient quantity, it can upset the sodium balance in the body. In most cases, salt replacement is not necessary as long as the diet is adequate. The practice of taking salt tablets has fallen out of favor because an appropriate amount of water must also be taken in at the same time, and this often does not happen. Consequently, the body receives too much sodium. It is more important to replace the lost water, keeping salt intake low. Potassium deficits are difficult to produce and it usually takes days of heavy sweating although intake of large amounts of salt can hasten potassium loss. It is rarely a significant problem.

Tremendous amounts of water can be lost through sweating, causing dehydration and upsetting fluid balances in the body. Recent evidence suggests a few facts about water intake. Cold water empties from the stomach quicker than hot, allowing a faster rate of intestinal absorption. Some studies show that small amounts of salt in the water may also increase stomach emptying. Quick emptying of the stomach simply allows it to be refilled sooner and hence more fluid can be taken in. Athletes require water at different rates and should be weighed before and after training activity to determine water loss and determine competition needs. Fluid intake can then be adjusted accordingly. More water can be replaced if there is free access to it during activities than if it is taken in at one or two break periods.

Glucose (dextrose) intake is also practiced by some athletes. Glucose is stored in muscles and liver. The muscle stores are the first to be used in activity followed by the liver stores. In endurance events (two hours or more), once the liver stores become used, blood glucose levels fall and fatigue begins. Glucose solutions will prevent exhaustion of liver stores if given during exercise. Many athletes take this immediately after endurance activities as well. It is generally accepted that honey is not absorbed as quickly as other forms of sugar.

Many electrolyte solutions are used by athletes. ERG, Gatorade, Body Punch and Body Ammo are four although many others are available. The ideal solution should contain salt and glucose with a water vehicle. It should be cold and have not more than 2.5 grams of glucose and 0.2 grams of salt in 100 milliliters of water. Most commercial solutions are more palatable but tend to contain more ingredients, which increases the osmolality of the solution and decreases stomach-emptying time. There should also be free access to the solution during and after activity.

37

In
Conclusion

We have attempted to present a practical book on foot care to the athlete, coach, trainer and interested professional. Sports medicine is a field where the various professions can work together to minimize injuries and maximize performance. Certain structural abnormalities which in the past would limit athletic potential have been described. Through scientific evaluation and treatment procedures, an improved understanding of conditioning exercises and suggestions on coaching methods, most athletes can achieve their optimum individual potential. It is important to remember that each individual sport develops certain body functions at the expense of others, producing a dynamic imbalance. Therefore, the athlete must condition opposing body structures in order to prevent overuse and imbalance injuries.

As podiatrists involved in the care of athletes, we have learned and are constantly learning about the biomechanics of each sport. We are happy to see that we can contribute to the welfare of athletes while doing no harm, and often allow the athlete to maintain good physical condition by resting the injured structures while substituting other aerobic activities. Because this attitude toward "ambulatory care" is not yet accepted by many professionals, we are often asked to treat injuries that are clearly out of our field of expertise. It is important to use the recommendations of this book as a guideline in the understanding of foot and leg disorders, and to seek professional attention from a podiatrist or sports medicine specialist when indicated.

We consider *The Foot Book* a necessary addition to the understanding of biomechanical factors in sports. We have been very pleased with our results in the care of specific foot injuries and in related lower extremity overuse syndromes, yet we feel there is a great deal more for us to learn about athletes and about sports medicine. If you have critical or constructive comments, questions or concerns, please contact us through World Publications or at P.O. Box 3964, San Rafael, Calif. 94902.

We hope that you reach your full potential and that you include the love of sport in your life.

Selected Readings

American Academy of Orthopedic Surgeons—*Symposium on Sports Medicine,* C.V. Mosby Co., St. Louis, Mo., 1969.

American Medical Joggers Association Newsletter, P.O. Box 4704, North Hollywood, Calif. 91607.

Brubaker, T.E., and James, S.L.—*Injuries to Runners,* Laboratory for Human Performance, University of Oregon, 1974.

Brachman, P.—*Mechanical Foot Therapy,* Edwards Bros., Ann Arbor, Mich., 1940.

Bruno, J.—"Gross Muscle Evaluation by the Podiatrist," *JAPA,* 57:309-315, 1967.

Cailliet, Rene—*Knee Pain and Disability,* F.A. Davis Co., 1973.

Ciba Pharmaceutical Co.—*Traumatic Disorders of the Ankle and Foot,* Summit, N.J., 1965.

Clancy, William G. et all.—"Achilles Tendonitis in Runners: A Report of Five Cases," *Sports Medicine,* March-April 1976.

Clancy, William G.—"Jogger and Distance Runner," *The Physician and Sports Medicine,* June 1974.

Close, J. R.—"Some Applications of the Functional Anatomy of the Ankle Joint," *JBJB* 38A:761-781, 1956.

Close, J.R. and Inman, V.T. *The Action of the Subtalar Joint,* Inst. of Engin. Research, University of California, Berkeley, Series II, Issue 24, May 1953.

Corrigan, A.B., and Fitch, K.E.,—"Complications of Jogging," *The Medical Journal of Australia,* 363, 1972.

Craig, T.T.—"Comments in Sports Medicine," *JAMA*, 231:333, 1973.

Dickinson, Arthur L.—"Nutrition," *Far West Ski News*, Nov. 15, 1975.

Dickson, F.D., and Diveley, R.L.—*Functional Disorders of the Foot*, J.B. Lippincott, Philadelphia, 1939.

Downer, Ann H.—"Ultrasound," *Athletic Training Magazine*, Vol. 10, No. 3, 138-139, Sept. 1975.

DuVries, H.—*Surgery of the Foot*, Ed. 2, Mosby Co., St. Louis, 1965.

Elftman, H.—"Transverse Tarsal Joint and Its Control," *Clinical Ortho.*, No. 16, 42-46, 1960.

Gamble, F.O., and Yale, I.—*Clinical Foot Roentgenology*, Williams and Wilkins Co., Baltimore, 1966.

Giannestrias, N.J.—*Foot Disorders: Medical and Surgical Management*, Lea and Febiger, Philadelphia, 1967.

Gray, H.—*Anatomy of the Human Body*, Ed. 28, Lea and Febiger, Philadelphia, 1966.

Hamblin, Gordon S., et al.—*A Podiatric Screening Program Involving 105 High School and College Wrestlers*, CCPM, 1975.

Harris, R.I., and Beathe, T.—"Short First Metatarsal, Its Incidence and Clinical Significance," *JBJS*, 31A:553-565, 1949.

Henderson, Joe, et al.—*The Complete Runner*, World Publications, Mountain View, 1974.

Hicks, J.H.—"Mechanics of the Foot: 1. The Joints," *J. Anat.*, 87:345-357, 1953.

Hiss, J.M.—*Functional Foot Disorders*, University Publishing.

Hlavac, H.F.—"Differences in X-Ray Findings with Varied Positioning of the Foot," *JAPA* 57:465-471, 1967.

Hlavac, H.F.—"Compensated Forefoot Varus," *JAPA*, 60:229-233, 1970.

Hlavac, H., and Schoenhaus, H.—"The Plantar Fat Pad and Some Related Problems," *JAPA*, 60:151-155, 1970.

Injured Athlete, The—American Academy of Podiatric Sports Medicine, c/o California College of Podiatric Medicine, San Francisco, Calif.

Inman, Verne T.—*The Joints of the Ankle*, The Williams and Wilkins Co., Baltimore, 1976.

James, S.L., and Brubaker, C.E.—"Biomechanics of Running," *Orthopedic Clinics of America*, Vol. 4, No. 3: 605-616, July 1973.

Jesse, John—*Strength, Power and Muscular Edurance for Runners and Hurdlers*, The Athletic Press, Pasadena, 1968.

Johnson and Johnson—*Therapeutic Uses of Adhesive Tape*, 2nd edition, New Brunswick, N.J., 1958.

Kelikian, H.—*Hallux Valgus, Allied Deformities of the Forefoot and Metatarsalgia*, W.B. Saunders Co., Philadelphia, 1965.

Lewin, P.—*The Foot and Ankle*, Lea and Febiger Co., Philadelphia, 1940.

Melillo, T.V.—"Gastrocneumius Equinus: Its Diagnosis and Treatment," *Proc. Res. Alumni Assn.*, California Podiatric Medical Center 1:37-58, 1972.

Morton, D.J.—*The Human Foot*, Columbia University Press, New York, 1935.

O'Donoghue, D.H.,—*Treatment of Injuries to Athletes*, 2nd edition, W.B. Saunders Co., Philadelphia, 1970.

O'Shea, John P.—*Scientific Principles and Methods of Strength Fitness*, 2nd edition, Addison-Wesley Publishing Co., 1976.

Root, M.L., Orien, W., Weed, J.H., Hughs, R.J.—*Biomechanical Examination of the Foot*, Vol. 1, Clinical Biomechanics Corp., Los Angeles, 1971.

Root, M.L., et al.—*Neutral Position Casting Techniques*, Clinical Biomechanics Corp., 1971.

Sgarlato, T.E.—*A Compendium of Podiatric Biomechanics*, California College of Podiatric Medicine, 1971.

Sheehan, G.M.—"Chondromalacia in Runners," *American College of Podiatric Sports Medicine Newsletter*, Vol. 7, No. 4, 1972.

Sheehan, G.M.—*Encyclopedia of Athletic Medicine*, World Publications, 1972.

Steindler, A.—*Kinesiology*, Charles C. Thomas, Springfield, Ill., 1955.

Subotnick, S.I., *Podiatric Sports Medicine*, Futura Publishing Co., Mt. Kisco, N.Y., 1975.

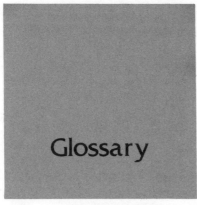

Glossary

—A—

Abduct—to move away from the midline of the body.

Abrasion—(cinder burn, floor burn, grass burn, mat burn, slide burn, strawberry), an injury from the scraping away of a portion of skin or mucous membrane through an abnormal mechanical process.

Abscess—a pus producing infection, usually staphylococcal.

Achilles tendon—large tendon that attaches in the back of heel. Actually includes the tendons of three muscles, the gastrocnemius, the soleus and the plantaris.

Acute—having a rapid onset with a short and relatively severe course.

Adduct—to move toward the midline of the body.

Adhesions—(sticking together) surface contact; a fibrous band or structure by which parts abnormally join together.

Aerobics (with air)—the exercise program designed by Kenneth H. Cooper, M.D., M.P.H., designed to get enough oxygen to all the areas where the food is stored, so that the two can combine to produce enough energy to provide oxygen to all tissues through long-term conditioning.

Anaerobic Exercise (Without Air)—exercise incurred during an oxygen debt, the "huff and puff" stage of vigorous exercise; used by competitive athletes to build up speed at the expense of creating large oxygen debts that must be paid quickly by stopping and recovering from the activity—e.g., wind sprints, interval training, the 100-yard dash; vigorous exercise causing the person to be out of breath resulting in an oxygen debt.

Analgesic—an agent that alleviates pain without causing loss of consciousness.

Anatomic stance position—the body is erect, elbows extended, palms facing forward, knees extended and facing forward, and feet in the normal angle and base of gait.

Anhidrosis—an abnormal deficiency in sweating.

Anterior—in front, forward.

Anterior tibial compartment syndrome—serious, severe shin splints with compression and destruction of muscle and nerve; also called Volkmanns ischemic contracture.

Apophysitis—inflammation in a growing area of the heel bone.

Arthritis—inflammation of a joint; may be caused by injury or metabolic problems.

Aspirate—the removal of fluids or gases from a cavity by suction.

Athlete's foot—a fungus infection of the skin of the foot; also tinea pedis, dermatophytosis, ring worm.

Athlete's heart—normal, healthy, efficient heart in well-conditioned athlete; apparent enlargement may be from ventricular hypertrophy and/or increased distensibility; returns to prior size after cessation of training.

Atrophy—decrease in size.

Avulsion—the tearing away forcibly of a part or structure.

Axis (es) of motion—line around which a part moves, controlled by the shape of the bones at joints.

—B—

Baseball finger—a ball hits your finger, bending it backwards or to one side, causing swelling and pain; in the foot, called "Turf-toe."

Benign—not death dealing (not malignant); favorable for recovery.

Bilateral—two sides or both extremities.

Blister—the separation of the outer layer of skin from the inner layer, with the intervening space becoming filled with a watery substance or blood.

Bone bruise—periostitis, stone bruise.

Boot-top fractures—fractures which occur higher up the tibia shaft as seen with rigid ski boots.

Bromhidrosis—odorous perspiration.

Bulla(ae)—primary lesions(s); fluid filled blister, larger than a vesicle.

Bunion—inflammation over the first toe joint (first metatarsal-phalangeal joint).

Bunionette—inflammation over the fifth toe joint (fifth meta-tarsal-phalangeal joint); also called tailor's bunion.

Bursa—a sac or sac-like cavity filled with fluid and situated at places in the tissues at which friction would otherwise develop; may be normal or acquired.

Bursitis—inflammation of the bursa or sac that absorbs the shock and reduces the friction between two structures—e.g., bursa between the heel and bone and achilles tendon.

—C—

Calcaneus—heel bone.

Calcaneal apophysitis (Sever's disease)—inflammation of growth areas at the back of the heel bone during adolescence, aggravated by trauma.

Callus—flat, horny overgrowth of epidermal skin.

Cartilage—a smooth, gristle-like tissue that protects the joints and becomes rough with joint arthritis.

Center of gravity—the weight center or concentration of weight of the body; it is the point at which all parts of the body exactly balance each other; it is the point in the body at which the three reference planes intersect; average location is in the pelvis just in front of second sacral vertebra. It is lower in women than in men.

Charleyhorse—soreness and stiffness in a muscle caused by overstrain or contusion; the term is usually restricted to injuries of the quadriceps muscle.

Chiropodist—old term for foot doctor; not officially used in USA since 1958.

Chondromalacia patella—softness of the kneecap from repeated stress; also called "runner's knee."

Chronic—persisting over a long period of time.

Cicatrix (scar)—a secondary lesion; fibrous tissue replacing normal tissue lost or destroyed.

Clubfoot—a gross foot deformity, usually congenital, especially talipes equino-varus.

Colic — acute abdominal pain or cramps.

Compensation—a change of structure, position or function of one part in an attempt by the body to adjust to or make up for the abnormal force of a deviation of structure, position or function of another part.

Condyle—prominent portion of bone.

Contusion—a bruise; an injury of soft tissues without a break in the skin.

Corn—a corn is a cone shaped, horny layer of skin which usually forms on the upper part of the toe or between the toes, in places at points of pressure and friction.

Cramps—pain or discomfort resulting from contractions or spasms in the muscles of the toes, calves, hamstrings, back, neck, etc.

Crepitus—a grating sound or sensation as a joint is moved through its range of motion; the term is sometimes used when soft tissues move roughly on each other.

Crust—a crust is a secondary lesion composed of dried serum, pus, or blood.

—**D**—

Dermatitis—inflammation of the skin.

Dislocation—the displacement of any part, usually a bone; separation of bones at joint.

Distal—farthest away from center of the body.

Dorsal—upper surface; top of foot.

Dorsiflexion—motion occurring on an up and down plane during which the distal part of the foot or the toes moves up or towards the leg bones.

—**E**—

Edema—swelling.

Eversion — motion which causes the plantar aspect of the foot (bottom) or part of the foot to tilt so as to face more away from the midline of the body.

Excoriation—a secondary skin lesion; loss of skin substance produced by scratching.

Exostosis—a bony growth projecting outward from the surface of a bone; spur.

Extension—straightening or movement of two parts away from each other at the joint.

Extensor tendon—tendon located on top of foot which lifts the foot or toe upward.

Extremity—the terminal portion (the foot and leg).

Extrinsic—that which originates from without (outside)—e.g., the muscles of the foot which originate in the leg.

—**F**—

Fabella—a small sesamoid bone sometimes present in the tendon of the lateral head of the gastrocnemius muscle. Often mistaken for fracture.

Fascia—a specialized firm connective tissue which covers and separates tendons and ligaments.

Fatigue fracture—a hairline bone break occurring after prolonged repetitive stress against firm resistance; no history of specific traumatic incident; also called stress or march fracture.

Femur—the thigh bone.

Fibula—smaller lateral bone of leg.

Fissure—a secondary skin lesion; deep linear crack or defect in the skin.

Flat feet—a depression or flattening of the inside or medial longitudinal arch of the foot, not necessarily pathologic.

Flexion—bending of two parts towards each other at the joint.

Football clip—lateral blow to the leg causing a side-to-side force on the knee.

Forefoot valgus—the forefoot or ball of the foot is turned out from the midline of the body in relationship to the rearfoot.

Forefoot varus—the forefoot or ball of the foot is turned inward in relation to the rearfoot.

Fracture—break in bone.

Frontal plane—this is a flat vertical plane passing through the body from side to side, dividing it into a front half and a back half; the cardinal frontal plane passes through the center of gravity and divides the body into equal but asymmetrical halves; all other frontal planes are parallel to the cardinal frontal plane.

Fungus—a vegetable cellular organism that subsists on organic matter; grows in moist, warm areas.

—G—

Ganglion (synovial hernia, cyst)—accumulation of fluid from a joint or tendon sheath.

Genu recurvation—hyperextensibility of the knee.

Genu valgum (knock knee)—deformity when knees together, ankles apart.

Genu varum—deformity with knees apart, ankles together.

Growing pains—abnormal spasms or pains in muscles from overuse, especially when at rest.

Gym itch—jock itch; usually caused by fungus or bacterial infection.

—H

Hallux—first (big) toe.

Hallux Limitus, Rigidus—limited or no movement at great toe joint.

Hallux valgus—lateral deviation of great toe associated with bunion.

Heat cramp—spastic contraction of a voluntary muscle sometimes precipitated by dehydration and salt depletion.

Heat exhaustion—(heat syncope, prostration)—state of shock with sweating, rapid pulse, low blood pressure, cool wet skin. Needs medical attention, water and salt.

Heat fatigue—transient deterioration in performance from exposure to heat and humidity, and resulting in a relative state of dehydration and salt depletion.

Heat stroke (sunstroke)—severe medical problem; failure of temperature regulation; mechanism under stressful conditions; dry skin, high fever, diminishing pulse.

Hematoma—a blood blister or tumor containing effused blood.

Hernia—the protrusion of a loop or portion of an organ or tissue through an abnormal opening.

Herpes simplex—a virus disease transmitted through contact with an infected person.

Hip pointer—iliac crest contusion.

Hydro-therapy—whirlpool; use of moving water for massage.

Hyperdrosis, hyperhidrosis—excess perspiration.

Hypermobility—any motion occurring in a joint during weight-bearing when that joint should be stable under such load.

Hyperpigmentation—a secondary lesion; abnormal darkening of the skin; colors within the skin due to external deposits, chemicals or tattoos, or produced by formulation of melanin in the basal layer of the epidermis; mole, freckle.

—I—

Ice therapy—use of ice to shrink swollen tissues.

Immunization—a disease-preventive measure in which the introduction of an appropriate antigen into the body stimulates the production of antibodies to a specific disease.

Incurvated—curving inward.

Inflammation—swollen tissues characterized by redness, heat, swelling and pain; initial result of injury and a part of healing.

Ingrown toenail—a large nail margin or a nail deformity where the nail pushes into the skin along the nail marging.

Intrinsic—that which originates from within (inside)—e.g., the muscles that originate within the foot.

Inversion—motion which causes the plantar (bottom) aspect of the foot or part of the foot to tilt so as to face more toward the midline of the body.

Ischemia—loss of blood supply/oxygen to tissue.

Isometric—a muscle contraction in which the muscle remains in partial or complete contraction without changing its length; muscle tension without movement.

Isotonic—muscle tension with movement.

—J—

Jogger's heel—heel trauma that comes about as a result of running on hard surfaces like asphalt or concrete.

Jock itch—fungus infection causing inflammation of the skin in the groin region.

Jumper's knee—result of extending the knees and jumping; frequently as seen by basketball players.

370

—K—

Kinesiology—the study of movement.

Knock-knees—with the knees together the distal parts of the large leg bones angulates out from the midline of the body.

—L—

Lace bite—painful inflammation over dorsum of foot, usually over prominent ridge of base of first metatarsal; usually from tight shoelaces.

Lateral—side away from midline of the body.

Leg—defined as area between knee and ankle.

Lesion—reaction of the skin to stress; takes many forms.

Lichenification—thickening of the skin with exaggeration of its normal markings so that the lines form a criss-cross pattern enclosing flat-topped, shiny, smooth, Y-sided facets between them.

Ligaments—non-elastic tissue which connect bone to bone.

Longitudinal arch—medial or inside portion of the foot from heel to ball of the foot.

—M—

Macule—a primary lesion; spot without elevation or depression—e.g., freckles.

Malleolus(i)—ankle bone(s).

Massage—physical manipulation of tissues to help blood supply and mobility.

Matrix—roots (growth area) of nail.

Medial—closest to middle line of the body.

Midfoot (lesser tarsus)—consists of the navicular, cuboid, and three cuneiform bones.

Morton's foot—foot with a short first metatarsal bone or excessively long second; also called Morton's toe, Morton's syndrome.

Morton's neuroma—swelling of nerve at point where branches of medial and lateral plantar nerve join and then separate to pass to adjacent sides of third and fourth toes; also called Morton's metatarsalgia.

Mycosis, mycotic—fungus, infected with fungus.

Myositis—inflammation of a muscle.

—N—

Neurologic—condition affecting a nerve.

Neutral position—the position of best function from which motions are smooth and predictable, measured for each individual; in the ideal normal foot, the neutral position is the same as the normal position; the objective of treatment for mechanical abnormalities is to support the neutral position and prevent compensation.

Neutral subtalar joint—the position of the talus over the calcaneus (rearfoot) resulting in maximum stability and functioning of the foot.

Nodule—a primary skin lesion; a sharply circumscribed lesion larger than a papule and firmer than normal surrounding tissue—e.g., fibroma, wart.

Normal (average) foot—a healthy-appearing foot without any apparent abnormality or loss of stability and function during gait that would cause it to stand out as unusual or out of the ordinary.

Normal (ideal) foot—the average foot which is structurally and functionally aligned during stance and gait when in the ideal neutral position, whereby the rearfoot is perpendicular to the supporting surface, the forefoot is perpendicular to the rearfoot, the heel bone is parallel to the leg bone, and the whole foot-leg-thigh moves as a unit when locked.

Normal foot—the term normal represents a set of circumstances whereby the foot functions efficiently and with stability under normal conditions as dictated by the norms of the surrounding community or society.

—O—

Orientation planes of the body—there are three reference planes of the body, each one perpendicular to the other two, corresponding to the three dimensions of space; they are the sagittal, frontal and transverse planes.

Orthoses—orthotic devices, appliances that support the foot in a neutral or more functional and stable position.

Overuse syndrome—that situation where the functional demands of the sport exceed the physical ability of the individual, resulting in a stress reaction at the weakest point in the structure; overuse implies "undercondition."

—P—

Padding—a pad can be any device or material used to supplement the body's own protective mechanisms.

Palliative—affording relief, but not cure.

Papule—a primary skin lesion; an elevated lesion—e.g., one degree lesion.

Paronychia—inflammation involving the folds of tissue surrounding the fingernails and toenails.

Patella—kneecap; a specialized sesamoid bone invested in a tendon.

Periostitis—bone bruise; blood between bone and bone covering.

Pes, pedis—latin term for foot.

Pes cavus—high-arched foot.

Pes planus—low-arched foot.

Phalanges—bones of the toes or fingers.

Physiology—the study of tissue function.

Plantar—bottom surface of the foot.

Plantar wart—verruca plantris; papilloma caused by virus infection on bottom of foot.

Plantarflexion—downward motion during which the distal part of the foot or the toes moves away from the leg bones.

Plaque (foot and ankle)—a primary skin lesion; large flat papule.

Podiatrist—foot healer.

Poliomyelitis—an acute viral disease characterized clinically by fever, sore throat, headache and vomiting, often with stiffness of the neck and back; in the major illness central nervous system involvement, causing drop-foot.

Posterior—back, behind.

Pronation (foot)—a three-plane motion consisting of simultaneous movement of the foot or part of the foot in the direction—away from the midline of the body, out and up; flattening of the foot to the ground; opposite of supination.

Prone—to lie face down, flat on the stomach.

Prophylactic—preventive.

Proximal—nearest the origin or center of the body.

Pulled muscle—trauma to a portion of the musculotendinous unit from excessive forcible use or stretch; strain.

Pump bump— (*retrocalcaneal exostosis*)—bony protrusion located on the dorsal lateral superior aspect of the heel bone or calcaneus due to excess motion of the rearfoot in the shoe.

Postule—a primary skin lesion; a lesion containing free pus; an infected vesicle.

—R—

Rearfoot (*greater tarsus*)—consists of the talus and the calcaneus.

Runner's knee—a condition known as chondromalacia patella, an irritation or roughening of the back surface of the knee cap.

—S—

Sagittal plane—this is a flat, vertical plane passing through the body from front to back, dividing it into a right half and a left half, the cardinal sagittal plane passes through the center of gravity and divides the body into equal symmetrical halves; all other sagittal planes are parallel to the cardinal sagittal plane.

Scale—a secondary skin lesion; a dry or greasy flake of epidermis; secondary lesion.

Scar—healed fibrous connective tissue; a secondary skin lesion.

Sesamoid—a bone invested in a tendon such as the kneecap, and the tibial and fibular sesamoid bones in the foot.

Shin splints—pain and discomfort in the leg from repetitive running on a hard surface or forcible excessive use of foot flexors.

Sign—observations and descriptions by the doctor of a patient's condition.

Spasm—a sudden, involuntary contraction of a muscle or group of muscles, attended by pain and interference with function.

Sprain—a tear in a ligament.

Spur—a projecting body as from a bone; exostosis.

Stitch—a vague term applied to any number of internal pains that occur while running.

Stitch-in-side—the rapid, severe pain which affects either the left or right side of many athletes. Thought to be a spasm of diaphragm muscle.

Strain—a tear in the muscle-tendon complex.

Strapping—a semi-rigid or elastic support that splints soft tissues and limits their function without completely immobilizing the part.

Stress fracture—partial crack in skeleton from overuse; also called fatigue or march fracture.

Subluxation—a displacement in the congruity of a joint; a slow, forcible dislocation.

Subtalar joint—the joint beneath the ankle which allows side-to-side motion of the foot.

Supination (foot)—a three-plane motion consisting of simultaneous movement of the foot or part of the foot in the direction—towards the midline of the body, in and down; opposite of pronation; similar movement at the wrist.

Supine—to lie face up, flat on the back.

Surfer's knee—inflammation of the bursa, caused by constantly kneeling on a surfboard; also called pre-patellar bursitis; housemaid's knee.

Symptom—observations and description by the patient of his condition.

—T—

Tendons—elastic tissue which connect muscles to bones.

Tendonitis (tendinitis)—tendon or tendon covering inflammation.

Tenosynovitis—inflammation between tendon and tendon sheath.

Tennis toe—blood blister, often quite painful, that develops under the big toenail from jarring.

Tetanus—an acute, non-aerobic infectious disease caused by a toxin produced in the body with tonic spasm of the masseter muscles causing lockjaw.

Thigh—anatomically defined as the area from the hip to the knee.

Tibia—largest bone in the lower leg.

Tibial varum (bowleg)—curving inward of the distal portion of the larger leg bone with the proximal portion acting as the pivot point or hinge.

Transverse plane—this is a flat, horizontal plane which passes through the body from side to side and from front to back, dividing it into an upper half and a lower half; the cardinal transverse plane passes through the center of gravity and divides the body into equal but asymmetrical halves.

Trauma—injury.

Trick knee—a torn meniscus (cartilage) in the knee joint that has never mended, causing the knee to buckle or suddenly to "lock."

Triceps surae—three calf muscles.

Tumor—a primary skin lesion; abnormal overgrowth of cells in a localized area; an enlargement or swelling which may be benign or malignant.

—U—

Ulcer—destruction of the skin extending beneath the epidermis; it always leaves a scar; a secondary lesion.

Unhappy triad—classic football injury from block on lateral side of knee with foot fixed to ground; inward rotation of thigh on an externally rotated leg, producing medial collateral sprain, medial menisus tear and anterior cruciate sprain.

—V—

Valgus—an abnormal fixed position in which the foot or part is tilted away from the midline of the body.

Valsalva maneuver—the practice of inhaling before a strenuous event; forcing the inspired air against the closed glottis so that it can't escape, thereby increasing the pressure within the chest cavity.

Varus—an abnormal fixed position in which the foot or part is tilted toward the midline of the body.

Vasoconstriction—a diminution in the size of a vessel leading to decreased blood flow to a part.

Vasodilation—a wider opening of the vessels leading to increased blood flow to a part.

Verruca—wart.

Vesicle—a primary skin lesion; a sharply circumscribed, small elevation containing clear, free fluid; tiny "blister."

Volkmann's ischemic contracture—see anterior tibial compartment syndrome.

—W—

Warm down—decrease vigorous activity to allow the muscles to dissipate waste products and maintain flexibility.

Wheal—a primary skin lesion; edematous circumscribed and slightly elevated superficial lesion which appears and disappears rapidly leaving no permanent changes; hives.

Index

Muscle length-tension ratio
(chart) — 243

-N-
Nerve injuries — 195-197
Nerves of feet-legs — 37-38
Neuromuscular
abnormalities — 66
Neuroma — 196-197
Neuroma (illus.) — 197
Normal foot — 12-38
Normal foot in stance
(illus.) — 14

-O-
Off-weight-bearing
examination — 48-49
One-foot test — 48
One-foot test (illus.) — 47
Orthoses — 289-320
Orthoses (chart) — 312
Orthoses, construction of
(illus.) — 286-288
Orthoses, effects of (illus.) —
313
Orthoses, rigid — 311-312
Orthoses, semi-rigid — 311
Orthoses, semi-rigid (illus.) —
311
Orthoses, soft — 310
Orthotic materials — 310-314
Overuse compartment
syndrome — 226-227

-P-
Padding — 298-309
Padding (illus.) — 293-297
Pads, varus heel and arch
(illus.) — 308

Pain responses — 140-141,
144-146
Planes of body — 20-21
Planes of body (illus.) — 14
Physical therapy — 335
Plantar fascia injuries —
187 191
Plantar fascia (illus.) —
188-189
Plantar flexion (illus.) — 28
Podiatrist, role of — 6-7
Poison ivy and oak,
treatment — 348
Posture (chart) — 47
Prevention of injuries —
251-360
Pronation syndrome — 69-71
Pronation (illus.) — 28-29, 57,
72
Psoriasis, treatment —
346-347

-R-
Rectocalcaneal exostosis
(illus.) — 193
Reflexology therapy — 340
Rolfing therapy — 339-340
Rotational
abnormalities — 83
Runner's knee — 236-237
Running (illus.) — 101

-S-
Sciatic nerve injuries —
244-247
Self-examination — 142-151
Shin splints — 227
Shin splints (illus.) — 230

381

About the Author

The Foot Book's editor and principal author, Dr. Harry F. Hlavac, is typical of the new breed of sports podiatrists in that he combines his professional and avocational interests.

Dr. Hlavac discovered jogging as a path to health when he was in his late 20s, 30 pounds overweight and already suffering from high blood pressure. His running led him back to vigorous good health and into long-distance running. He is a veteran of two of the country's most prestigious races, the Boston and Pike's Peak Marathons.

The doctor's running brought him into contact with injured athletes and gave him a special understanding of their problems. As a result of his growing number of athletic patients, he founded the Sports Medicine Clinic at the California College of Podiatric Medicine (CCPM) in San Francisco.

Dr. Hlavac currently directs the Sports Clinic, in addition to serving as an associate professor of biomechanics at the CCPM. He conducts his private practice in Mill Valley, Calif., and is director of research and development at Sports Safety, Inc. He is a member of several running clubs in the San Francisco Bay Area, including the Tamalpa Runners.

Harry Hlavac was born in 1944 and grew up on Long Island, N.Y. He did his undergraduate study at Bucknell University and the University of San Francisco, and holds a doctor of podiatric medicine degree from the California College of Podiatric Medicine

384

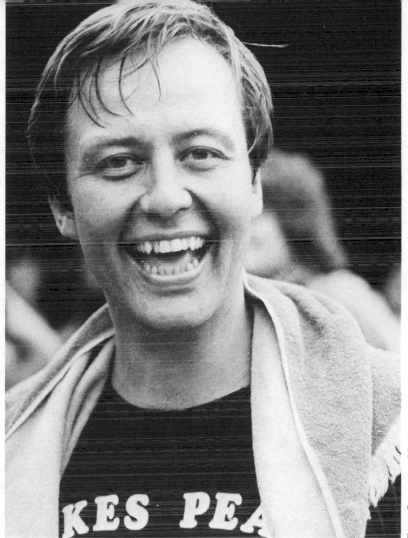

and a master of education degree (in educational psychology) from Temple University.

Dr. Hlavac is the medical columnist for *Nor-Cal Running Review* and a contributor to *Runner's World*. He assisted *RW* with its 1976 Special Shoe Issue, and *Soccer World* with its 1977 shoe evaluation.

The doctor is executive secretary of the American Academy of Podiatric Sports Medicine, a fellow of the American College of Foot Orthopedists, and a member of the American Podiatry Association, American Medical Joggers Association and the National Jogging Association, among other medical and sports-related groups.